A Matter of Principles?

A Matter of Principles?

Ferment in U.S. Bioethics

EDITED BY

Edwin R. DuBose

Ronald P. Hamel

Laurence J. O'Connell

*A book from the Park Ridge Center
for the Study of Health, Faith, and Ethics*

TRINITY PRESS INTERNATIONAL

Valley Forge, Pennsylvania

First Published 1994

Trinity Press International
P.O. Box 851
Valley Forge, PA 19482–0851

Library of Congress Cataloging-in-Publication Data

A matter of principles? ferment in U.S. bioethics / edited by Edwin
 R. DuBose, Ronald P. Hamel, Laurence J. O'Connell.
    p. cm.
  "A book from the Park Ridge Center for the Study of Health, Faith,
and Ethics."
  Includes bibliographical references and index.
  ISBN 1-56338-081-1
  1. Medical ethics—United States. 2. Bioethics—United States.
I. DuBose, Edwin R. II. Hamel, Ronald P., 1946–   .
III. O'Connell, Laurence J. IV. Park Ridge Center (Ill.)
R724.M2654 1994
174'.2'0973—dc20
                                      94-33
                                      CIP

Printed in the United States of America

94   95   96   97   98   99   10 9 8 7 6 5 4 3 2 1

Contents

Part One
PRINCIPLISM IN U.S. BIOMEDICAL ETHICS

Part Two
PRINCIPLISM AND ITS CRITICS

FOREWORD

This is a book about an *ism.* In our language, *ism* is a suffix that can do quite different things to the word to which it is fixed. Often, it turns a perfectly respectable word into something suspicious. In his classic *Modern English Usage,* under the heading "worsened words," Fowler notes that "changes in the meaning of words, and still more in their emotional content, often reflect changes of opinion about the value of what they stand for." His first examples of worsened words are *imperialism* and *colonialism.* This collection of essays about the neologistic *principlism* reflects a change of opinion about the value of principles as the intellectual framework for bioethics. For the first decade of its existence, scholars in bioethics valued principles; but almost all the authors of these essays see principlism as too fragile, too constrained a structure to sustain the large issues that bioethics must consider. Even the one advocate of principlism, its fond father, James Childress, offers but a measured and mild defense, seeing merit in the views of his opponents.

Curiously, none of the astute commentators on principlism says much about where it came from. How did bioethics go principlist? A little history might be helpful. Bioethics, by almost everyone's assessment, started in the late 1960s or early 1970s. Even if, as I have suggested, the birth of bioethics was the establishment of the Seattle Artificial Kidney Patient Selection Committee in 1960, its growth into a scholarly field of study certainly did not begin until a decade later when the Hastings Center and the Kennedy Institute were established, a few individuals were appointed to medical faculties, a literature in scholarly and professional journals sprouted, and conferences began to convene.

In order to understand how bioethics became principlist, one must return to those early days. A very few scholars, most fresh out of graduate school, found themselves attracted to the study of moral and ethical questions posed by the progress of scientific medicine. Several senior scholars — theologian James Gustafson and philosopher Hans Jonas, for example — had commented on these questions to some extent. Joseph Fletcher was already a popular author, and Paul Ramsey opened the decade of the seventies with his magisterial *Patient as Person*. At the beginning, however, most of those who would be designated ethicists arrived with freshly minted doctorates in philosophy, theology, or religious studies. In order to understand how bioethics became principlist, it is necessary to appreciate the ideas that they brought to this new endeavor and to know something of the state of the academic study of ethics during the era of their education. Those of us who were in on the creation were not trained as bioethicists — there was no bioethics; we were educated as philosophers and theologians in the academic philosophy and theology of the 1960s and gradually turned those disciplines to the work that in time became bioethics.

The topics that attracted our interest, and the interest of many among the public and the professions, were varied: experimentation with human beings, genetic engineering, organ transplantation. Behind these particular topics was the awareness that science was bringing great changes to medicine and that the social, political, and financial climate in which medicine was practiced was changing. How would these changes affect our values and our perception of human nature and the human condition? The phrase "moral and ethical implications" began to appear in discussions and commentaries on these changes. One by one, people whose scholarly work identified them as interested in the "moral and ethical implications" of things were invited to participate in those discussions. In 1968, Ralph Potter, professor of religious ethics at Harvard, was appointed to the Beecher Committee of the Harvard Medical School to Examine the Definition of Brain Death; in the same year, Michael de Bakey asked Kenneth Vaux, theologian at the Institute of Religion at Texas Medical Center in Houston, to join him on "Meet the Nation" to talk about heart transplants; in 1971, I, a moral theologian, was appointed to the first federal body to review the "ethical, moral, legal, economic, sociological, and psychological implications" of a new medical technology, the totally implantable artificial heart. In those same years, Dan Callahan, a philosopher, and Robert Veatch, trained in religious studies, were asked to initiate teaching in medical ethics at Columbia College of Physicians and Surgeons; Dan Clouser, a philosopher, became the first regular ethics professor in a modern medical school; and Warren Reich and LeRoy Walters, both in theology, were brought to Georgetown University by André Hellegers to open the Kennedy Center for Ethics. We few had somehow become, by choice or by chance, the commentators on the changing scene of biomedical science and medical practice. And it happened that the language of our commentary was ethics.

In those years, the language of ethics was not easy to speak or understand. Everyone uses the language of ethics, calling some things bad and others good, some actions right and others wrong. Scholars since the dawn of philosophy have tried to write the grammars and dictionaries of that language. Yet as scholars often do in the name of precision or clarity, they change the idiom and even create other vernaculars that are not easily understood by the native speakers. From Plato's vision of the good to Kant's categorical imperative to Rawls's reflective equilibrium, scholarly ethics represents not one language but many, and they are only loosely related.

Those of us who studied philosophical or theological ethics in the 1960s heard several distinct accents. In the philosophical world, several decades of clipped and dry speech, unmodulated by emotion or passion, had been spoken almost exclusively. This was the language of the linguistic analysts and the metaethicists. They were concerned almost exclusively with the form of moral discourse, not about its substance. Scholars at that time commonly distinguished metaethics from normative ethics, which admittedly dealt with the justification of ethical beliefs and statements. It was much more intellectually fashionable, however, to penetrate the meaning of ethical words like *ought* than to dwell on the murky question, "What ought I to do in this moral crisis?" Many of us who read the moral philosophy of that era learned the vocabulary and grammar of metaethics which contained such monstrous words as *nonnaturalism* and *noncognitivism* and R. M. Hare's *phrastics* and *neustics*. This language had little to do with such emerging questions as "Now that science is on the verge of cloning humans, should we do it?" or, more urgently, "How do we protect the rights and welfare of the human subjects of biomedical research without curtailing scientific and medical progress?" Indeed, Hare himself, at one of the early conferences on bioethics, admitted as much, saying, "perhaps the only contribution of the philosopher to the solution of these problems [in medical ethics] is the clarification of the logical properties of tricky words like wrong" (Hare 1977).

In the theological world, a very different language was spoken. There people wondered how the absolute command of God and the difficult imperatives of Jesus could be realized in the weak and sinful human community with which God had covenanted. The overarching doctrines of Christian faith (such as creation and redemption) had implications, it was thought, for the life of humans in the modern world: how could we work from these visions of faith to directions about the form of life and society? Protestant theologians criticized the prevailing "social gospel," which in their eyes had become a secularized and sociologized ethic that substituted liberal rationalism for the powerful and even apocalyptic judgment of God on a sinful world. Catholic theologians grew skeptical of the rationalistic rules of the natural law and their authoritarian interpretation by the hierarchy; they sought to revive an ethics based on the imitation of Christ and the command of love. We neophyte philosophers and theologians learned these languages and spoke them, imitating the accents of the great teachers — Moore, Ayer, and Stevenson in philosophy, Barth, Niebuhr, and Häring in theology.

We could have attempted to analyze the new science and the new medicine in the terms of the languages we had learned. But we gradually realized that, if we did, our words would be uttered largely in vain. The philosophical ethics of that era had very little to say about the substantial content of moral decision and action. Theological ethics used terms that were incomprehensible to many who were not believers or were believers of another sort. We had to find an idiom that, at one and the same time, expressed substantive content and was comprehensible to many listeners. Although there were no consultations among us, no convocations to debate the issue, and no conspiracy to create an *ism*, almost all of us drifted away from the philosophical and theological languages of our intellectual tutelage. Like strangers in a strange land, we had to devise new forms of communication among ourselves, with our scientific and medical colleagues, and with the public.

In those years, the arid ground of philosophical ethics was watered by some streams. A few philosophers like Frankena, Baier, and Brandt remained more interested in normative ethics than in metaethics. They had recognized that the then-popular metaethical theses of emotivism and prescriptivism evacuated ethics of all objectivity and so worked to restore some semblance of rational order to moral discourse. Ethics, they proposed, could be conceived as a coherent system of principles derived from cultural morality which could be corrected and justified by reference to one or several moral theories. Several moral theories, indeed, the very idea of moral theory, had won favor among the normative ethicists during the previous several decades. In the 1930s, C. D. Broad suggested that careful reading of the great moral philosophers would reveal that beneath their multifaceted reflections on morality two basic systems of ethics prevailed, namely, the teleological and the deontological. In the first of these, a single principle, utility, ruled; in the latter, a set of principles having certain formal characteristics was invoked. John Stuart Mill provided the best example of the former, while Immanuel Kant represented the latter. In both, however, principles, and the attendant idea of obligation, were seen as the center of formal ethical discourse.

This version of normative ethics was prevalent in the 1960s. Even in philosophy departments where the humble discourse of normative ethics was considered philosophically uninteresting, whatever was said about normative ethics was articulated in terms of principle and theory. In theological ethics, the sublime discourse about grace and sin was supplemented by the same normative ethics. Courses in Christian ethics and moral theology often used William Frankena's convenient little volume *Ethics* as supplementary reading to the great tomes of Karl Barth and Bernard Häring. Thus at the beginning of bioethics, the embryonic ethicists found some guidance away from the arid land of metaethics and out of the prophetic but parochial land of religion. The guidance was the language of theory and principle.

Even that guidance was sketchy and vague. The word *principle* and its equivalent in other languages signify many things of relevance to morality. There are many other words of equal importance in moral discourse: ideals, obligation, virtue, duty, rights, and so forth. Most of the great authors in ethics had written of principles, but few had made them the sole focus of moral attention, and those few who did used the term in rather different ways. Kant's *Grundsätze* and Bentham's principle are hardly the same in concept or function. Thus in the 1960s there was no fully formed principlist approach to ethics. Yet the suggestion that ethics could be rebuilt by attention to a critical system of principles was attractive. I recall the impression made upon me by John Rawls's 1957 article "Outline of a Decision Procedure for Ethics," in which he wrote, "Perhaps the principal aim of ethics is the formulation of justifiable principles which may be used in cases wherein there are conflicting interests to determine which of them should be given preference" (Rawls 1957). As embryonic ethicists in the world of biomedicine, we were ready to "formulate justifiable principles" for the new and unusual cases that science and medicine were laying before us.

If we return to the dictionary definitions of *ism,* we find two meanings that are not in themselves derogatory. The *Oxford English Dictionary* notes that the suffix forms a noun of action from a verb, giving *baptism* from *baptize* as an example. In a sense, the normative ethics of principles served a similar purpose. Those of us who had initiated the study of bioethical issues found ourselves pressed to turn reflection into action. We were asked not only to ruminate on the problems but to advise how they should be managed in the world of practice and public policy. The idea that a clear statement of principle could serve as the premise of a practical syllogism, whose conclusion was a choice or a recommendation, was attractive. If the normative ethic of principle and theory became a principlism, it was in part because we, unlike the pure scholars whose works we had read, had to contribute to decision and action. Our ism, like baptism, was an initiation to life.

The *Oxford English Dictionary* gives us one more definition: "ism," it states, "forms the name of a system of theory or practice" as in Protestantism, Buddhism, Platonism, and Toryism. These "isms" are certainly not, for their adherents, "worsened words" but cherished affiliations. Some of the essays in this collection suggest that principlism in bioethics has this meaning: somehow a system of theory and practice with principles as its creed has come into being, and that system has its devoted adherents. The somewhat sarcastic allusion to the "Georgetown mantra" of four principles intimates this: just as religious devotees chant sacred words, so the principlist ethicists invoke principles to address difficult moral dilemmas and exorcise paradoxes.

It may be that the normative ethics of theory and principle has become a system, a doctrine, an orthodoxy. I must admit that it appears so. The appearance comes, I think, not merely from the intellectual proclivities of the first bioethicists: it took an act of Congress to move academic notions into public discourse and to make principles into the doctrine of principlism. In 1974 Congress passed the National Research Act (Public Law 93–348), which established the National Commission for the Protection of Human Subjects of Biomedical and Behavioral Research. The law mandated: "The Commission shall (i) conduct a comprehensive investigation and study to identify the basic ethical principles which should underlie the conduct of biomedical and behavioral research involving human subjects, (ii) develop guidelines which should be followed in such research to assure that it is conducted in accord with such principles..." (202[a][1][A]). I do not know who wrote the words "basic ethical principles" in that public law (probably the first time they ever appeared in U.S. legislation!). Whoever it was used commonsense words that would resonate in the minds of theologians and philosophers.

Congress had also ordered the commission to produce within four months a report on research involving the human fetus. The commissioners (of whom I was one) turned full attention to that subject, leaving the "basic ethical principles" task for later. As we were working through our other specific charges (research with children, prisoners, and the mentally infirm), we asked philosophers and theologians to help us with the "comprehensive investigation and study to identify the basic ethical principles." During 1974–75, we considered a variety of views. I recall a fruitful meeting of three commissioners and several of our philosophical consultants in the study of my home in San Francisco: the study was a small room on the roof, which Stephen Toulmin had named The Belvedere. On February 13–16, the full commission met at the Belmont Conference Center in Elkridge, Maryland, to deliberate on the final form of the "ethical principles" report. That meeting produced the *Belmont Report* (which I, recalling that San Francisco meeting, prefer to call the *Belvedere Report*).

The commissioners and their consultants ruminated and argued: at one time, as many as seven principles were considered; at another, a single principle was proposed. In the end, we settled on three basic principles: respect for persons, beneficence, and justice. We did so because these three are profoundly rooted in the moral traditions of Western civilization, are implied in many of the codes and policies about human experimentation that had been previously published, and seemed to reflect the commissioners' own deliberations as they worked through the particular issues of research with fetuses, children, prisoners, and so on. A paper submitted by one consultant, philosopher H. Tristram Engelhardt, Jr., had adumbrated, in slightly different form, the eventual statement of the commission, and commissioner Karen Lebacqz, a theologian, was influential in their final formulation. At the same time, the statement of principles was created not by philosophers and theologians working with the tools of their intellectual trade but by a group of twelve commissioners, of whom only two were ethicists. The principles were not arcane statements of scholars. They were spoken by and intended to speak to persons of moral sensitivity, and we hoped that they would be understood beyond the commission — in the Congress that had ordered their preparation, by the scientists and researchers that would be guided by them, by the regulators that had to enforce them.

The *Belmont Report,* published for comment in the *Federal Register* in 1976 and officially promulgated in 1978, had a broad impact. It became the classic principlist statement, not only for the ethics of human experimentation but for bioethical reflection in general. Perhaps this was a mistake. Since the report was designed to meet the ethical problems posed by the use of human subjects, it bore the marks of the problems and practices, and indeed, of the abuses, in that field of endeavor. Still, the succinct statement of principles caught on and was generalized. Tom Beauchamp (who had participated as a consultant in the drafting of the *Belmont Report*) and James Childress reworked the three principles into four, separating beneficence and nonmaleficence, and explained them somewhat differently than the commission had in its brief document. (In saying "reworked," I do not imply that they merely picked up what the commission had created; their own thinking contributed to the commission's work and, as Tom Beauchamp has suggested elsewhere, predated it.) Their book, *Principles of Biomedical Ethics*, became, as this volume demonstrates, the principal theoretical statement of the new field of biomedical ethics.

The "basic ethical principles," whether the three of the *Belmont Report* or the four of Beauchamp and Childress, gave the scholars in this new field something that their own disciplinary traditions had not given them: a clear framework for a normative ethics that had to be practical and productive. They provided a focus for the broader, vaguer, and less applicable general reflections of philosophers and theologians of the era. In their simplicity and directness, they gave us a language to speak with our new audience, the physicians, nurses, and others in health care. As Christine Cassel — who was my student in those early days — says in this volume, "Principlism gave clinicians the vocabulary with which to discuss the previously inchoate moral gut feelings."

Bioethics became principlist, then, for several reasons. First, the first bioethicists found in the style of normative ethics current at that time, the style of theory and principle, a *via media* between the arid land of metaethics and the lush but generally inaccessible visions of theological ethics. Second, the *Belmont Report* was a foundational document that met the need of public-policy makers for a clear and simple statement of the ethical basis for regulation of research. Third, the new audience of doctors and medical students had to be led through dilemmas and paradoxes by ideas and language that clarified rather than complexified the issues.

Has all this made the normative ethics of theory and principle into a system that is equivalent to an orthodoxy? Is principlism — like Calvinism, Jansenism, communism — an all-encompassing doctrine that tolerates no departures from faithful practice? Can one be a nonprinciplist bioethicist? The essayists in this volume strongly affirm that a nonprinciplist bioethics is possible and necessary. I think they are right. Of course, some might say, Jonsen became a heretic some time ago, when he and Stephen Toulmin resuscitated medieval and Renaissance casuistry for use in bioethics. Still, I would think that most of the original bioethicists would not be averse to the theses of these essays. Indeed, Childress admits that he and Beauchamp become casuists when they examine cases. Even though the educational background of the pioneers made the principlist approach attractive to them, and even though the approach has proven useful for those in education and in public policy, it is a truncated version of the moral life. Those who read the great classics of ethical literature and contemporary authors like Hampshire, Williams, MacIntyre, Nussbaum, and Murdoch know this. Principlism is not, in my view, an orthodoxy but a utilitarian abbreviation of moral philosophy and theology that served the pioneers of bioethics well and may continue to be useful.

The authors of these essays are, with a few exceptions, the second generation of bioethicists. They bring fresh insights and different visions both to the old problems and to the new ones that press on bioethics relentlessly. They have profited from the resuscitation of moral philosophy that Stephen Toulmin described in his frequently cited "How Medical Ethics Saved the Life of Moral Philosophy." Moral philosophy has rejoined the world of action, and moral theology has been liberated from moralism. Methods like hermeneutics, phenomenology, and narrative enliven both, and perspectives from feminist and ethnic experience challenge them both. Just as the normative ethic of principle and theory contributed to the creation of bioethics, these will contribute to its evolution.

The essays in this book rightly insist that ethics consists of more than principles. Yet the state of ethical reflection in the days when bioethics was being born, together with the demands both of public policy formulation and of communication with health professionals, explains how principles came to occupy the center of the new field of biomedical ethics. The new perspectives will expand and enrich the field. At the same time, they too will have to meet the demands of policy formulation and practical, clinical decision making. I shall watch their work with interest.

ALBERT R. JONSEN

REFERENCES

Hare, R. M. 1977. "Can the Moral Philosopher Help?" In *Philosophical Medical Ethics*, ed. Stuart F. Spicker and H. Tristram Engelhardt, Jr. Dordrecht and Boston: D. Reidel.

Rawls, John. 1957. "Outline of a Decision Procedure for Ethics." *Philosophical Review* 66:177–97.

ACKNOWLEDGMENTS

The completion of this volume has been a collective effort. We would like to thank Hal Rast, director of Trinity Press International, for his encouragement and support throughout this project and for his understanding in its concluding phase; Jon Sande, a former research assistant at the Park Ridge Center, for his creative energies and insights in shaping the project; Rose Luciano for her untiring administrative efforts and her work on correspondence and text processing; Susan Messer for her patient and skilled editing of the manuscripts and Loretta Faber for her attentive proofing; Park Ridge Center editors, Barbara Hofmaier and Sandy Pittman, for giving the manuscript a final read; John Kilner and Stephen Hudson, for their help with a final proofing of the manuscript; our research assistant, Agnes Coveney, for her patience in the painstaking work of checking incomplete citations; and a "special thanks" to our colleague, Trecy Lysaught, for her most helpful suggestions on the Introduction and her invaluable assistance with last-minute text processing. We are also indebted to the participants in the original "case conference": Patricia Benner, Kenneth Boyd, Paolo Cattorini, Larry Churchill, James Drane, Dietrich von Englehardt, Renée Fox, Hernan Fuenzalida, Diego Gracia, Henk ten Have, Johannes Huber, Kathryn Hunter, Peter Kemp, Karen Lebacqz, Fernando Lolas, Patricia Marshall, William F. May, Richard McCormick, Thomas H. Murray, Angela Schneider-O'Connell, Pinit Ratanakul, Warren Reich, David Thomasma, Stephen Toulmin, Guido Van Steendam, Charles Vella, and Richard Zaner.

THE EDITORS

INTRODUCTION

A fairly widespread perception exists, both within and without the bioethics community, that the prevailing U.S. approach to the ethical problems raised by modern medicine is ailing. Principlism is the patient. The diagnosis is complex, but many believe that the patient is seriously, if not terminally, ill. The prognosis is uncertain. Some observers have proposed a variety of therapies to restore it to health. Others expect its demise and propose ways to go on without it.

Broadly considered, this volume attempts to "map" a phase in the development of U.S. bioethics. More specifically, it represents a "case conference" on principlism, consisting mainly in a variety of assessments of principlism and U.S. bioethics (diagnoses) and discussions of alternative approaches to the practice of biomedical ethics (therapeutic options). The volume concludes with three reflections on the future of principlism and its alternatives (prognoses).

Since its emergence some thirty years ago, bioethics in the United States has employed several methodologies. Principlism — the use of moral principles to address issues and resolve case quandaries — has come to dominate. Although their versions differ, two major proponents of principlism have been Robert Veatch in *A Theory of Medical Ethics* (1981) and H. Tristram Engelhardt, Jr., in *The Foundations of Bioethics* (1986). Even more influential have been Tom L. Beauchamp and James F. Childress, whose *Principles of Biomedical Ethics* (1979) is now in its fourth edition. Perhaps more than anyone else, Beauchamp and Childress have shaped the teaching and the practice of biomedical ethics in this country. *Principles of Biomedical Ethics* is a standard text in courses and a virtual bible to some practitioners.

The ethical framework they provide, or some version of it, shapes much of the discussion and debate about particular bioethical issues and policy, whether in the academy, the literature, the public forum, or the clinic. It is also widely employed at the bedside to resolve dilemmas about patient care. *Principles of Biomedical Ethics* consists mainly in the explication and subsequent application of two major ethical theories (rule-deontology and rule-utilitarianism) and four principles (respect for autonomy, beneficence, nonmaleficence, and justice). As medical ethicist Albert Jonsen has noted, "these four principles have become the mantra of bioethics, invoked constantly in discussions of cases and analyses of issues" (Jonsen 1991:32). There can be little doubt that the principlism of Beauchamp and Childress has made important contributions toward establishing an identity and providing a language for biomedical ethics, fostering its development, successfully grappling with perplexing issues and formulating public policy, and improving patient care.

Recently, however, theoreticians and practitioners of bioethics, as well as observers and critics outside the field, have found principlism (and thus to a considerable degree, U.S. biomedical ethics) to be ailing. Careful observation of symptoms and examination of the patient have led them to diagnose a range of problems. Some have found that the principles enunciated in Beauchamp and Childress's version of principlism function neither as moral theory nor as practical guides for determining a morally correct course of action. At best, these critics charge, principles serve as a checklist of considerations worth taking into account when addressing an issue. At worst, they "obscure and confuse moral reasoning by their failure to be guidelines and by their eclectic and unsystematic use of moral theory." Consequently, when moral agents apply principles, the critics claim, they are not applying a well-developed unified theory but rather diverse and even conflicting accounts. This they believe to be perilous for moral argumentation (Clouser and Gert 1990).

Other critics are troubled by the paramount status principlism accords to the "value complex of individualism," with its emphasis on autonomy, self-determination, and individual rights. This, some believe, has led principlism to neglect "the skein of relationships of which the individual is a part, the sociomoral importance of the interdependence of persons, and of reciprocity, solidarity, and community between them" (Fox 1989:229). As a result, socially oriented values, virtues, and issues are relegated to secondary status.

Still other observers have noted, and some deplore, the secularity of both U.S. bioethics and principlism. As bioethics moved increasingly into the public arena, occupying the attention of the media, the courts, and the legislatures, it felt compelled to speak in a way that respected the pluralism and secularity of American society. To do so, bioethics turned to an ethics of "universal principles" based on reason (such as autonomy, beneficence, and justice) and on concepts and language from the American legal tradition (such as rights, self-determination, and informed consent).

This development muted the distinctive voice of religion and theology in biomedical ethics, in spite of the fact that in its early days, the emerging field was dominated by religious and medical traditions. Even religious ethicists working in the area more often than not spoke and continue to speak the language of principles rather than their own religious language, especially when engaged in public discourse. Critics believe that the exclusion of religious and theological discourse from biomedical ethics calls into question religious thinkers' vocational commitments, denies the loyalties and identities of particular communities, deprives the field of the accumulated insights and wisdom of religious traditions, and relegates the enduring questions of meaning inherent in the experience of illness and the pursuit of health to the outer fringes of bioethics (Callahan 1990; Campbell 1990; Kass 1990; Verhey 1990).

Principlism generally understands itself as applied ethics, that is, the application of general ethical principles and rules to illuminate and resolve moral problems. Some critics, however, question whether biomedical ethics should even be conceived as applied ethics and whether applied ethics is appropriate and adequate to the clinical setting or whether it is in fact "foreign and ill-fitting." Edmund Pellegrino and David Thomasma, for example, argue that the ethics of biomedicine, or preferably "clinical ethics," arises out of the very practice of medicine and the nature of the doctor-patient relationship. It is not something external to medicine, imported to resolve dilemmas. Dilemmas are resolved not by applying principles but by attending to a whole complex of factors particular to the clinical relationship and deciding on the basis of analogy with other cases (Clements and Snider 1983; Green 1990; Jonsen and Toulmin 1988; Pellegrino and Thomasma 1988).

Still other observers have recognized additional symptoms of principlism's malaise and have diagnosed additional problems. Some maintain that principlism neglects patient narratives and the contextual dimension of cases. Others believe it is preoccupied with quandaries to the neglect of virtue and thus displays a narrow interpretation of the moral life. For yet others, principlism is too rational and does not make space for emotion or take sufficient account of the notion of care in relationships. Or it is too Western, too American, too white, too middle-class. Principlism would seem to be seriously ill.

Faced with this complex of symptoms and problems, the Park Ridge Center, in December 1990, convened (in the words of James Wind in his Afterword) "a most unusual case conference to examine this most unusual patient." Committed to an interdisciplinary approach, the Center assembled a team of twenty-seven health care professionals, sociologists, anthropologists, ethicists, philosophers, and theologians from the United States, Europe, Asia, and Latin America. With this team, the Center tested "a diagnosis that the reigning approach to the ethical problems of modern medicine [in other words, principlism] was inadequate and was causing something analogous to the iatrogenic disease that can occur when physicians intervene...[causing]...side effects that were harmful to patients, caregivers, and society at large" (Wind, Afterword). Upon confirming the diagnosis, the team began to probe a variety of treatments.

This collection of essays is a follow-up to the 1990 "case conference." It might be considered a "documenting" of that conference. Approximately half of the contributors were part of the original case conference; the other half were invited in as "consultants" afterward. Nearly all participated in a second meeting in October 1991, where they presented the substance of their observations and received feedback from the team. The culmination of two years of consultation, writing, conversation, and revision, these essays can be read as a patient's "chart." They give something of the patient's history (Part 1), and then move through diagnoses (Part 2) and treatment alternatives (Part 3) to prognoses (Part 4).

Part 1, "Principlism in U.S. Biomedical Ethics," offers a sociological overview of the current state of bioethics in the United States and a defense of principlism by one of its major proponents. Renée Fox maps bioethics as it appears in the early part of this decade. After noting the ways in which the field continues to grow and to become institutionalized, she identifies issues that have been the focus of attention, reflection, and debate in the bioethics community. Fox observes that despite the diversity of problems and issues, bioethicists' approach to them has remained relatively unchanged. The conceptual framework provided by principlism has gained hegemony.

Fox sees bioethics as currently in a time of ferment and incipient change. Most striking to her is the critical assessment of bioethics and of principlism, coming both from within and from without the bioethics community. Much of this criticism is occurring, she believes, because of what principlism has become at the hands of individuals less skilled than its originators. It concerns her that some are rejecting principlism and are proposing alternative approaches without knowing whether or how they might be fruitfully combined or integrated. In addition, these alternative approaches continue to be dominated by philosophy and display no greater reliance on the insights, knowledge, and methodology of the social sciences than does principlism. Ultimately, Fox is unsure how much the current ferment will alter the foci, social organization, conceptual framework, mode of inquiry, ethos, and worldview of biomedical ethics over the course of the 1990s.

James Childress's essay is an apologia for his version of principlism. He responds to many of the major questions raised about principlism — the source and justification of moral principles, their relationship to particular cases, their relative weight and strength, their relative priority in situations of conflict, principlism's alleged leaning toward liberal individualism, its preoccupation with quandaries and with procedures and regulations, and its neglect of the religious dimension.

He concludes that the critics "have not dislodged principles from a central place in the structure of biomedical ethics." At least some principlist approaches, he believes, with modifications and revisions, appear to withstand the most serious challenges. Furthermore, they may not be so different from some alternatives being proposed, particularly casuistry. Critics of principlism must pay greater attention to the diversity of principlist perspectives and to what each actually claims about the interpretation and function of principles. At the same time, however, principlists should attend more thoughtfully to challenges to their approaches and be willing to modify their frameworks as appropriate. Childress maintains that the most defensible principlist frameworks envision bioethics as principle-guided, not principle-driven.

Although Childress's essay could have been placed at the conclusion of this volume to serve as something of a refutation of what has preceded, we wanted readers to have Childress's rebuttals in mind as they move through the major critiques of principlism. Against this background, readers will be better able to judge the validity and success of the assessments of principlism offered in this volume as well as the possible alternatives.

Part 2, "Principlism and Its Critics," consists of six assessments of principlism from a range of cultural and social perspectives — Western European, Asian, Latin-American liberationist, African-American, feminist, and religious. These diverse angles of vision on the "patient" are meant to be suggestive rather than exhaustive.

It was obviously not possible to include in one volume all cultural perspectives on principlism, nor even the variety of views within any given group or area. There would be, for example, many ways of viewing principlism from a feminist perspective. While most contributors in this section offer an explicit critique of principlism, Márcio Fabri dos Anjos focuses more on the characteristics of his own approach, offering an implicit critique through contrast.

The section begins with Henk ten Have's essay. Ten Have finds

U.S. principlism problematic for three reasons. First, in focusing on the application of principles, norms, and rules, principlism lacks a more encompassing critical, theoretical perspective on its own practical activities. Second, insofar as applied ethics is a phenomenon of a particular culture, principlism cannot be accepted as the timeless and univocal norm for bioethics it claims to be. Finally, by appealing to abstract moral theories and principles, principlism fails to attend sufficiently to the inescapable particularities of the clinical setting, and the importance of the lived experience of health care professionals and patients. Relationships in health care are not timeless, acultural, or abstract; persons are always persons-in-relation, steeped in tradition, and participants in a particular culture.

Ten Have calls for biomedical ethics to be reconnected with both a general philosophical standpoint and the concrete practice of medicine. In doing so, he points toward a new conception of U.S. bioethics, one that illuminates and clarifies the complex interaction between moralities internal and external to medicine as they bear on health care practices. But this conception will entail a careful study of the morality internal to clinical practices, an analysis of the external morality (the social ethos) that influences health care practices and debates about medical ethical issues, and development of new theoretical perspectives (philosophies or histories of medicine) on health care practices.

The next several essays illustrate ten Have's claim about the importance of cultural context. Pinit Ratanakul observes that Theravada Buddhism both is and is not sympathetic to principlism. On one level, Theravada Buddhism appreciates principlism's formulation of moral principles as guidelines for moral decision making. Buddhism teaches above all the importance of purity of heart and other virtues for the attainment of *nibbana,* the supreme goal of human existence. However, people are creatures of mixed motivation. Hence, they need principles to guide them toward right action, to assist in the production of good *kamma,* and to generate purity of heart.

But Theravada Buddhism parts company with principlism in its conception of the person. Unlike principlism, Buddhism does not view the person as isolated from his or her social context. Even though the individual is autonomous in Buddhism, in the sense that he or she must strive individually for purity of heart and is held responsible for his or her actions through the cycle of *kamma,* each person exists in relation to others. Thus, one's *kamma* affects the entire community. The individual does not exist primarily in isolation from others but rather in social contexts. In such a view, social duties and obligations carry more weight than individual rights. Ratanakul warns that U.S. biomedical ethics is in danger of slipping into an egoistic orientation with a strong affirmation of self-centeredness under the name of inalienable individual rights.

Finally, in Theravada Buddhist ethics principles such as nonmalefi-cence, beneficence, and justice are superseded by the moral principle of compassion. Buddhist compassion is neither an *emotional* identification with the suffering of others nor a vicarious bearing of another's pain in one's own self. Rather, as Ratanakul explains, compassion radiates from the *mind* as a result of the realization that all beings are self-less and are consequently equal with one another. Ratanakul claims that compassion as a moral principle must be given central place in bioethics because compassion is frequently given as the motive for entering medicine and is most called for and called upon where people are the most vulnerable to pain and suffering.

Working within the context of liberation theology, Márcio Fabri dos Anjos contrasts U.S. bioethics with a Latin-American liberationist bio-ethics that is inspired not by theoretical reflection but by questions about social, economic, and political oppression. Dos Anjos claims that in a liberationist bioethics, the *locus* from which one initiates ethical re-flection is not an ethical theory or a list of principles but rather one's network of social relationships, the people whom one values and the problems to which one gives priority. This approach brings into bio-ethics the larger community of persons of which one is a part and raises the question of what society does to discover the root causes of suffering and death, especially of the poor and excluded. The challenge, therefore, for U.S. bioethics is not whether the application of principles to cases sheds adequate light on concrete problems, but whether it helps trans-form the unjust situations of the poor and marginalized into a more just configuration, one that indeed may give preferential treatment to the concerns of the poor.

Dos Anjos asks how a bioethics of principlism can connect with the basic questions that come out of the experience of people who are wrestling with the meaning of human life and its ultimate end, as well as the deeper meaning of suffering. He is concerned that U.S. bio-ethics separates itself from social ethics and from the concerns of justice, and warns that the hospital ethicists might become "co-opted by an anti-ethical system."

Cheryl Sanders observes that Beauchamp and Childress's *Principles of Biomedical Ethics* lacks any discussion of the perspective, thought, or experience of African Americans as theorists or participants in the American health care system. She charges the authors with marginaliz-ing race and religion and of devaluing the African-American community and its belief systems. But Sanders argues for a unique African-American perspective in bioethics — one based on such norms as the value of community, the importance of religion, the ethics of virtue, and the weight given to personal experience. This would only solve part of the problem, however. In addition, those in bioethics and health care must appreciate the injustice, insensitivity, and irresponsibility that mark a racist European-American ethos. If the essentially racist matrix of U.S. bioethics is not recognized, the particular contributions that African Americans can make to U.S. bioethics will be ignored by the dominant ethos. Principlism's essentially European-American ethos presents other problems. Although it trumpets objectivity and universalism, principlism in fact represents a cultural parochialism that overlooks the potential contributions of a holistic, inclusive, and spiritual ethos. Consequently, it fails to posit a body of knowledge that is intellectually rigorous and universally applicable cross-culturally. Moreover, Sanders believes that the dominant European-American ethos and the values that it fosters may render U.S. bioethics exclusive, inflexible, and materialistic, re-sulting in a bioethics in which praxis and principle too easily become divorced from each other. In order to be adequate, U.S. bioethics must reflect not only the thought of European-American philosophers, but also the particularity and universal elements of the African-American experience.

In presenting a feminist critique of principlism, Christine Gudorf out-lines the social and political presuppositions of a health care system that has engendered and continues to support principlism. Gudorf criticizes principlism for one foundational defect: that the specific moral princi-ples it invokes regulate and maintain an unjust social system oppressive to women and other marginalized groups.

From the perspective of a feminist ethics, an adequate bioethics must include only one principle: the promotion of the common good of all persons in the community *as persons,* not relative to their assigned so-cial roles. This principle has at least two theological implications. First, like Latin-American liberation theology, it stresses a preferential option for the poor and the marginalized. Second, it challenges principlism's prevailing assumption that principles reveal truth about a moral di-lemma. Gudorf argues that the divine message comes through stories in which relational criteria reveal more of truth. Lived experience should not be captive to principles or rules divorced from the life experience in which they are embedded. In the end, Gudorf proposes a qualified type of principlism, one that emphasizes the option of marginalized people, substitutes individual integrity and responsibility for autonomy, and emphasizes social and relational principles (wellness, responsibility, mutuality, and community).

According to Courtney Campbell, principlism not only reflects a particular view of ethics, it also entails a view of the moral self. The current controversy over the status of principlism in bioethics is concerned in part about moral discourse across communities and whether principles themselves validly express transcommunal moral values. This quest for a common ground of moral discourse tends to favor a moral point of view generated by detached, abstract reflection that marginalizes the religious or spiritual self. In a rich and powerful essay addressing the question of the relevance of religious perspectives for bioethics, Campbell develops an analogy between principlism and moral law to exhibit some theological limitations of principlism. He then draws on the moral meanings of prophecy for insight into those limitations and a renewed appreciation of the spiritual self, which he believes is an ingredient in any work of bioethics.

Campbell describes the possibility of a distinctive religious presence in bioethics. Like the prophets, the bioethicist calls the community to expose hypocrisy, to preserve and remember the values embedded in its history, and to embody the promise of bioethics. Unlike the detached reflection of the principlist, which requires a sense of critical distance otherwise unavailable to those immersed in everyday life, a prophetic witness in bioethics *recovers* by *remembering* the inherited, generally accepted norms of a moral community embedded in a moral culture of which medicine is a part. Such norms can serve as a powerful source of insight and critique. But too often the critical edge of such norms can be diminished by a subtle shift from critique to legitimation, a danger Campbell sees with principlism's focus on procedures to secure agreement among friendly strangers. This danger can be avoided if bioethicists attend to the role of prophetic witness. Campbell believes our moral selves are constituted not only by reason, will, embodiment, and sociality, but also by a distinct capacity for self-transcendence and a concern for the common human questions of meaning that arise in the practice of medicine.

From these assessments of principlism and diagnoses of its ailment, we move to a consideration of "treatment alternatives" in part 3, "Currents in U.S. Biomedical Ethics." While recognizing the intellectual power and cogency of principlism and its many contributions to biomedical ethics, the contributors to this section believe that the prognosis for principlism as it is currently articulated and as a single, unified approach is grim. Each suggests an alternative treatment that either replaces principlism entirely (though retaining a role for principles as well as insights from principlism) or complements it, filling it out and providing correctives for its ills. The "new currents" included in this volume —

phenomenology, hermeneutics, narrative, virtue, and casuistry — are by no means exhaustive, but they seem to us to be the approaches that receive the most attention (with possibly the exception of an "ethics of care") and that, perhaps, offer the greatest promise.

The central point in Richard Zaner's essay is clear: clinical ethics is an exercise in the phenomenology of the illness experience, addressing the complex set of relationships that flow directly from that experience. Physician and patient are wrapped up in the web of their own interactions, interpreting each other from their respective points of view. The phenomenological ethicist, on the other hand, clears a neutral zone — what phenomenologists call an epoché — in order to create an unbiased perspective on the situation. The ethicist focuses on the relationship itself, *for its own sake.*

For Zaner, clinical ethics, as a phenomenological enterprise, explores the concrete ways the participants *themselves* experience and understand *their* situation and endow its components with *meanings of their own.* Having exposed the particular meaning each participant attaches to the clinical encounter, the ethicist establishes the ground for shared understanding and informed action on ethical issues.

Drew Leder focuses upon the *interpretive* nature of the bioethical situation in his essay. Drawing on classical hermeneutical theory, Leder likens the clinical situation to a narrative text that is open to multiple interpretations. The ethicist as hermeneut approaches a case with a sense of respect for its "otherness" and allows it to speak its own "truth(s)." Although the ethicist cannot shed her own prejudgments and expectations, she recognizes that they always remain provisional and open to challenge as the complexities of the case unfold. The basic dynamic of bioethics, then, is understood as an ongoing circle of experience-reflection-experience.

Leder argues against a "top down" methodology that would impose uniform abstract principles on diverse situations. He insists that the rich complexity of actual cases demands openness to a variety of interpretive perspectives, a range of complex and comprehensive readings, including religious renderings. The ethicist as hermeneut assists the participants in a case to tell and retell, interpret and reinterpret their own stories. This enhances the likelihood of achieving consensus and mutual understanding in the face of ethical dilemmas.

In her essay, Rita Charon singles out narrative knowledge and practice as central in considering and resolving biomedical ethical cases. Charon echoes the words of J. Hillis Miller: " 'The moral law gives rise by an intrinsic necessity to storytelling. . . . Without storytelling there is no theory of ethics.' "

Charon describes how narrative's form of "knowing-in-telling" supersedes the popular principlism by taking us beyond a "formalist sanitization" to the essence of a case. The story line of any given case far exceeds the simple facts. It evokes crisscrossing vectors of personal, social, historical, and psychological meaning. The fundamental elements of narrative production — recognition, formulation, interpretation, and validation — are used to tap into these wider dimensions and elucidate the ethical dimensions of a case. This, according to Charon, contributes to the trustworthiness of medical ethics because it more adequately resonates with the experience of patients, doctors, nurses, families, and others who live through the case together. It is a more solid, richer basis for action.

James Drane premises his approach on the conviction that in many situations character and virtue are more important than methodologies of moral reasoning, rules, principles, rights, and the like. A character or virtue approach to bioethics focuses on the kind of person who makes a decision or acts in a certain way. The driving forces of ethical analysis are inner realities like motivations, dispositions, intentions, and attitudes. Thus, the descriptive thrust of this approach focuses on the character traits of the good doctor, while its normative agenda attends to justifying a certain content of the inner being of a good doctor.

Although Drane does not make a case for an exclusive ethics of intrinsic virtue or character, he rejects the notion that ethical analysis and informed moral choice can be guided by extrinsic, formal principles alone. Drane precisely draws the bottom line: "refocusing attention in mainstream biomedical ethics on character and virtue will considerably broaden the ethical playing field beyond what the mainstream principles approach identifies as biomedical ethics. Integrating the inner being of the doctor into a biomedical ethics of acts and rules will enhance it as a form of applied philosophy without diminishing any of the power of the mainstream principles approach."

Finally, in his essay, Stephen Toulmin uses the term *casuistry* to refer to direct analysis of particular cases in clinical medicine. Indeed, according to Toulmin, attention to particular cases is the heart of clinical ethics. Overarching ethical theories are helpful only to the extent that they throw incidental light on particular cases. Clinical ethics, Toulmin maintains, actually operates on a *pre*theoretical level that is more basic than that of any theoretical axiom or principle. The ethicist becomes a medical casuist. The task is straightforward: "to refer difficult cases arising in marginal or ambiguous situations to simpler, more nearly paradigmatic examples, and to consider how far the simpler examples can guide us in resolving the conflicts and ambiguities that awaken our moral perplexity."

Rooted as he is in the particular, Toulmin dismisses generalized bioethical theories or boilerplate principles as virtually irrelevant to the practical needs of medicine. Perhaps the following chapters will help us assess the validity of his apodictic claim!

What impact are these alternatives likely to have on principlism and U.S. bioethics? What is the prognosis for principlism? Part 4, "Horizons in U.S. Biomedical Ethics," offers three reflections — one by a bioethicist, one by a physician, and one by a theologian — that address these very questions.

According to Larry Churchill, the problem in U.S. bioethics is not the use of principles per se but the tendency toward an exhaustive reliance on them. He reads the essays in this volume as midcourse corrections, as ways to rearticulate and reaffirm the power of principles in ethics without becoming captivated by them. Each ethical mode of thought, including principlism, has its own assets and liabilities. To reject the contributions that principles make to ethical reflection and to turn to another approach would merely replace one dogma with another. Churchill hopes to separate the abuses of principlism from the enduring value of principled thinking in ethics.

Churchill locates the source of the abuses of principlism in the appetite that it serves — the human need for moral assurance and certainty in an uncertain world. This moral anxiety, combined with the importance of principles in ethical judgments, leads to overextensions and distortions associated with principlism, such as the claim that while moral customs are culture bound and subjective, principles transcend particular societies and historical circumstances and are, thereby, more objective. Only in isolation from actual events and people, only as categorical abstractions, can principles be thought of as truths independent of the histories and traditions of individuals and communities. Instead, principles should be seen as instruments for interpreting moral facets of situations and as guides to action; abuses of principles occur when we shape circumstances to fit a favored principle. The desire for the security and certainty of principlism is part of the human need to think that we are good people who can know and do the right thing in a morally ambiguous world. In response to the temptation of principlism, we ought not to replace judgments with principles but attempt to recapture moral agency and with it, a more robust cultural context for our ethical lives.

Christine Cassel also attempts a midstream analysis of the present state of U.S. bioethics. Drawing on her experiences as a clinician, she notes how bioethics has remarkably affected her profession over the last fifteen years. Before the emergence of principlism, physicians had no way to articulate their moral concerns. The success of principlism was due to its adoption by clinicians. Principlism gave them a vocabulary, logical categories for previously inchoate moral feelings, and a means to resolve moral uncertainty in a given case. Principlism was a "safe harbor" for physicians during a period of rampant change in the ethical understanding of the delivery and financing of clinical care in the United States.

As medicine and clinical care enter the 1990s, it is clear to Cassel that principlism does not explain the full complexity of moral problems and human interactions. She argues that it may now be time for a theory of communicative ethics, which she interprets as simply saying that we can expect imperfect results from ethical choices. Striving for the best among imperfect results is admirable, especially when strict adherence to principles does not allow for the negotiation and compromise essential to the sharing of power and the framing of decisions in specific contextual realities. As a clinician, however, she worries about how well new understandings of bioethics will translate into the daily practice of medicine. Up until now, principlism at least has helped clinicians to make decisions and understand the reasons for them. She hopes the efforts to work out new models of bioethics will enable clinical practitioners to find greater meaning in their work in the face of the challenges to come.

The challenges to and changes in the professional life of medicine that concern Cassel also provide the focus of Richard McCormick's essay. Refusing to represent himself as "the" theologian speaking for a whole discipline, McCormick offers the personal reflections of "one who tries to approach and view matters from a theological perspective." In doing so, he aims not to draw out explicit theological themes from the various essays but to point out factors in U.S. health care that foster problematic perspectives (identified with principlism) that bioethics should be challenging.

McCormick does not think that the diagnoses of and correctives offered to principlism are aimed at the proper target. For him the current dissatisfaction with principlism is a superficial response to the major transformation occurring in U.S. health care, namely, the displacement of the culture of medicine as a profession. McCormick sees the critique of principlism as indicative of deeper longings and losses, a symptom of a deeper malaise. He fears that the changes recommended in the various essays are not likely to occur unless the practice of medicine itself changes. McCormick identifies five forces that shape the practice of medicine but that are generally overlooked in discussions of bioethics, let alone principlism. Cumulatively, these forces are undermining the culture that makes medicine a profession. In this, medicine is losing its soul.

McCormick calls on bioethics to confront these forces honestly and effectively and here raises the theological focus of his reflection. In the Christian understanding, the encounter between persons has a certain structure, a charge to people to remember that in fulfilling their secular duties of daily life they " 'see Christ in all men whether they be close to us or strangers.' " Infusing medical practice with this perspective can nourish, protect, and support the medical encounter as a truly human encounter, full of possibility for transforming the lives and labors of participants. When that encounter becomes a business, it not only introduces a disharmony into the heart of the medical art, it displaces the grace that is a source of healing and growth for both physician and patient.

We close with an Afterword by James Wind. He addresses a theme that was not sufficiently addressed by most of the contributors to part 3, namely, the possible role of religion and theological reflection in the new currents or "therapeutic alternatives." This was a primary concern of the project and reflects the mission of the Park Ridge Center. As noted earlier, religious considerations and religious discourse have been virtually excluded from the discourse and practice of biomedical ethics. The development of alternative approaches provides an opportunity to re-examine whether and how the religious dimension can be taken into account and even contribute to biomedical ethics. The lack of sustained attention to this topic in these essays suggests a continuing hesitancy to allow the religious and theological through the door. Much still needs to be done to create space for them.

•

Bioethics has been fortunate in finding such powerful and expressive allies in the areas of phenomenology, hermeneutics, the philosophies of casuistry and virtue, as well as literary criticism. The ability of bioethics to absorb the insights of such divergent fields is indicative of both the breadth of the enterprise and the increasing sophistication of its practitioners. The foregoing "therapeutic options" give clear evidence that bioethics is on the brink of substantial development and, perhaps, better health.

The criticisms leveled at principlism can hardly be characterized as a condemnation of the earlier phase of bioethical inquiry. Rather, they recognize principlism's commitment to the moral significance of the medical encounter. More important, they reflect attempts to surface and better understand the complexity and density of human moral experience. The phenomenological and hermeneutical approaches highlight the need to recognize that all experience is subject to interpretation. There are both subjective and objective dimensions in every situation. Phenomenology brackets subjectivity in an attempt to penetrate the situation itself, for its own sake. This clearing process allows for the emergence of meanings that can be analyzed and shared. Similarly, the hermeneutic approach underscores the bipolar or circular character of human experience by stressing the need to accept the "otherness" in every situation that should be engaged as a partner in respectful dialogue. These approaches point to the relative superficiality of the principles approach. Human experience cannot be easily captured and directed toward informed moral choice through the simple imposition of abstract principles and rules.

The narrative approach provides another way into human experience and the moral dilemmas that characterize it. It reminds us that individuals achieve identity and intimacy by telling and following stories, just as entire cultures define their values and membership through myth and epic. Each situation that the ethicist encounters has a narrative dimension. The narrative is an inextricable part of life. The richness of story and its capacity to elicit meaning that goes beyond mere facts make the narrative approach a powerful complement to the abstractness of formal principles. Like the phenomenological and hermeneutical approaches, it demands a fuller account of human experience and provides a way to find it.

The virtue-based approach to bioethics shifts the field of ethical analysis away from rules, principles, rights, and the like. Indeed, it even refocuses the field away from the contextual questions important to the phenomenological, hermeneutical, and narrative approaches. Rather than emphasizing the application of extrinsic principles or the thick context of experience, it focuses upon the inner being of persons, considering the moral qualities that one brings to a given situation. Moving away from other approaches that emphasize certain forms of objectivity, a virtues-based approach concentrates more upon the ethical competencies, the character of the participants.

Medical casuistry turns entirely away from the theoretical perspectives of the other approaches we have considered. It claims to operate on a *pre*theoretical level in resolving ethical issues. It centers on particular insights accumulated in the course of concrete experience. In assembling paradigmatic cases, the casuist creates a common ground for comparison and contrast. The casuist approach to bioethics does provide important information, but its intuitionist tendencies render it suspect. In many ways, it occupies the opposite end of the spectrum from principlism.

The similarities and differences among the various approaches to bioethics lead us to an unavoidable conclusion: The moral dimensions of human experience cannot be captured by a single approach. The approaches to bioethics that we explore here are different paths to a common ground. Each method aims at unpacking the dense layers of human experience in an effort to achieve shared insight and to promote informed action. Each in its own way suggests that, although principlism is valuable, it also has serious limitations. This is not surprising since the breadth and depth of human experience will always exceed the reach of any single philosophical or theological system. The commonalities and differences between and among phenomenological, hermeneutical, narrative, virtue-based, and casuistic approaches to bioethics underscore the need for a variegated approach to ethical dilemmas. Each alternative moves beyond principlism by providing access to different provinces of meaning and alternative paths of action in the face of moral ambiguity. Each should be mined for its respective strengths. In the end, U.S. bioethics should be healthier for this endeavor.

EDWIN R. DuBOSE
RONALD P. HAMEL
LAURENCE J. O'CONNELL

REFERENCES

Beauchamp, Tom L., and James F. Childress. 1979. *Principles of Biomedical Ethics*. New York: Oxford University Press.

Callahan, Daniel. 1990. "Religion and the Secularization of Bioethics." *Hastings Center Report* 20 (July/August): 2–4.

Campbell, Courtney. 1990. "Religion and Meaning in Bioethics." *Hastings Center Report* 20 (July/August): 4–10.

Clements, Colleen D., and Roger Snider. 1983. "Medical Ethics' Assault upon Medical Values." *Journal of the American Medical Association* 250 (21 October): 2011–14.

Clouser, K. Danner, and Bernard Gert. 1990. "A Critique of Principlism." *Journal of Medicine and Philosophy* 15, no. 2 (April): 217–36.

Engelhardt, Tristram H., Jr. 1986. *The Foundations of Bioethics*. New York: Oxford University Press.

Fox, Renée. 1989. *The Sociology of Medicine*. Englewood Cliffs, N.J.: Prentice-Hall.

Green, Ronald. 1990. "Method in Bioethics: A Troubled Assessment." *Journal of Medicine and Philosophy* 15, no. 2 (April): 179–97.

Jonsen, Albert. 1991. "Of Balloons and Bicycles, or The Relationship Between Ethical Theory and Practical Judgment." *Hastings Center Report* 21 (July/August): 14–16.

Jonsen, Albert, and Stephen Toulmin. 1988. *The Abuse of Casuistry*. Berkeley: University of California Press.

Kass, Leon. 1990. "Practicing Ethics: Where's the Action?" *Hastings Center Report* 20 (January/February): 5–12.

Pellegrino, Edmund, and David Thomasma. 1988. *For the Patient's Good*. New York: Oxford University Press.

Veatch, Robert. 1981. *A Theory of Medical Ethics*. New York: Basic Books.

Verhey, Allen. 1990. "Talking of God — But with Whom?" *Hastings Center Report* 20 (July/August): 21–24.

Part One

Principlism in U.S. Biomedical Ethics

THE ENTRY OF U.S. BIOETHICS INTO THE 1990s

A SOCIOLOGICAL ANALYSIS

Renée C. Fox

Introduction

At the inception of the 1990s, several intellectual events signaled the entry of U.S. bioethics into a new stage of development. First, *Strangers at the Bedside,* by David Rothman (1991), the first scholarly history of bioethics in the United States, was published and reviewed appreciatively though critically by participants in that history, and by others. Second, theologian-bioethicist Albert B. Jonsen held a September 1992 conference at the University of Washington, Seattle, in celebration of what he deemed the thirtieth anniversary of the field. This was more than a "commemoration," he wrote to the fifty "pioneers" of bioethics whom he invited to attend; it was also a "serious effort to create . . . the history of the bioethics movement put together by those who have lived through the three decades of [its] development."[1] Third, a revised edition of the *Encyclopedia of Bioethics*, scheduled to appear in the fall of 1993, was in its final stages of preparation when this conference took place.[2] Its "Statement of Purpose" underscored the fact that since the 1978 publication of its first edition "a number of key scientific, intellectual, legal and cultural factors [had] worked a profound change in bioethics." Finally, it was at this time (1991–1992), too, that the Park Ridge Center launched its project on "the changing foundations of bioethics." The project was triggered in part by the Center's perception that "there [was] an increasing lack of satisfaction with the dominant conceptualization and methodology of bioethics in the U.S., and [that] efforts to develop alternatives [were — and should be] under way."[3]

These events marked the "coming of age" of bioethics — a field that within a remarkably short period had expanded so greatly on the American scene that it was characterized as "an American growth industry" by theologian James M. Gustafson (Gustafson 1990:126; 1991:1–5). As Gustafson pointed out, bioethics was neither an isolated nor a purely intellectual happening. It was a central part of a broader ethics movement that, in his opinion, had "produced important achievements," but "still [had] a way to go" before fulfilling what he took to be its aims — "increased moral responsibility by persons and institutions and a more just social order in which the common good is realized" (Gustafson 1991:5).

The historic atmosphere in which the self-proclaimed thirtieth anniversary of bioethics took place was more than celebratory. It was also considered to be an occasion for stocktaking: an opportune time to examine and interpret the genesis, definition, and *raison d'être* of the field; to delineate and reflect on the evolution it has undergone; and to discuss, appraise, and, if need be, alter its conceptual framework, mode of inquiry, and ethos in order to enlarge its ethical approach and cultural view, and make it more applicable to social praxis and social change.

This essay will focus on some of the distinguishing intellectual, social, and cultural characteristics of U.S. bioethics in the early 1990s — at a juncture in its development that those in the field regard as a time both of consolidation and of transition. Observations will be made on what has changed in the organization and outlook of this American variant of bioethics over the past three decades. Observations will be made as well on what has *not* changed despite the growth and progressive institutionalization of the field and the self-conscious efforts it is currently making to modify some aspects of its cognitive and sociocultural framework. The essay will also contain reflections on where the field seems to be going, and why.

Continuing Growth and Institutionalization of U.S. Bioethics

During the past decade, the social role of the *ethicist* — "a word that was not in our vocabulary 25 years ago" (Gustafson 1991:3) — has continued to develop and gain prominence. It has become a full-time occupation in many milieux, rather than an occasional or part-time intellectual activity. This evolution has occurred in conjunction with the escalating philosophical, professional, and public interest in moral problems encountered in various spheres of American social life: in a wide gamut of professions; in science and technology and the research they entail; in academia; in the sphere of business and corporate functioning; in both the legislative and judicial branches of the polity; in the mass media; and in matters pertaining to the family, to the environment, and to the conduct of warfare, among others.

As has been true since the 1960s, the greatest amount of ethical attention is concentrated on moral issues associated with medicine, especially the questions and quandaries around which the domain of bioethics has crystallized. By 1990, these "ethicizing" activities were conspicuous and pervasive enough to impel *New York Times* columnist and social critic Russell Baker to write a seriously humorous essay about "the new kind of bird...called an 'ethicist,' " and the phenomenon of "ethicizationism...in America" (Baker 1990). In the same year, the *New York Times Sunday Magazine* devoted its cover story to the role and "new profession" of medical ethicist (Bouton 1990).

Both as a multidisciplinary field and as an occupation, U.S. bioethics is firmly established and widely recognized at the beginning of the 1990s. Organizations engaged exclusively or primarily in bioethical research, teaching, writing, publishing, consulting, and advising have proliferated, exhibiting greater diversity as their numbers have increased. The three associations that virtually founded the field of bioethics — the Hastings Center, the Society for Health and Human Values, and the Kennedy Institute of Ethics at Georgetown University — are still of central importance. They are nuclei of a network of intellectuals who have been the chief shapers of the foci and discourse of bioethics from its commencement. During the second half of the 1980s, however, several more recently created centers and associations attained new eminence and influence in the field — most notably, the Park Ridge Center for the Study of Health, Faith, and Ethics in Chicago, the Poynter Center for the Study of Ethics and American Institutions at Indiana University, the Center for Biomedical Ethics at the University of Minnesota, the Society for Bioethics Consultation, and the American Society of Law and Medicine. As will be seen, there is evidence that their perspectives and emphases are helping to effect some of the changes that are occurring in the outlook of bioethics.

The continuing growth and institutionalization of U.S. bioethics is manifest in other ways. The number of universities and medical and nursing schools with undergraduate, graduate, and postdoctoral programs and curricula in bioethics has steadily increased, along with the repertoire of short-term bioethics courses and seminars offered for credit at meetings, or under the auspices of professional societies and groups. The array of medical and nursing associations that maintain an active interest in the field has expanded, too. Local, national, and international conferences on general and specific bioethical topics abound. The journals that specialize in the presentation of bioethical materials have also multiplied.[4] Especially "during the past several years," writes LeRoy Walters, editor of the *Bibliography of Bioethics*, "there has been a veritable explosion of literature on bioethical issues" (Walters and Tamar 1991:3). Each annual volume of the *Bibliography* has contained more entries than the one before, reaching 2,500 new citations in its Volume 17, 1991 edition.

Extensive and prominent mass media reporting of happenings relevant to bioethics continues as well. Bioethical events are highly newsworthy. They are closely followed and considered important enough to be recurrently assigned to particular journalists with bylines, who have established reputations in this area. Periodically, bioethical stories become front-page news and foci of major television and magazine reportage. These are generally woven around identified individuals who are viewed as personifications of dramatic, often tragic bioethical issues of societal significance. During 1991, for example, Nancy Beth Cruzan and Helga Wanglie, who were being sustained in persistent vegetative states on life support systems; Marissa Ayala, who was conceived by her parents to be a bone marrow donor for her sister Anissa; and Kimberly Bergalis, who contracted HIV infection from her seropositive dentist, were all elevated to this kind of human-interest and morality-play status by the media. The Cruzan, Wanglie, and Bergalis cases were associated, too, with another strongly institutionalized bioethics phenomenon: the ever-increasing attention that state and federal legislatures and courts devote to bioethical problems.

Also during the early 1990s, bioethics made significant inroads into areas of health and medicine that formerly lay on its periphery. The most notable instance of such expansion was the growing "merger of bioethics and epidemiology" that occurred (Weed 1991). Numerous meetings, articles, commentaries, and special issues of professional journals were devoted to "ethics in epidemiology." These were not only concerned with the role of values in epidemiology and the development of guidelines and a code of professional conduct for epidemiologists. They also dealt with the theoretical and epistemological, and the social, cultural, and moral implications of conducting research on whole populations and entire communities, in local, national, and international contexts (Dickens, Gostin and Levine 1991; Fayerweather, Higginson, and Beauchamp 1991).

A more commercial indicator of how far-reaching and entrenched the "bioethicization" of American medicine had become by the beginning of the 1990s was the widely circulated promotion flyer announcing that an "interActive" software computer program, entitled DR. ETHICS (for both Macintosh and IBM platforms), now exists. Not only was it billed as a program that gives access to a large collection of codes of medical ethics, to federal regulations on research with human subjects, and to the correct forms for writing up the ethical aspects of a research grant. In addition, it was claimed, the program "can analyze the ethical implications of case studies in clinical medicine." "Whether you are a medical ethicist, physician, researcher, academician, student, lawyer, nurse, chaplain or any other type of 'health care professional,'" the advertisement declared, "DR. ETHICS will be an indispensable tool."[5]

Private bioethics companies have been established, too, such as the Bioethics Consultation Group, Inc., in Berkeley, California. Founded in 1986 by John Golenski, a Jesuit priest, who also directs it, by 1992 the firm had a staff of fourteen and a number of major hospital groups as its clients, including the Kaiser Permanente health maintenance program, with its 6.5 million members and thirty-six institutions in sixteen states and the District of Columbia. Father Golenski's work as a consulting medical ethicist is so extensive that, according to reports, he logs some 10,000 airline miles a week, helping hospitals to set up in-house ethics committees and teaching nurses, doctors, and other health care workers how to deliberate and resolve difficult bioethical questions (Phalon 1992).

At this stage in its institutionalization U.S. bioethics is displaying two countervailing organizational tendencies. On the one hand, the centrifugal movement to create specialized bioethical societies has gained momentum. A strong drive in this direction comes from persons and groups engaged in what is known as clinical ethics or ethics consultation, who are called upon to apply their professional expertise to identifying, analyzing, and helping to resolve ethical problems that arise in clinical care in the hospitals and other health care settings. Increasingly, clinical ethics consultants do their work at the patient's bedside and in conjunction with hospital ethics committees, which they often chair or co-chair (LaPuma and Schiedermayer 1991). Although "there is not a uniform vision" of what is described as this "emerging field," there is a growing consensus regarding the distinctive role of ethics consultants and the need for a "consolidated identity" among them (O'Connell 1991). This is apparent in the foundation of the Society of Bioethics Consultation in 1987; in the way that the field has flourished since then as "the forum of choice" for those interested in this developing subfield of bioethics; in the joint "consensus panel" that the Society for Bioethics Consultation and the Society for Health and Human Values have agreed to form in order to study and produce a "white paper" on "questions of standards, accreditation and credentials" for "clinical ethics education and consultation" (Frader and Arnold 1992); in the series of national conferences on ethics consultation in health care which have been held since 1985; and in the creation of two specialty journals: the *Journal of Clinical Ethics* and the *Cambridge Quarterly of Healthcare Ethics: The International Journal for Healthcare Ethics Committees.*

Impetus for identification as a separate field is also present among participants in bioethics who are involved in the sphere of literature and medicine. The year 1991 was a watershed time for this development. The *Literature and Medicine* journal marked its tenth anniversary with the publication of a "retrospective" volume of essays. The volume surveyed and summed up the first decade of work in this interdisciplinary subfield and suggested an agenda for future research, writing, and teaching in which it might engage. Inside the Society for Health and Human Values (which has played a seminal role in fostering the connections among medicine, literature, and bioethics),[6] proposals for the formation of a professional society around these specialized interests are being contemplated.

Interacting with these forces and counterbalancing them were the centripetal efforts made to create a national organization for bioethics — an American Association of Bioethics. The proponents of this organization view it not only as a means of coordinating the array of groups engaged in bioethical activities in the United States, and of increasing the communication between them, but also as a way of advancing the professional status and quality of bioethics as a field.

On November 11, 1991, "representatives of a number of institutions and organizations active in bioethics" convened at the New York Academy of Medicine to "discuss the need and practicality of [this] kind of very broad grouping of bioethicists" (Battin and Wikler 1992). The meeting was put together by Daniel Wikler (professor in the program in medical ethics at the University of Wisconsin Medical School and in the university's department of philosophy); the Academy and its president, physician Jeremiah A. Barondess, "acted in a catalyzing and host capacity."[7] Its participants included members of three kinds of organizations: freestanding bioethics centers, institutes, and societies; university-based bioethics programs; and major medical, nursing, and hospital clinical societies (such as the American Medical Association, the American Nurses Association, and the American Hospital Association). A planning committee composed of nine members — three representatives from each of these so-called bioethics "estates" — was elected. In turn, that committee met on March 8, 1992, at the Park Ridge Center in Chicago, where they agreed on a proposal to found a membership organization of bioethics that would coordinate the meetings of existing societies, hold plenary sessions, and act as an information bank and clearinghouse. For the time being, however, they would have no role in credentialing bioethicists or in taking public stands on bioethical issues.

Margaret P. Battin, a University of Utah philosophy professor, and several of her colleagues were designated to operate an interim structure, undertaking a needs assessment survey, establishing an electronic bulletin board, and publishing the directory of graduate and postdoctoral programs in bioethics and medical humanities formerly prepared by the Center for Biomedical Ethics at the University of Minnesota. Upon approval of this proposal by a number of organizations actively engaged in bioethics, a founding meeting of the new national organization of bioethics was held in New York City in the spring of 1993. However, the boards of the American Society of Law and Medicine, the Society for Bioethics Consultation, and the Society for Health and Human Values decided not to affiliate themselves with the American Society of Bioethics for the time being. Instead, they agreed to hold a joint meeting of their three organizations in the fall of 1994 in Pittsburgh.

The movement to create an American organization accompanies, and is partly associated with, an initiative previously taken by Daniel Wikler, in conjunction with philosophers Peter Singer and Helga Kuhse: the creation of an International Association of Bioethics, whose inaugural congress was held on October 5–7, 1992, in Amsterdam. One advantage of bringing a national organization of bioethics into being was that it could "facilitate American involvement in international forums and organizations, such as the fledgling International Association of Bioethics" (Battin and Wikler 1992). This is an organizational expression of a general intellectual resolve of the American bioethics community to be more "attentive" to what *Encyclopedia of Bioethics* editor Warren T. Reich terms "international perspectives and dimensions" than it has been in the past (a trend I discuss later in this essay).

A major set of institutional developments on which U.S. bioethical associations have been seeking more national and international collaboration in the 1990s are the composition, nature, purposes, and procedures of health care ethics committees. This has been precipitated by the greatly expanded number of these committees established during the past few years, and by the realization that they have become the principal loci of "hands-on" bioethical activity at the institutional level — in hospitals, nursing homes, hospices, rehabilitation centers, and other health care facilities.

An organized impetus to break through the relative isolation and localism in which such ethics committees previously operated — and to link them in a national and international network through which they can regularly exchange ideas and experiences about the educational, policy formation, and case review functions they serve, and their relations to patients, families, the community, and the courts, as well as to their own institutions — has become manifest in such events as the first annual congress of Healthcare Ethics Committees held on April 5–7, 1991, in San Francisco. Entitled "Ethics Committees at Work in the 1990s: Expanding the Circle," and cosponsored by the Hastings Center and the International Bioethics Institute, the Congress featured open forum discussions on substantive and procedural issues generated by committees "around the country." The invitational brochure that it issued included a statement by the President of the Board of Directors of the International Bioethics Institute (William A. Atchley, M.D.) asserting that the "need for a place and time for ethics committees to come together is so great that we are committed to making this Congress the first of a continuing series." The International Bioethics Institute has also launched an official journal "designed to meet the needs of professionals serving on healthcare committees": the *Cambridge Quarterly of Healthcare Ethics*.

The Chief Concerns of U.S. Bioethics in the Early 1990s

 From its earliest days to the present, American bioethics has focused its gaze on a particular cluster of advances in biology and medicine, and on the actual and potential problems to which these scientific, technological, and clinical developments have contributed. What the bioethical perspective views as troublingly double-edged forms of medical progress has remained remarkably constant. Developments in genetics, in artificial means of reproduction, in birth and population control, in life-support systems, in the implantation and transplantation of human tissues and organs and the deployment of artificial organs, and in the capacity to modify human behavior or thought have been consistent centers of scrutiny and discussion. Within these biomedical parameters, certain issues concerning human experimentation (especially informed consent), the moral status of patients and their rights, physicians' responsibilities and duties, medical decisions at the beginning and end of life, and the allocation of scarce medical resources have been continual bioethical preoccupations (Fox 1974; Fox 1989). The tenacity of these patterns notwithstanding, the amount of consideration accorded to different biomedical phenomena and issues has fluctuated over the course of the several decades of the field's existence; and from time to time, new medical occurrences and moral quandaries have been added to the roster of bioethical concerns.

Death and Dying

At the debut of the 1990s, certain medical modalities and "promptings of moral uneasiness" (Gustafson 1990:126) have become focal points of U.S. bioethical discourse and debate. Foremost among these are a constellation of medical predicaments and moral issues that concern death and dying. They are variously expressed as "the right to die"; "death with dignity"; the "withholding," "forgoing," "withdrawal," and "refusal" of "life-sustaining treatment"; "advance directives"; "passive euthanasia"; "active euthanasia"; and "assisted suicide." To a significant degree, these preoccupations are rooted in the collective interest in death and dying and anxiety about them that have been evident in the United States since the 1960s. A number of developments have triggered this interest: medical, scientific, and technological advances; the power to prevent and cure many infectious diseases and to sustain biological life; the greater prevalence of chronic illness; the increasing numbers of elderly persons in the population; and what sociologist Otto Pollak has described as "the shadow of death over aging" (Pollak 1980).

Life-and-death issues have increasingly become matters of public concern, appearing more frequently, prominently, and evocatively in the courts and the media. Especially striking is the escalation of individual and public fear of how suffering at the end of life, in a state of terminal illness, can be augmented and sustained by the capacity of modern medical technology. The raised consciousness and ferment surrounding death and dying have converged with the broad affirmation of individual rights in American society during this period, and with organized efforts to expand the scope of these rights. The most conspicuous part of this process is the articulation and active espousal of a "right to die" — that is, the right to exercise control and decision-making influence over the conditions of one's own death.

However, the chief death-and-dying-centered bioethical discussions of the 1990s are not simply continuations of what has gone before. With the advent of the '90s, U.S. bioethicists have devoted a great deal of attention to the implications of a series of events that have brought the issues involved to a new stage of development. Primary among these events are the following:

- The U.S. Supreme Court's June 25, 1990, decision in the case of Nancy Cruzan — the first "right to die" case that it accepted out of the fifteen-year-long series of disputes concerning what medical interventions should be used to sustain lives, who should make this decision, and on what grounds, that had been deliberated by state courts since the landmark Karen Ann Quinlan case in 1976.

- Two cases — those of "Baby L" and of Helga Wanglie, which surfaced in 1990 and 1991 respectively — in which the families involved wanted to continue intensive treatment that the hospitals wished to discontinue. The "Baby L" and Helga Wanglie situations represented the obverse of most of the prior "right to die" cases — those of Nancy Cruzan and Karen Quinlan included — in which families petitioned for the withholding of life-sustaining treatment that medical care institutions were reluctant to stop.

- The passage of the Patient Self-Determination Act by the U.S. Congress in October 1990 (which took effect on December 1, 1991) that requires hospitals, nursing homes, hospices, managed care organizations, and home health agencies participating in Medicare or Medicaid to advise patients on admission of their right to accept or refuse treatment, to execute an advance-directive instrument (such as a living will or durable power of attorney), and to document whether the patient has done so.

- Three attempts — in the states of California, Oregon, and Washington — to make "physician aid in dying" legal when terminally ill, conscious, mentally competent patients request physician assistance in ending their lives in as dignified, painless, and human a fashion as possible. The 1991 Washington State Initiative 119 proposal to legalize physician-assisted suicide made its way to the ballot, constituting the first time in the United States that such an issue became the subject of a statewide referendum. In November 1991 it was defeated by a margin of only 8 percent. One year later, in November 1992, California's Proposition 161 was rejected by a small, 54–46, majority of voters.

- The continuing repercussions of the January 1988 publication by the *Journal of the American Medical Association* (*JAMA*) of the "Debbie" case, a first-person account, written by an unnamed physician, about how during his residency in the field of obstetrics and gynecology, at the request of a young woman hospitalized with metastatic ovarian cancer to "get this over with," he administered a lethal injection of morphine to her ("It's Over, Debbie," 1988).

- The subsequent publication of a signed article by Dr. Timothy E. Quill, in a March 1991 issue of the *New England Journal of Medicine*, describing how he facilitated the suicide of a longtime patient ("Diane") in the final stages of acute myelomonocytic leukemia, by putting her in touch with the Hemlock (voluntary euthanasia) Society and providing her with a prescription for the barbiturates with which, at a time of her own choosing, she ended her life (Quill 1991). After the publication of his article, Quill was investigated for his role in Diane's death by the prosecuting attorney for the City of Rochester, where he is on the staff of Genesee Hospital, and by the New York State Department of Health. Although in the end they did not seek either a criminal indictment against him or a revocation of his medical license, the debate about this case continues.

- The highly publicized "medicide" crusade which Dr. Jack Kevorkian, a retired Michigan pathologist and self-declared "death specialist," has waged since 1990. He is committed to helping gravely ill persons kill themselves, either by a lethal injection of potassium chloride or by inhaling carbon monoxide through a mask, with the assistance of homemade, so-called mercitron devices that he invented. From June 1990 (when he aided Janet Adkins, a Portland, Oregon, woman with Alzheimer's disease, to end her life) through December 1992, Dr. Kevorkian helped in the suicides of eight women whose ailments included multiple sclerosis, breast and lung cancer, heart disease and emphysema, amyotrophic lateral sclerosis, and an unspecified pelvic disorder. His medical license was suspended in 1991; and on three occasions he was indicted for murder, but the charges against him were dropped by the presiding judges who noted that assisted suicide was not a crime in Michigan.

  On December 15, 1992, Michigan Governor John Engler signed legislation specifically intended to stop Dr. Kevorkian, as well as to wrestle with the more general moral question of assisted death. The law, which temporarily criminalizes assisted suicide for a maximum of twenty-one months, making it a felony punishable by up to four years in prison and a $2,000 fine, was originally supposed to go into effect on March 30, 1993. While the ban is in operation, a commission will study assisted suicide (already a crime in 22 other states) and make recommendations to the Legislature which will have six months to act before the law's penalties expire. Speaking through his lawyer, the undeterred Dr. Kevorkian issued a public statement that "there [would] be several deaths" prior to the time the law went into effect. Over the course of the two months following the passage of this law, during January and February 1993, Dr. Kevorkian helped seven more gravely ill persons to die: four men and three women, five of whom suffered from cancer (of the bone, neck, breast, ovaries, and pancreas), one from multiple sclerosis, and one from congestive heart disease. Kevorkian publicly alleged through his lawyer that the accelerated pace of suicides over which he was presiding was triggered by the increasing numbers of seriously ill persons seeking his assistance before March 30. In an effort to stem this "last minute flurry" of suicides, on February 25, 1993, the Michigan Legislature passed another law that put the state's ban on assisted suicide into immediate effect.

After keeping a low profile for several months, Dr. Kevorkian assisted in a suicide on May 16, 1993. On August 4, 1993, he assisted in still another suicide. Kervorkian publicly acknowledged his role and invited prosecutors to press charges. On September 9, 1993, a judge ordered him to stand trial but allowed him to remain free on bond; later the same day, Kevorkian attended his eighteenth suicide. On October 11, 1993, Kevorkian was ordered for a second time to stand trial and warned that he might be jailed.

On October 22, 1993, for the nineteenth time, Kevorkian helped someone to commit suicide, this time in the doctor's own home. Newspapers quoted Dr. Kevorkian as saying that he was going to jail now, something he had wanted for two-and-a-half-years.

- The publication in 1991, and ascension to best-seller status, of *Final Exit,* by journalist Derek Humphry, an active euthanasia proponent and organizer and former president of the Hemlock Society (Humphry 1991). Not only does the book encourage terminally ill persons to plan their own death when they decide that meaningful life is over. It is also a "how-to" manual, providing detailed instructions about both "self-delivering" and doctor- and nurse-assisted ways of ending one's life — for example, by using certain doses and combinations of lethal drugs, attaching a hose to a car exhaust, tying a plastic bag over one's head, or undergoing self-starvation.

By and large, American bioethicists' commentaries on these happenings have supported the U.S. Supreme Court's *Cruzan* decision affirming the right of competent patients to refuse life-sustaining treatment, including the forgoing of artificial nutrition and hydration which the Court did not distinguish from other forms of treatment. In connection with both the *Cruzan* case and the Patient Self-Determination Act, bioethicists have urged the use of advance directives, emphasizing that they should be accompanied by face-to-face discussions between patients, their physicians, families, and close friends about the use of life-sustaining treatments, and about patients' values and preferences in this regard (Annas, Arnold, Aroskar, et al. 1990).

The U.S. bioethical community has responded more skeptically to the Supreme Court's holding that Missouri could require the continued treatment of a patient in a persistent vegetative state, like Nancy Cruzan, unless there was "clear and convincing," rigorous proof that she had explicitly authorized termination of treatment before losing the capacity to make decisions. In the opinion of jurist-ethicist George Annas, for example, the *Cruzan* decision "virtually casts in stone the post-Reagan Court's general view that although citizens have personal constitutional rights, the state can restrict them as long as the restriction furthers a legitimate state interest and is not 'irrational.' " "It is cold comfort," he goes on to say, "when the Court concludes that no other state need follow Missouri's lead.... [I]f the state of Missouri can inflict its will on Cruzan and her family, none of us are safe from states that wish to control our health care decisions and our deaths" (Annas 1990a:672).

Almost all U.S. bioethicists have "recoiled at the grossness of [Dr.] Kevorkian's [suicide-machine] method" (Pellegrino 1991:3118) and expressed "profound disturbance" over the "exhortative" and "propagandistic" way in which Derek Humphry's *Final Exit* instructs persons suffering from terminal illnesses on how to commit "rational suicide" (Wolf 1992). Nevertheless, these occurrences, the initiatives taken in several states to legalize physician-assisted suicide, and the strong medical, professional, and public responses to them have elicited soul-searching among bioethicists about the fact that "[t]oday, the power of medicine to sustain life is often a source of fear rather than solace," and "[s]uddenly, the 'perils of the soul' and our secret fears are associated with sustaining life rather than facing death" (O'Connell 1991: vi). Moreover, some bioethicists regard what they interpret as a societal movement toward legitimizing active euthanasia and assisted suicide as such a profound "cultural shift" that it "could become *the* major public policy debate of the 1990s."[8]

Regardless of where they stand on the issue of active euthanasia and assisted suicide, most American bioethicists regard *Final Exit* and its popularity, the Kevorkian death device, and legislation like Initiative 119 and Proposition 161 as indicators of the failure of the "medical establishment" to "confront the overuse of medical technology that merely prolongs the dying process" and to "accept the necessity of allowing people to die when their time has come" (Hamel 1991). Yet despite their shared critique of the medical profession's highly technological and relentlessly cure-oriented approach to dying, their consensus about patients' rights to elect or refuse treatment, and their mutual conviction that concerted efforts should be made to provide more humane terminal care, bioethicists are deeply divided about active euthanasia, especially in its physician-assisted form. "[R]ekindled by the possibility of its acceptance as a social policy" (Pellegrino 1991:3119), debate about this option and the age-old questions it has raised occupies a great deal of intellectual and emotional space in the American bioethics arena of the early 1990s. These are questions about what a moral doctor and society ought ideally to be; about individual choice and responsibility to others; about the significance of pain and suffering, illness and healing; about good and evil; about the meaning of human life, its fullness and finitude; and, ultimately, about the "why" of death itself.

Bioethicists realize that these issues are not only medical and philosophical but also religious in nature. Yet much of their discussion is phrased in secular biomedical and ethical language, with only occasional reference to faith traditions.[9] The infrequency with which they invoke the concept of hospice care, its emphasis on pain control, and the way it ministers to the psychological, social, and spiritual needs of dying patients and their families is also striking. Bioethical discussion acknowledges that both the right to refuse life-sustaining treatment and the decision of individuals to take their own lives involve and profoundly affect others — above all, medical caretakers, family members, and friends (Hamel 1991). Still, bioethicists have not challenged the appropriateness of affixing such an individualistic, autonomy-ridden title as the "Patient Self-Determination Act" to the legislation that authorizes advance directives. Philosopher Daniel Callahan comes closest to doing so in his vehement statement that when euthanasia "can only be effected by the moral and physical assistance of another," such as in the case of physician-assisted suicide, it is "a mutual, social decision between two people, the one to be killed and the other to do the killing" (Callahan 1992:52). Nevertheless, Callahan continues to characterize it as a form of self-determination, albeit one that in his view has "run amok" (Callahan 1992:55).

However, it is primarily within the framework of U.S. bioethical discourse about death and dying, termination of treatment, and euthanasia in the early 1990s that a new concern has emerged. This is what Daniel Callahan identifies as the still "immature" concept and problem of "medical futility" — namely, "whether it is possible to say, on scientific grounds alone, that some kinds of medical treatment will be futile, or useless, for some kinds of patients," and "whether, if some treatments are judged by physicians to be futile, there is an obligation on their part to tell patients (or their families) that is the case, letting them make the final decision" (Callahan 1991:31).

An embryonic medical futility debate began to develop around two well-publicized cases. The first was that of "Baby L," a two-year-old girl, blind, deaf, quadriplegic, profoundly retarded, gastrostomy-fed, subject to recurrent bouts of pneumonia, cardiopulmonary arrests, and daily seizures, who required repeated cardiopulmonary resuscitation and constant mechanical ventilation for survival. The child's mother insisted that the mechanical ventilation and cardiovascular support be continued, while the medical team unanimously believed that this would subject "Baby L" to additional pain and suffering without affecting her underlying condition or its ultimate outcome (Paris, Crone, and Reardon 1990). The second case (which received much more attention from the media as well as from bioethicists) concerned Helga Wanglie, an 85-year-old woman who tripped over a rug and broke her hip in December 1989. Wanglie underwent a series of treatments in a succession of acute care, rehabilitation, and nursing facilities, during which time she had several cardiopulmonary arrests. For over a year, until she died in July 1991, she remained unconscious, in a persistent vegetative state, and was maintained on a respirator and fed through a tube. In June and July of 1990, physicians suggested that Wanglie's life-sustaining treatment be withdrawn, saying that it was not benefiting her and that they did not want to give medical care that they considered "futile." Her husband, daughter, and son insisted on continued treatment.

In both the "Baby L" and Wanglie cases, the medical centers involved turned to the courts to settle the disputes. The guardian *ad litem* for "Baby L" appointed by the court found a pediatric neurologist consultant willing to accommodate the parents' desires, to whom the child's care was transferred. (Two years later the little girl, who required intensive home care 16 hours a day, was still alive.) In *Wanglie*, the court affirmed that Mr. Wanglie was the most suitable and best qualified of guardians for his wife, thereby denying the hospital's petition to replace him with a more "independent" conservator. Life-sustaining treatment was continued, but only three days after the judge's decision, Helga Wanglie died of multisystem organ failure resulting from septicemia.

Around these cases, especially that of Mrs. Wanglie, animated bioethical discussions on a number of issues have occurred. In particular, bioethicists have debated whether it is appropriate at this early stage in the framing of the concept of futility to ask the courts to make treatment decisions that override the wishes and beliefs of patients' families (Callahan 1991:34).

However tentative and ambiguous the idea of medical futility may still be, it has become an important concept of U.S. bioethics in the 1990s.[10] " 'Futility' is one of the newest additions to the lexicon of bioethics," declare physician-ethicists Robert Truog, Allan Brett, and Joel Frader, who have strong reservations about "the rapid advance of the language of futility into the jargon of the field" (Truog, Brett, and Frader 1992:1560, 1563). The fact that it intersects with the increasing bioethical emphasis on setting and accepting limits to medical progress has enhanced its significance (Callahan 1989; 1990a; 1990b). As philosopher Nancy S. Jecker and physician Lawrence J. Schneiderman astutely observe, although the concepts and connotations of medical futility and health care rationing differ in important ways, "[i]t seems more than coincidental [that in] recent years" these ideas have "gained prominence in the medical literature and in legal and clinical settings" and have "suddenly" become foci of "ethical debate" (Jecker and Schneiderman 1992:189).

This new bioethical preoccupation is unsettling to the philosophers, physicians, jurists, and members of the media who are reporting, pondering, and debating it. They are concerned about how "elusive" and "ambiguous" the concept of futility is — how difficult it is to define it and achieve a working consensus about its meaning. At the same time, they are wary about reducing it (and the gravity of making clinical decisions on behalf of critically ill patients that it entails) to "universally applicable principles" (Truog, Brett, and Frader 1992:1563). In any case, they wonder, "Who should decide when medical treatment is...futile?" Physicians? patients? their families or surrogates? "society" more broadly? Under what circumstances, in what combination, and by what process? (Jecker and Pearlman 1992:1140; Truog, Brett, and Frader 1992:1560, 1563). These commentators also express disquietude about the value assumptions that assertions of futility may "camouflage" — judgments about "comparative worth," for example, as well as about "the allocation of resources" (Truog, Brett, and Frader 1992:1563).

The diffuse unease that such bioethics futility-watchers are experiencing as this notion gains ascendancy also emanates from the challenge to quintessentially American values and beliefs that it represents. Not only does it run counter to the American conception of "limitless medical progress" in which "every disease should be cured, every disability rehabilitated, every health need met, and every evidence of mortality vigorously challenged" (Callahan 1990b:1811). In more far-reaching ways, it also contravenes the most energetic and optimistic "dare greatly," "strive mightily," "we shall overcome" constituents of the U.S. American worldview.

Abortion and Artificial Means of Reproduction

Some European observers view this concentration on death and dying as an American pattern. They contrast it with what they characterize as a tendency for European bioethics to be more preoccupied with beginning-of-life issues — especially abortion, artificial means of reproduction, and research on the embryo (Nau 1991).

Nonetheless, U.S. bioethicists continue to be acutely concerned about what they consider the "most contentious issue ... of moral choice ... that [American] society faces": the national struggle with abortion.[11] At the commencement of the 1990s, a great deal of the bioethical commentary about abortion has involved monitoring and appraising the consequences and implications of the July 1989 U.S. Supreme Court ruling on *Webster v. Reproductive Health Services.* In the view of most bioethicists, the Court's support in this case of a Missouri law barring the use of public hospitals or clinics for abortions "signaled a retreat" from its 1973 *Roe v. Wade* decision that "there is a fundamental constitutional right of privacy broad enough to encompass a woman's decision to have an abortion" and that "the state's interests in abridging the exercise of this right are related to the stage of pregnancy" (Annas 1989a:1200, 1202).

Although technically the Court made no changes in *Roe,* the separate opinions on *Webster* written by a plurality of the judges "ignored the right of privacy altogether"; "made it clear that they no longer believe[d] the [pregnancy] trimester scheme of *Roe* to be tenable"; and indicated that they were "ready to permit states to regulate heavily, and perhaps even prohibit outright, most abortions at any point in pregnancy" (Annas 1989a:1202). Furthermore, bioethicist-observers have been troubled by the "dramatic increase in the agitation ... on the subject of abortion" (Park Ridge Center 1990:4) that has ensued, opening up an increasingly bitter and politicized "clash of absolutes" (to use jurist Laurence H. Tribe's phrase) between the "prolife" and "prochoice" positions and movements that have formed around the abortion controversy. Some bioethicists are worried about the "number of tangentially related issues" that have become "captive" of the escalating abortion debate: the persistent moratorium on federal funding of fetal tissue transplant research for one, and the effective campaign to keep RU-486, the French antiprogestin drug that interferes with uterine implantation of fertilized eggs, off the United States market, for another (Charo 1991:43).

U.S. bioethicists grope for a "middle-ground" way (Lichtenberg 1990) of defusing, if not resolving, this intensifying conflict in American life — a way, as Roger Rosenblatt puts it, to have a society that "permits but discourages" abortion (Rosenblatt 1992). They note that such a "formula" would be congruent with what public opinion polls have consistently shown over the past twenty years: that rather than subscribing to either of the absolutist opposing views of abortion, the majority of Americans are deeply ambivalent about it.

Occasionally, the bioethical literature tries to place the abortion issue and its solution in a larger societal perspective — linking them with the fact that among Western countries, the United States has one of the highest pregnancy rates, percentages of unwanted pregnancies, and average number of abortions, and that it is "women who are poor, unmarried, under 25 years of age, and representative of minority communities [who] are more likely to have abortions than women who are not" (Capps 1990:6). Implicitly, at least, this raises the question of what connections exist between the approximately 1.6 million abortions that are performed each year in the United States and the society's deficiencies in providing adequate shelter, nutrition, education, employment, and medical and child care to women of disadvantaged social, ethnic, and racial backgrounds.

On June 29, 1992, the U.S. Supreme Court issued its long awaited ruling on the Pennsylvania abortion case, *Planned Parenthood v. Casey.* By the narrowest of margins, in a sharply split 5–4 decision, the Court reaffirmed what it defined as the "essential holding" of *Roe v. Wade:* "that it is a constitutional liberty of the woman to have some freedom to terminate her pregnancy." This is a "rule of law and a component of liberty," they stated, that "we cannot now repudiate." At the same time, invoking the portion of *Roe* that established the "state's important and legitimate interest in potential life," the Court permitted some new state restrictions on abortion that did not, in their opinion, impose an "undue burden" on the abortion decision by creating a substantial obstacle to the woman's exercise of the right to choose. Specifically, it upheld the requirements of a twenty-four-hour waiting period; medical counseling on alternatives to abortion; girls under eighteen years of age obtaining the consent of a parent or the approval of a judge before getting an abortion; and doctors or clinics performing abortions making statistical reports to the state. However, it struck down a provision obliging a married woman to tell her husband of her intention to have an abortion. The Court commented on the fact that national "divisiveness" over abortion "has grown only more intense"; and there was both "anger and anguish" (Greenhouse 1992:1A) in the language the judges used to express how they felt about being "under fire" in the midst of all the political pressures and counterpressures surrounding it. Although U.S. bioethicists did not react to the Court's decision by leaping into print to discuss it, there is every reason to suppose that they will continue to be as concerned with this national controversy as they have been throughout the history of bioethics.

Along with the abortion debate, U.S. bioethicists have carried their involvement with the new reproductive technologies into the 1990s. Still, the focus lacks the intensity it had in 1987–88, when the Superior and Supreme Courts of the State of New Jersey were deliberating on parental custody and visitation rights in the case of "Baby M," a child born under a surrogate parenting contract between William Stern and Mary Beth Whitehead, who had been artificially inseminated with his semen.

Much of U.S. bioethical reflection on the new, noncoital means of reproduction is still concerned with Alexander Pope's question, "To whom related, and by whom begot?" As a consequence of in vitro fertilization, embryo transfer, artificial insemination, and surrogacy, for example, it is "possible for a child to have five 'parents': a genetic and rearing father, and a genetic, gestational, and rearing mother" (Elias and Annas 1986:62). The ongoing bioethical discussion about these methods is catalyzed in part by the recurrent appearance in the courts of cases involving issues associated with reproductive technology: the status and disposition of frozen embryos produced during an in vitro fertilization procedure and, especially, the status and rights of the so-called surrogate mother, who is the gestational carrier of a child (Annas 1989b; Annas 1991).[12] As numerous bioethical commentators continue to state, the development and deployment of these artificial means of reproduction raise fundamental biological, social, and moral questions about our conceptions of the family, parenthood, the child, lineage, legitimacy, and identity (Elias and Annas 1986; Macklin 1991).

Bioethicists write thoughtfully about how difficult it is to determine what and who "counts as family" in today's society. They express wariness about adopting notions of the family and relatedness that are too determined by genetic- or gestational-based biology, by traditional custom, or by law and contract (Annas 1991; Macklin 1991). Increasingly in the 1990s, American bioethical discussion about the new reproductive technologies has also recognized that feminist thinkers and writers generally oppose these methods, primarily on the grounds that "both by reinforcing sex-role stereotypes in which a woman's worth is dependent on her reproductive capacity and... by reinforcing the power of men in the reproductive sphere," they are likely to "undermine women's freedom in the long run" (Lebacqz 1991:12–14). However, the bioethical literature is more inclined to tackle "the question of how artificial means of reproduction affect our understanding of the family" (Macklin 1991:11) than to examine the uncertainty and lack of consensus in American society about what we mean by a family, who we are, and how we are related. And only rarely is it suggested that a "disquieting aspect" of "the intense concern" about "the fate of frozen embryos" and the "occasional children born of forms of technology that have outstripped our social consensus" may be that it helps divert attention from the "great many children in this country [who] die of neglect, abuse, or preventable disease" (Angell 1990:1202).

Organ Transplantation

> "Organ Procurement: Supply, Demand — and Ethics"
> As scientific developments improve success rates, the number of patients who could benefit from organ transplantation has increased dramatically. Yet the supply of transplantable organs falls well short of demand. What can we do to increase the number of available organs? And what sorts of social and ethical considerations must our proposals take into account? ...

This statement, excerpted from the announcement of a conference held in 1991 on "ethical dimensions" of the current situation in organ procurement and "suggestions for increasing the supply of transplantable organs"[13] expresses the major thrust of the bioethical attention paid to organ transplantation in the United States during the late 1980s and early 1990s. The arrival of a new immunosuppressive drug on the scene — cyclosporine — helped to precipitate a so-called transplant boom. Cyclosporine's ability to forestall the immune system from defensively rejecting tissue and organ transplants emboldened many American physicians and medical centers to enter the field, to transplant a wider spectrum of organs, singly and in various combinations, and to do a greater number of retransplants. This expansion of organ transplantation and the exuberance that fostered it have made it harder to procure enough organs for the growing lists of transplant candidates. What is perceived as a serious "organ shortage" and a crisis about how to allocate scarce organs most fairly has generated an array of strategies to obtain more donated organs and to decide who should receive them

(Fox and Swazey 1992: chaps. 3 and 4). As noted, this is the set of problems with which U.S. bioethics has become principally involved.

By and large, American bioethical commentary has not critically examined two of the basic beliefs undergirding the dramatic escalation of transplants during the past decade: namely, that organ transplantation is unequivocally and unconditionally good; and that the more organs given, acquired, and transplanted, the better the situation is, both medically and morally. Most U.S. bioethicists implicitly accept these premises and unquestioningly assume that it is the dearth of organs donated rather than an excess of transplants performed that has given rise to urgent concerns about "supply," "demand," and "shortfall." As their vocabulary suggests, in the free-enterprise, supply-side economics-infused American value climate of the 1980s and early 1990s, bioethicists, like transplanters and health policy analysts, have progressively moved away from the "gift of life" framework within which organ transplantation was originally defined, toward a market-oriented and commodified conception of the acts of giving and receiving that it entails.

More than a linguistic change is involved, however. For increasingly, various types of market systems (especially futures markets) and regulated financial compensation and incentives are being proposed as inducements to motivate cadaveric organ donation. In turn, these developments (along with the use in medical research of human organs, tissues, cells, and body fluids that could yield products of marketable value) have stimulated bioethical thinking and metaphysics-like debate about the nature and meaning of the human body: What is the relationship of our embodiment to "the humanness of our human life" and to our personhood? Where is our human identity "located"? And is our body our own, individual property over which we have dominion, or do we hold it in stewardship or trusteeship as a gift — "whether or not there be a giver" (Kass 1985:101–2, 283)? The discernible shift that is occurring in the direction of "organs for sale," their biological reduction to "mere body" and "thingness" and a *homo economicus* conception of the human person worries some bioethical thinkers — practically, morally, and existentially — more than it does others (Childress 1989:101, 110; Childress 1992; Fox and Swazey 1992: chap. 3; Kass 1985:99–127, 276–98; Kass 1992; Levine 1986; Murray 1987).

Another phenomenon that has been evoking bioethical unease and discussion in the United States since the mid-1980s is the "generation of human beings to serve as transplant donors" (Kass 1992:85). Concretely, this entails the decision by parents to conceive an infant with the hope that he or she will prove to be a suitable, matched bone marrow donor for another one of their children whose illness (usually leukemia or lymphoma) would otherwise result in imminent death.

In 1990–91, the moral issues surrounding bringing a baby into the world for this purpose surged into prominence. The Ayala family, whose nineteen-year-old daughter Anissa was slowly dying of chronic myelogenous leukemia, publicly announced that after failing to find a compatible bone marrow donor for her within their own family or through private bone marrow registries, they had conceived a child on the one-in-four chance that the baby's tissue type would match Anissa's. The ensuing debate over "the permissible limits of one of our most powerful instincts, the one that leads us to fight for the life of our children" (Quindlen 1991) made a media celebrity of Anissa Ayala (who was the subject of a June 17, 1991, *Time* magazine cover), and of her baby sister Marissa, born in April 1991, who indeed proved to be a compatible donor. The bone marrow withdrawn from Marissa when she reached the age of fourteen months and infused into her sister Anissa seems to have been life-saving.

On March 23, 1992, *Time* announced that Ayala "now plans to marry her longtime boyfriend and start a support group for other cancer patients" who, in her words, "don't have the closeness my family and I have" ("A Sister Is Saved" 1992). One year and one day after she received her transplant, on June 5, 1992, Anissa's marriage to Bryan Espinosa took place. Two-and-a-half-year-old Marissa was her flower girl. She "shared her wedding day with the little sister who made it possible," reported the media that extensively covered the occasion. "When you see Marissa walking down the aisle as a flower girl," Anissa's physician, Rudolf Brutoco, was quoted as saying, "you have to realize that either girl wouldn't be here without the other" ("A Life-Saving Sibling Helps Once More" 1992).

The "happy ending" notwithstanding, bioethical opinion has been divided over how morally acceptable such a utilitarian act of science and love is. Questions have been raised about the impact this act may eventually have on the sense of identity and the reason for being of the donor child, who did not consent to be used in this way and might not have agreed to the transplant if she had been able to choose (Kearney and Caplan 1992).

A much sharper and deeper split exists among American bioethicists regarding the use of anencephalic infants (born with the rapidly fatal absence of most of the brain other than its stem) as organ sources for infants and young children awaiting transplantation. This split has been apparent each time an attempt has been made over the past twenty-five years to procure and transplant organs from such infants (Churchill and Pinkus 1990). Two cases in particular highlighted these differences. The first concerned the Loma Linda (California) University Medical Center, which in July 1988 called a moratorium on the controversial protocol under which it had been the only center in the United States with an active program for obtaining organs from anencephalic infants for transplantation (Peabody, Emery, and Ashwal 1989). The second concerned the unsuccessful medical and legal quest in March 1992 by Laura Campo and Justin Pearson, the parents of a baby girl (Theresa Ann) born with only a brain stem, to donate her organs for transplant. The kind of bioethical dispute that these events elicited in the glare of the media and the Court attention they received suggest that the differences between U.S. bioethicists on matters as basic as their views of personhood, "aliveness," death, the human community, and the good society may be greater than in the past.

One group of bioethical thinkers feel strongly that the parents of an anencephalic infant should be able to make something positive and meaningful from their tragedy by donating their baby's organs to other children who may live on because of them. This group goes so far as to say that "if even a single life could be saved" through this act of parental donation, it is "worthy" as well as "rewarding" (Truog and Fletcher 1990). But waiting until all activity in the brain stem of anencephalic infants ceases and spontaneous breathing stops — the criteria of total brain death — is likely to damage their transplantable organs. In contrast, providing the infants with intensive care, as was done under the Loma Linda protocol, tends to preserve their brain stem along with their other organs, making the occurrence of brain death unlikely.

This conflict has impelled some bioethicists who advocate the use of anencephalic infants as organ sources to argue that "no relevant distinction can or should be made between anencephaly and brain death" (Truog and Fletcher 1989). They propose further that the Uniform Anatomical Gift Act or the Uniform Determination of Death Act be revised to make anencephaly a variant of brain death, in order to allow organ removal from anencephalic infants who have brain stem activity and are still breathing spontaneously. This proposal to make "the condition of anencephaly...a special case in which removal of the organs for transplantation should be permitted without regard for the criteria of brain death" (Truog and Fletcher 1989) rests on another set of assumptions made by those who advocate it. In their view, because such infants lack virtually all integrative brain function, they are not "alive as persons"; rather, they are "living non-persons" without the activity of the higher brain that "makes us human" (Cefalo and Engelhardt 1989; Zaner 1989; Kolata 1992). Among these bioethicists, some regard anencephaly as the "congenital counterpart" of the persistent vegetative states in which persons like Karen Ann Quinlan and Nancy Beth Cruzan languished. Ethicist John Fletcher, for example, is so committed to promoting the idea that people in this state, along with anencephalic infants, should be considered dead, that he has publicly revealed the existence of a clause in his living will stating that when his higher brain permanently ceases to function, even if activity in his brain stem persists, he wants his organs to be "quarried" for transplantation (Kolata 1992).

Another group of bioethicists strongly oppose this way of thinking about anencephalic infants, their parents, their involvement in organ donation, and the definition of death. The fact that donating their anencephalic infant's organs for transplantation could provide meaning and consolation for stricken parents, they say, does not necessarily make it justifiable (Churchill and Pinkus 1990:155–57). Furthermore, these bioethicists take a stand against any attempt to "alter statutes and re-categorize anencephalic infants as 'dead,' 'nonpersons,' or in some other way remove them from moral and legal protections and deny them a locus in the human world" (Churchill and Pinkus 1990:165; Annas 1987; Shewmon et al. 1989). Even though such infants probably cannot experience pain, these bioethicists are concerned about the harm and the wrong done to the infants if their organs are taken, especially in the face of the conceptual confusion and emotional disquietude that currently surround the concept of brain death.

They are plagued by the "slippery slope" implications — a slippery slope, they contend, that is "real," not just hypothetical. For, they point out, the Loma Linda team "received from 'good' physicians several referrals [of infants as organ donors] with less severe anomalies [than anencephaly], such as 'babies born with an abnormal amount of fluid around the brain or those born without kidneys but with a normal brain'" (Shewmon et al. 1989:1775). Finally, they raise searching questions about the profound damage to the humane and moral foundations of the entire society that could result from such "overly aggressive efforts to increase the supply of donor organs" (Evans 1990) if this leads to placing "greater value on meeting the needs of organ recipients than on protecting donors, respecting the rights of persons, and protecting the vulnerable" (Churchill and Pinkus 1990:165).

Acquired Immunodeficiency Syndrome (AIDS)

The AIDS epidemic has been called a "total social phenomenon" (Bosk and Frader 1991:150), so "freighted with social and cultural meaning...[that] it will have long-term, broad-ranging effects on personal relationships, social institutions, and cultural configurations" (Nelkin,

Willis, and Parris 1991:1). Still, the preponderance of U.S. bioethical discussion devoted to it during the late 1980s and early 1990s has been more narrowly concentrated on questions about the role responsibilities, rights, and exemptions of physicians and other health care workers.[14] Initially, these questions crystallized around the uncertainties, risks, and dangers of caring for persons who are infected with the human immuno-deficiency virus (HIV) or with AIDS. They have also focused on the reactions of anxiety, fear, avoidance, and repugnance that patients who have this protean, communicable, as yet incurable, and lethal disease can elicit in health professionals. Deep feelings of aversion to the way of life of some persons with HIV infection or AIDS — especially those who are gay or are intravenous drug users — along with concern about infecting themselves or family members have contributed to the reluctance with which many medical professionals approach their care. As a consequence, the "duty to treat or the right to refuse" (Daniels 1991) became a preoccupying bioethical question as the 1980s progressed, with a sharp focus on whether physicians have an unqualified obligation to treat patients with AIDS.

Both ethicists and medical spokespersons have enunciated an almost unanimous moral stance on these matters. They affirm that physicians have a fundamental responsibility to "provide competent, sensitive, and compassionate care to all patients" (Association of American Medical Colleges 1988); that refusing to treat patients with AIDS or evading doing so violates the very nature of the profession and the commitment to care selflessly for the sick on which it is grounded; that the work of a doctor, including ministering to those with AIDS, entails accepting some personal risk "without panic or avoidance" (Cooke and Sande 1989:1337); but that the risks in taking care of AIDS patients (or persons with other contagious diseases) should be prudently handled through the employment of protective measures in the clinical setting, within the framework of well-designed and well-observed programs of infection control (Cooke and Sande 1989; Daniels 1991; Emanuel 1988).

In 1991, however, bioethical attention shifted from "dangerous patients" to "dangerous doctors" and other health care personnel, when the media made it known that five patients had contracted HIV infection from a seropositive dentist. Among them, twenty-three-old Kimberly Bergalis, by her repeated appearances and pronouncements throughout the tragically fatal course of her disease (including her testimony to the U.S. Congress just prior to her death), dramatically personified the vulnerability of patients to HIV infection from health care workers, the widespread fear and indignation that the public felt about this ironic possibility, and their expectation that measures be taken to protect them against the risk. As the Centers for Disease Control struggled to develop acceptable guidelines for preventing the transmission of HIV to patients, bioethical commentary addressed the challenge of morally articulating an approach that would "protect patients while minimizing disruptions to patient care" and "respecting the privacy and livelihood of health care workers" (Lo and Steinbrook 1992:1100, 1105).

The Human Genome Project

Finally, with the advent of the 1990s, the implications of the U.S. Human Genome Initiative to characterize, map, and sequence the human genome or gene set have become important centers of bioethical activity. As sociologist Howard L. Kaye has written, "[a]pplause and a collective sigh of relief greeted the announcement in 1990" that as much as five million dollars of the project's budget would be set aside for studies of ethical, legal, and social issues that may arise from the application of knowledge about gene structure and function and the genetic aspects of human disease that may be obtained as a result of the genome research. For, "[m]indful of past experience with the atom and other revolutionary research that were put to uses that were not fully anticipated, scientists and administrators now seemed to be preparing to grapple with possible uses and abuses of their work while it was underway" (Kaye 1992:77).

In 1991, as many as nineteen ethics programs dealing with the genomic-code undertaking were being sponsored by the Project (Zylke 1992:1715). A list of the ethical concerns with which these groups have been dealing — often in workshop and conference form — would include these: the historical "shadow of eugenics that looms over human genetic research" (Kevles 1992:68) and the potential for its revival; the phenomenon of "homemade eugenics" — couples deciding what kinds of children they do and do not want to have — that the advance of human genetics and biotechnology has already made possible (Kevles 1992:75); the issues of fairness in the use of genetic information and of opportunities for genetic discrimination on the basis of this information by insurance companies, employers, the criminal justice system, educational institutions, the military, and adoption agencies, among others; the ways in which knowledge of relevant genetic information might be used to label and stigmatize particular individuals, families, or racial and ethnic groups, and create a "genetic underclass" (Dreyfuss and Nelkin 1992:334); questions about the privacy and confidentiality of individual genomic information, its ownership, control, and conditions of disclosure; and the bearing of the commercialization of products from the Human Genome Initiative on intellectual property rights, scientific collaboration, and accessibility of data. In addition, certain conceptual and philosophical ramifications of the human genome undertaking are also being broached: its potential impact, for example, on ways of thinking about health and disease, identity and personhood, individuality and freedom of will, and community and responsibility.

Whatever forms bioethical reflection on the human genome endeavor is taking, only rarely is a voice heard that goes beyond these issues and challenges the underlying assumptions of the Project itself. Sociologist Howard Kaye considers this lack one of the most insidiously worrisome aspects of the debates that the U.S. Human Genome Initiative is both eliciting and supporting. "To think in terms of 'implications' and 'logical consequences' [of the Human Genome Project]," he writes, "is to suggest that certain facts or propositions about human social behavior are so inseparably entwined with certain facts or propositions about biology that if the biological statement is true, the social statement follows necessarily" (Kaye 1992:78). It is to fail to raise sufficiently penetrating questions about the fact that "[m]any of the prominent scientists involved believe that the logical consequence of unlocking the gene's secrets will [require] nothing less than a fundamental change in our understanding of human nature ... a transformation of how we understand ourselves: from moral beings, whose character and conduct is largely shaped by culture, social environment, and individual choice, to essentially biological beings, whose 'fate,' according to [the former] project head James Watson, 'is in our genes' " (Kaye 1992:77). In Kaye's view, this "forgetting of the kind of beings we are" and "our construction of a new self-definition seemingly sanctioned by the biological sciences" constitute a highly reductionistic and deterministic "dehumanization in thought" that is dangerously seductive in this period of "cultural crisis and moral uncertainty" in U.S. society and the West, when we are individually and collectively "[c]onfused about who we are, ... how we should live," and where we are going (Kaye 1992:80, 84).

Whether one agrees with Kaye's interpretative analysis, it exemplifies what James M. Gustafson characterizes as "prophetic moral discourse": it tends to be more "macro," "general," and "passionate" than the discourse that predominates in U.S. bioethics; more concerned with "meaning and significance" in a "larger cultural and human context"; more likely to lay bare "assumptions that seem not to be radically challenged by scientists and clinicians"; and more intent on "peer[ing] through ... immediate and confined things ... to describe

a profound malady...that is a threat to the whole of humanity"
(Gustafson 1990:130–36).

Major Characteristics of the Discourse
and Outlook of U.S. Bioethics

As the foregoing suggests, the discourse of U.S. bioethics retains many
attributes that it has displayed since the inception of the field. The
concrete moral problems and solutions, critical choices, and alternative
courses of action (in particular medical research and care circumstances)
are usually discussed in technical, unemotional, nonmetaphorical language, and in a rigorously rational, formal, largely deductive mode of
argumentation framed by a "relatively small set of concepts" (Gustafson
1990:127) — chiefly the principles of respect for autonomy, beneficence,
nonmaleficence, and justice, and the derived rules of truthfulness, privacy, confidentiality, and fidelity (Beauchamp and Childress 1979, 1983,
1989).

A number of converging factors have reinforced and enhanced these
intellectual and linguistic characteristics of U.S. bioethical thought over
the years. To begin with, its regnant paradigm, currently referred to
as "principlism," was chiefly fashioned and codified by philosophical ethicists, working out of an Anglo-American analytic and secular
philosophical tradition. What has become the *"locus classicus* for this
tendency within contemporary bioethics" (Wikler 1991:238) — a veritable " 'Bible' of academic medical ethics" (Hoffmaster 1991:219) — is
Tom L. Beauchamp and James F. Childress's *Principles of Biomedical
Ethics,* now in its fourth edition (1979, 1983, 1989, 1993). Beauchamp
and Childress used this approach, working in a flexibly systematic
way, to "illuminate the cases and policies that they discuss" (Wikler
1991:239–40). Furthermore, implicit in Childress's perspective are la-
tent theological assumptions such as the prominent theological theme in
Quaker thought (Childress's tradition) of " 'answering that of God in
every person' " through respecting all persons as equals, and an *"agape*
or love of neighbor" commitment to "preventing and removing harm
from others as well as doing good toward them" (Campbell 1989:119,
121, 127). But in the "less expert hands" of the multitude of persons untrained or poorly educated in philosophical or theological ethics
who are participants in U.S. bioethics, the deployment of the "principle
approach" is often so formulaic that it has been portrayed as a mechanically applied, ritually intoned, "mantralike" form of analysis (Clouser
and Gert 1190:219–20; Wikler 1991:239–40).

Several factors have helped to give this simplified, "stripped-down" version of principlism hegemony in U.S. bioethics: first, the multidisciplinary nature of the field; second, the public status of the bioethical debates taking place in a pluralistic, religiously resonant but secularized society that is undergoing what observant social critics describe as a fragmenting cultural process of separation and individuation (Bellah et al. 1985); and third, the acutely felt need under these conditions for "a single, common, comprehensive, and coherent way" of addressing and resolving moral problems and quandaries (Blake 1992:7). In this regard, the "mantra-driven" form of principlism (Wikler 1991:240) serves as a fundamentalistic *lingua franca* — "a moral Esperanto" constructed around the limited ethical precepts about which consensus can be presumed (Verhey 1990:24).

As has been true from the outset, the agenda of U.S. bioethics is more reactive than initiatory. To a striking extent it responds to the predominating political, economic, and value orientation of the society, which it tends to reflect rather than criticize or challenge. The "topicality" of bioethics — especially its temporal, empirical, and thematic synchronization with the popular "bioethical sound bites" carried by the news media (Wikler 1991:248) and with the announcement of new legislation and judicial decisions relevant to bioethical issues — is one manifestation of this pattern. Still another is the notable degree to which U.S. bioethical discussion has been increasingly conducted in the materialistic, free enterprise, supply-side economics vocabulary, keynoted by the Reagan and Bush presidential administrations.

This vocabulary is apparent, for example, in the "shift away from the traditional view of health care as a social good that is exempt from market forces and towards a view that health care is an economic commodity subject to the influence of supply, demand, and price. Concepts like *cost containment, competition, consumer attitudes*, and *capitation arrangements* presently shape the discussion of health care in the United States" (O'Connell 1987:286). The same shift is visible in the concern about the allocation of scarce, expensive resources for advanced medical care, research, and development that has increasingly preoccupied U.S. bioethics since the 1970s; in the elevation of cost containment to the status of a bioethical moral imperative (Fox 1989:230); and in the arguments gaining momentum in U.S. bioethical circles in favor of defining "human body parts" as private property and increasing the "supply" of transplantable organs by creating financial incentives for donation, such as "futures markets" in cadaveric organs (Kass 1992).

The economically individualistic and private-entitlement premises on which these concerns and proposals rest, coupled with the paramountcy accorded to autonomy and self-determination in the ethos of U.S. bioethics, bend the field away from an emphasis on responsibility to the community and the larger society. Furthermore, it removes the field from a conception of social justice that pays special attention to the plight of the poor, the disadvantaged, the victims of social prejudice and discrimination. Consider, for example, the following scenarios:

> When the acquired immunodeficiency syndrome (AIDS) first appeared in 1981, it was considered a disease of homosexual and drug-using men. Only later did it become evident that AIDS could also strike children and women. But attention to infection with the human immunodeficiency virus (HIV) in these groups still lags behind the attention given to the disease in men....
>
> Although we are making advances in the treatment of HIV infection, we continue to be reluctant to undertake widespread HIV-antibody testing of pregnant women.... Despite the medical uncertainties, the practical complexities, and the ethical conundrums of routine screening, these problems pale before the problems of the delivery of effective care to HIV-infected pregnant women and their children. Most women and children with HIV infection are urban, poor, and members of minority groups. The cities in which they reside face the most serious economic problems in the current recession. The combination of a chronic, ultimately lethal disease with serious economic hardship and family and social disintegration has made the daily care of these patients almost impossible. The difficulties of caring for women and children with HIV infection places in stark relief the fact that many citizens in this nation do not have access to medical care. Thus, the greatest problems that health professionals face in regard to this group of patients are not the clinical uncertainties so much as the lack of simple, basic necessities: housing, access to medical care, money for drug treatment, and social support for families in which someone is seriously ill....
>
> [W]hile we make sophisticated scientific advances, we continue to neglect the simple things. We can only hope that one day the nation will finally summon up the energy and the will to do what we already know how to do: to provide shelter, social support, and access to medical care for all who have this infection, no matter what their social class or ethnic or racial background. (Heagarty and Abrams 1992)

•

John Kingery, 82, physically helpless, emptied of memory by Alzheimer's disease and holding a bag of diapers, was abandoned in his wheelchair at an Idaho dog track the other day. "Proud To Be An American" were the words on his sweatshirt....

These abandonments are common enough nowadays, according to an agent of the old-people's lobby, to constitute a trend which they call "granny dumping."

I was forced to dwell on [this story that] got big [press] play across the country...at the very moment the posturing of Presidential candidates was at one of its seasonal peaks....

Contemplating the possibility of being granny-dumped, there in the wheelchair, holding the bag of diapers, "Proud To Be An American," I wonder if our politicians might be numb to furies seething among Americans....

Wake and look, gentlemen. There's trouble out here. People sleeping in streets. Terrorists killing for fun, money and revenge in filthy, ruined cities. Millions with no medicine, no doctor. The desperate young are abandoning helpless, hopeless Granny.

Some indignation must be voiced, some conviction about public morality expressed, some principles articulated. "Electability" is a shabby substitute for the passion that hates seeing the old county poorhouse revived as a dog track.... (Baker 1992)

•

... [M]edical indigence is a silent, largely invisible epidemic.... Most insured Americans are like the torturer's horse, minding their own business while somewhere, in another part of the forest, the uninsured poor suffer.... As long as these vulnerable people are subject to the whims and prejudices of payers, providers, and society, we are all at risk.... The medically indigent represent the risk of moral rot at the heart of our society, born of a callousness about those whose suffering we cannot see and therefore do not acknowledge.... Should we continue to treat the most fragile members of our society as strangers, we will not be acting like the torturer's horse; we will be the torturers. (Friedman 1989)

These at-once indicting and exhortative statements were written by two physicians involved in the care of women and children who are HIV-infected, a journalist/social critic, and a medical writer who is an independent health policy analyst. The fact that none of the articles from which they are excerpted was authored by a bioethicist or published in the bioethical literature has a relationship to the slant and style of the field. It is congruent with the already noted disposition of U.S.

bioethics to think on a "micro" level; to interpret social good in an individualistic, nontranscendent way; and to use "objectifying," image-free language drawn from or influenced by the logical positivism and legalism of its controlling paradigm. It also coincides with the conservative disinclination of U.S. bioethics to advocate social change that might call upon fortunate persons and groups in the society to generously forgo some of their advantages in order to help others who are deprived.

The restricted social and cultural scope and vision of U.S. bioethics is associated, too, with several other major attributes of its approach: its concentration on small-scale, immediate medical quandaries and regulatory questions; its pronouncedly secular outlook, despite the fact that some of its early shapers were theologians or religious ethicists (Callahan and Campbell 1990; Marty 1992b); and the relatively insignificant part that social science and scientists have played, or been invited to play, in its development (Fox 1989:237–39; Marshall 1992).

The focus of U.S. bioethics on "moral quandaries in narrowly circumscribed circumstances and [on] questions of public regulation" (Verhey 1990:21) emanates from the problem-solving role that it has been asked and is willing to assume in clinical and policy-making settings. This role has also encouraged the management and systematic reduction of complexity and uncertainty in order to dispel conflict, foster consensus, and facilitate purposive action. Furthermore, because the field has great "public interest, commanding the attention of the courts, legislatures, the media, and professional societies," it is under both internal and external "pressure . . . to frame the issues, and to speak in a common secular mode" (Callahan 1990c:3).

But the progressive secularization of U.S. bioethics over the three decades of its existence has involved more than abiding by the American constitutional principle of maintaining a separation between church and state; respecting the essentially pluralist nature of the society; and trying to avert the sorts of deep, unresolvable, potentially bitter moral conflicts that many Americans believe the public expression of religious convictions and debate about religious differences may unleash (Callahan 1990c:3–4; Marty 1992b:74–75). U.S. bioethics emerged in the late 1960s and early 1970s, during a period of tumult in religious communities and the society at large, when secularism "crested as a social movement" on the American scene — a movement in which some theologians figured prominently (Wind 1990:18). In addition, the academic milieux in which the majority of U.S. participants in bioethics — whether philosophers, theologians, physicians, or lawyers — received their professional training, and in which many now work, are "resolutely secular" institutions (Callahan 1990c:3) that "nurture and reward secular habits of thought" (Wind 1990:18). Partly as a consequence of these patterns, "most religious ethicists entering the public practice of ethics," writes physician-philosopher Leon Kass, "leave their special insights at the door and talk about 'deontological vs. consequentialist,' 'autonomy vs. paternalism,' 'justice vs. utility,' just like everybody else" (Kass 1990). In common with other professionals engaged in bioethics, they define their religious beliefs as private matters. When they apply their ethical analyses to clinical contexts, and especially to the public policy domain, they generally cordon off what they regard as their personal religious convictions and remain largely silent about them.

Thus reflection on basic and transcendent aspects of the human condition and on enduring questions of meaning that are integral to health, illness, and medicine have been relegated to the borderlands of bioethical concerns:

> The conception of human beings; their birth, survival, and growth; their physical, emotional, and intellectual capacities and development; sexuality; aging, mortality, and death — the very quality of their lives — are core foci of health, illness, and medicine. Our "coming in," our "staying in," and our "going out" are continuously linked with our health and illness concerns and with the medical care that we seek and receive.... The experience of illness and the practice of medicine also summon up critical problems of meaning — fundamental questions about the "whys" of pain; suffering, accident and *angst*; the limits of human life; and death; and about their relationship to evil, sin, and injustice. (Fox 1988:573)

What philosopher Simone Weil has called these "ponderable imponderables" are described by moral theologian Courtney S. Campbell as "problems [that] cannot be solved but must still be faced" (Campbell 1990:7). For the most part, however, U.S. bioethicists have not faced these problems. They have left them out of the bioethics repertoire or, as theologian Stanley Hauerwas would contend, they have deliberately and steadfastly excluded them (Hauerwas 1986).

The secular rationality of U.S. bioethics in combination with its autonomous individualism has contributed to the narrowing of its outlook in still another way. It downplays communal values and qualities of the heart, like caring, kindness, devotion, compassion, generosity, service, altruism, sacrifice, and love. These values involve recognizing and responding to close and distant others in a self-transcending way — to "neighbors" and "strangers," members of future generations in distant lands, as well as "sisters" and "brothers" who inhabit this time and this familiar place.

The "disappearance or denaturing of religion in [the] public discourse" of U.S. bioethics (Callahan 1990c:4) has also contributed to its flatness. It is devoid of the images and symbols, narratives and memories that are associated with both religion and literature, as it carries on its reflections in a language that "aspires...to a kind of detached neutrality...and a culture-free rationalistic universalism" (Callahan 1990c:4).

This latter commitment of U.S. bioethics to "identify and apply moral principles that all people can and must hold independently of their particular communities and histories" (Verhey 1990:21) is one of the primary sources of another enduring characteristic of the field: its tentative and strained relationship to the social sciences. As anthropologists Patricia A. Marshall and Richard W. Lieban point out, a key concept of social science, especially of anthropology — the notion of "cultural relativism" — has had a profoundly constraining influence on interdisciplinary exchanges between the two fields (Marshall 1992:56; Lieban 1990:221–22). Sociological and anthropological insistence on studying societies and cultures on their own terms, by recognizing and respecting the differences in their values, beliefs, and worldviews runs counter to the "culture-free universalism" that U.S. bioethics espouses. For example, social scientists have attempted to examine the effects of cultural variations on the ethicality of medical research methods in non-Western societies (Christakis 1988). Some philosophers and physicians in U.S. bioethics have repeatedly responded with intellectual and moral criticism:

> The concept of cultural sensitivity in research is appealing. It suggests the sophistication of the researcher, an absence of ethnocentricity, and an appreciation of the values of other cultures. Appeals to cultural sensitivity, however, are no substitute for careful moral analysis. We see no convincing arguments for a general policy of dispensing with, or substantially modifying, the researcher's obligation to obtain first-person consent in biomedical research conducted in Africa. (Ijsselmuiden and Faden 1992:833)

In this passage, a prominent American philosopher, Ruth R. Faden, and her coauthor, South African physician Carel B. Ijsselmuiden, imply that "cultural sensitivity" — their term for cultural analysis — is not only very different from "careful moral analysis," but that admirable though it may be, it has little bearing on "the development of ethical theory and practice of medical research in Africa" or elsewhere (Ijsselmuiden and Faden 1992:833).

The monistic conception of a globally applicable, transcultural set of moral precepts is responsible, too, for the general failure of U.S. bioethics to recognize how Western and distinctively American its philosophical principlism is. For example, the Thai Buddhist philosopher Pinit Ratanakul points to the "preoccupation of U.S. bioethics with the individual...his rights,...and his claims on society and others more than on his responsibility for himself and for society" — "a mark of American culture," he comments, that "is not prevalent in many Asian cultures" (Ratanakul 1991).[15] In placing greater value on the autonomous self than on the self in relation to others and the community, U.S. bioethics has also enhanced the standoff with regard to the social sciences. In addition, something like a "three culture split" is involved in the propensity of U.S. bioethics to regard the social sciences as a "third culture," an "intermediary sort of...sub-area" (Geertz 1983:158) between the "two cultures" of the sciences and the humanities, with the social sciences falling short of the "full scientificness" of science and the humanism of the humanities (Fox 1989:238).[16]

Still, metathinkers like Leon Kass periodically break through the field's confines to make such macrosocietal interpretations as this one:

> ...In the twenty-five years since I began thinking about these matters, our society has overcome longstanding taboos and repugnances to accept test-tube fertilization, commercial sperm-banking, surrogate motherhood, abortion on demand, exploitation of fetal tissue, patenting of living human tissue, gender-change surgery, liposuction and body shops, the widespread shuttling of human parts, assisted-suicide practiced by doctors, and the deliberate generation of human beings to serve as transplant donors — not to speak about massive changes in the culture regarding shame, privacy, and exposure. Perhaps more worrisome than the changes themselves is the coarsening of sensibilities and attitudes, and the irreversible effects on our imaginations and the way we come to conceive of ourselves. For there is a sad irony in our biomedical project....We expend enormous energy and vast sums of money to preserve and prolong bodily life, but in the process our embodied life is stripped of its gravity and much of its dignity. This is, in a word, progress as tragedy. (Kass 1992:85)

These more-than-ethical themes that have appeared and reappeared in U.S. bioethics (often despite rather than because of the field's explicit agenda) concern basic questions of definition and identity, values and beliefs, and ultimate ends: What is life? What is death? What is a person? A child? A parent? A family? What are the essences of humanhood? Who are my brothers, my sisters, my strangers, my enemies? What is "natural," and what is "artificial"? How vigorously should we intervene in the human condition? When should we desist or refrain from doing so? How should we think and feel and act in the face of the uncertainty, risk, and error inherent to illness and medicine, as to all human endeavors? The nature of these motifs and their steadfastness, it seems to me, indicate that " 'bioethics is not just bioethics' and [that it] is more than medical" (Fox and Swazey 1984:338).

"Using biology and medicine as a metaphorical language and a symbolic medium," U.S. bioethics is publicly grappling with collective problems of orientation and identity that are both urgent and fundamental, "in a greatly changed and changing society and world" (Fox and Swazey 1984:360). Bette-Jane Crigger, the (anthropologist) editor of the *Hastings Center Report*, calls this "cultural shadow work...on a grand scale":

> [T]hose moral debates in bioethical idiom — abortion, termination of treatment, euthanasia, allocation of resources, and all the rest — do a great deal of cultural shadow work. In talking about the nature of personhood, and particularly about the boundaries of agency, for example (as so many of our debates do at base), we continually renegotiate the social order. In ways that we do not fully intend and could never control, our discourse is part of the even more complex shadow work that will bring (perhaps already has brought) a new culture into being. Not that we truly choose the transformative role, of course. The shadow work goes on, and we are inevitably a part of it. (Crigger 1992)

The Future of U.S. Bioethics:
A Time of Ferment and Incipient Change

One of the most striking features of the U.S. bioethics scene is the self-criticism that currently pervades it. This reflexive critique is centered on the paramountcy that has been accorded to the value-precept of autonomous, self-determining individualism, and on the domination of the field by the paradigm of "principlism." The most recent literature is filled with phrases like "autonomy unbounded," "self-determination run amok" (Callahan 1992), "tyranny of rules" (Childress 1992:12), and "brandishing principles" (Clouser and Gert 1990:219). K. Danner Clouser and Bernard Gert's vivid portrayal of "throngs of converts to bioethics awareness" ritually chanting the "beneficence...autonomy

...justice...mantra [of the] 'principles approach'" (Clouser and Gert 1990:219–220) is repeatedly quoted.

The castigating of bioethical individualism and principlism also has a "mantra-like" quality as does the repertoire of prescribed alternatives that are being recited. Casuistry, virtue ethics, narrative ethics, hermeneutics, and phenomenology are all being advocated as philosophical systems that could correct, complement, broaden, enrich, or counterbalance the primary conceptual and methodological framework in which U.S. bioethics has proceeded until now. Proposals to elevate the values of caring, solidarity, reciprocity, trust, and love above the principles of autonomy, beneficence, nonmaleficence, and justice are repeatedly set forth. Enjoinders to incorporate feminist, literary, religious, social scientific, contextualist, relational, subcultural and cross-cultural perspectives and interpretations more fully into U.S. bioethical thought and health care proliferate. Detailed, thickly descriptive case stories about medically relevant moral and existential problems, humanely and feelingly told by the ill persons, families, and health professionals living the events — or by the ethicist as participant observer, ethnographer, and witness — are being held up as antidotes to the abstract, impersonal, and static character of a positivist medical ethics of principles.

The formal, principles-centered bioethics that has prevailed, some are contending, replicates the attributes of the "modern, bureaucratic medicine...practiced by strangers for strangers" that unfortunately is widespread in the United States (Hauerwas 1992:43; Siegler 1992:68). Declarations are also being made about the insufficient attention that U.S. bioethics has paid to issues of racial justice — to "poverty, homelessness, inequity and racism [that] are rife" in the society (Loewy 1992:8). And statements of resolve to address these larger social and moral problems more actively are being issued by associations like the Society for Health and Human Values. Conviction seems to be mounting, too, about the responsibility of bioethics to broaden its scope beyond concern with human health care to include the welfare of animal communities and of ecosystems in its orbit.[17]

As the foregoing suggests, the critical stocktaking and impetus for change come primarily from inside the U.S. bioethical community, spearheaded by an array of bioethical organizations and of scholars and professionals engaged in bioethics. There is some division of labor in this process. For example, along with the social justice initiatives the Society for Health and Human Values is taking, it plays an important part in linking bioethics and the humanities, especially in the area of literature and medicine. In contrast, the Society for Bioethics Consultation, whose membership is principally composed of individuals conducting clinical ethical consultations, emphasizes the value of detailed, empathic interpretations of cases based on what philosopher and jurist Susan Wolf has termed "the lived experiences of real people" (Wolf 1992:32). And the Park Ridge Center's major commitment is to relating "health, faith, and ethics" in an intellectually as well as religiously ecumenical way, "keep[ing] together...story and principle, narrative and reflection, cases and concepts...the concrete and the abstract" (Marty 1992a:9).

The U.S. bioethical community is also challenging its controlling paradigm through the work of its individual members and their forceful articulation of premises, methodology, and outlook. For example, Albert Jonsen and Stephen Toulmin "speak" this way for the "new" casuistry; James Drane and Alasdair MacIntyre for virtue ethics; Richard Baron, Ronald Carson, and Larry Churchill for hermeneutics; Richard Zaner for phenomenology; Margaret Farley and Karen Lebacqz for a feminist perspective; Courtney Campbell, Ron Hamel, and David Smith for a second generation of theologians bringing religion to bear on medical ethics; and Barry Hoffmaster, Bruce Jennings, and Patricia Marshall for the role of the social sciences in bioethics.[18] In addition, an increasingly prominent network of relatively young physicians, directly involved in clinical ethics, who are also trained in clinical epidemiology and biostatistics — such as Robert Arnold, Joel Frader, Bernard Lo, John LaPuma, David Schiedermayer, Mark Siegler, and Stuart Youngner — have been conducting and publishing first-hand, survey research-based quantitative studies of the attitudes and behavior of patients, physicians, and nurses in hospital contexts like intensive care units, emergency and operating rooms, and organ transplant programs where medical ethical questions and decisions of life-and-death import frequently occur.[19]

At the same time, the U.S. bioethics community is being confronted with criticisms from outside its fold. Some of these criticisms focus on what are felt to be the pedantic, "tweed-clad," and olympian ways in which U.S. bioethicists deal with painful, often tragic, medical and human dilemmas, and on their professional dominance as ethics experts. Here, for example, are two instances of external critique:

> **To the Editor.** — I feel compelled to reply to the recent *JAMA* review of my [Henry A. Shenkin, M.D.] book, *Medical Ethics: Evolution, Rights, and the Physician,* by Dr. [David] De Grazie.
>
> Much of my intent was to challenge the medical ethics establishment on two grounds. First, they continue to eschew an empirical approach to the subject; and second, they continue to ignore the fact that down in the trenches, most physicians are pretty good seat-of-the-pants ethicists...(Shenkin 1992.)

[A] slim book called *Final Exit*...written by Derek Humphry, a British journalist and euthanasia proponent,...has hit the best-seller list in the United States where suicide is still taboo but fear of twilight life tethered to feeding tubes or respirators is widespread....

It is not surprising but nonetheless disappointing that *Final Exit* has come under attack by ethicists and others who piously fear that its prescriptions for suicide for the terminally ill will be abused by the merely downhearted. Thus newspaper accounts of the book quote "experts" worried that it will get into the hands of the mentally ill without offering them the opportunity for what is a favorite US pastime — "counseling." (editorial in *Nature*, 15 August 1991)

The ironic allusions to U.S. society and culture quoted above (*"Final Exit:* Euthanasia Guide Sells Out" 1991) are related to another major criticism to which U.S. bioethics has become increasingly subject: the contention that it is excessively, and in certain respects, objectionably American. Historically (for reasons that have not received the attention they merit), bioethics emerged as a phenomenon and achieved professional and public prominence in the United States at least a decade earlier than in most countries.[20] In Europe, Asia, and Latin America, culturally and societally different versions of bioethics have developed more slowly — in some instances, against vehement resistance, as has been dramatically the case in the former Federal Republic of Germany, where an "antibioethics" movement exists (Schöne-Seifert and Rippe 1991). By the early 1990s, a variety of non-U.S. forms of bioethics had become sufficiently mature to represent systematic contrasts to the "North American standard" model, which was being increasingly criticized outside as well as inside the United States. For example, Sandro Spinsanti made the following comments in an essay review of what is considered to be "a handbook of Mediterranean bioethics":[21]

Many roads lead to bioethics; many heritages flow into this new field. Diego Gracia has come to the discipline through three kinds of interests: philosophy, the history of medicine, and the theory of medicine....Specific bioethical problems are embedded in a broader philosophy of medicine which is informed by an understanding of its historical roots and by an understanding of human beings as both natural and cultural beings....

Diego Gracia voices the dissatisfaction of Europeans (the Latin world in particular) with standard North American bioethics and wants to bring to Anglo-Saxon bioethics the reform it needs by

incorporating elements of the great traditions of medical humanism, the history of moral philosophy, and secular reflection on law
and politics....

As a dialectical integration of this distinctly European sensibility, Gracia also suggests a Mediterranean bioethics, whose goals
would be, not to ensure a minimal level of morality, but to look
for the best solution to the problems of daily living in the field
of health care. He invites us to move in the direction of acquiring
habits and qualities — that is, virtues. The Mediterranean countries can contribute to the bioethics movement by bringing to it
their concern for the understanding of the person, for the active
role of the family in managing situations of conflict, and for trust
as the foundation of the physician-patient relationship. (Spinsanti
1992:74–75)

There is, however, a certain trendiness in the outpouring of internal and external criticism that is being directed against "autonomy" and
"principlism" at the inception of the 1990s. Despite the verbal bashing
they are undergoing, they continue to be robustly central to the operating ethos of U.S. bioethics. Furthermore, even in areas of bioethical
concern, such as genetics, where because the ethical implications extend
"beyond the individual to family members and even potential family
members," there is a heightened "sense that the current emphasis on
individual autonomy may not be an appropriate paradigm," "no consensus on alternative models" exists (Glass 1992). Rather, many other
approaches are being advocated without a guiding idea about whether
or how these perspectives might be fruitfully combined or eventually
integrated.

Although the field "prides itself on its multidisciplinary orientation"
(Marshall 1992:5), it is still dominated intellectually by philosophy and
philosophers. Notwithstanding the renewed interest in the relationship
between religion and bioethics, the overriding secular humanism of
U.S. bioethics has not been dispelled. Nor has the field yet approached
greater reliance on social science insights, knowledge, and methodology. Instead, as anthropologist Patricia Marshall observes, "for the most
part, bioethicists and social scientists live and work in segregated academic areas," and "rarely is there any real exchange of intellectual
'juices'" between them.[22] To a notable degree, the efforts that U.S.
bioethics is making to become more cross-cultural in its outlook, to
emphasize "how individual stories are embedded within particular communities" (Davis 1992:13), and to use "thick ethnographic description"
(Geertz 1973) for richly and caringly interpreting cases (Davis 1992) are

all going forward with minimal recourse to pertinent anthropological and sociological literature, and little contact with the social scientists who authored it.

In addition, the greater hermeneutical richness to which the field aspires rarely extends to its public policy discourse. The logico-rational, legalistic, economically driven, and secular "common language" that most U.S. bioethicists continue to use in this sphere can and often does "wring the life out of" their public discussions.[23] They have paid less attention to the impoverishment of the concepts and vocabulary they employ when addressing public policy questions (and to the origins and consequences of this impoverishment) than to what they now consider the problematically restrictive ways in which they have discussed and written about bioethical issues for each other (Hamel 1993).

How much the ferment occurring in and around U.S. bioethics will alter its biomedical and health care foci, social organization, conceptual framework, mode of inquiry, ethos, and worldview over the course of the 1990s is difficult to discern. It is made all the harder by the integral relationship that exists between the evolution of U.S. bioethics and the values and beliefs, the identity and destiny of the society in which it is rooted. This is where the metameaning as well as the future development of U.S. bioethics ultimately lies.[24]

NOTES

I would like to thank Nicholas A. Christakis, Willy De Craemer, Judith P. Swazey, Howard L. Kaye, Stuart J. Youngner, and Charles L. Bosk for their careful and helpfully critical reading of this essay.

1. Letter from Albert J. Jonsen, February 7, 1991. Influenced in part by his role as Chairman of the Department of Medical History and Ethics in the School of Medicine of the University of Washington, Seattle, as he explained in his letter, Jonsen "decided to date the birth of bioethics in the United States on November 2, 1962, the date of the appearance of Shana Alexander's *Life* article, 'They Decide Who Lives and Dies.'" Alexander's article told the story of the Seattle Committee whose task was to select and unselect patients for dialysis, in an era when dialysis machines and access to them were very scarce. The Seattle Committee was set up soon after Dr. Belding Scribner, the inventor of the shunt that made chronic intermittent hemodialysis possible, and a member of the University of Washington medical faculty, placed the first patient with end-stage renal disease on chronic dialysis. Alleging that the publication of Alexander's article has "as good, or better claim of birthrights than any other," Jonsen made it the commemorative event around which his "Birth of Bioethics" conference was organized. Some (this author included) would consider Jonsen's version of the early history of bioethics a revisionist interpretation.

2. The second, revised edition of the *Encyclopedia of Bioethics*, like the first, was produced under the general editorship of Warren T. Reich, and published by Macmillan Publishing Company.

3. "Voices in U.S. Bioethics: A Cross-Cultural Appraisal and Response," unpublished working paper of the Park Ridge Center.

4. The *Hastings Center Report* retains its flagship status as a bioethical periodical; but it has been joined by numerous other publications that are wholly or heavily involved in bioethics, like the *Journal of Medicine and Philosophy*, and newer periodicals such as the Park Ridge Center's *Second Opinion* and the *Kennedy Institute of Ethics Journal* (launched in 1986 and 1991 respectively), that have considerable influence. In addition, coverage of bioethical issues and developments has become a regular feature of a host of science and medical journals, including *Science,* the *New England Journal of Medicine*, the *Journal of the American Medical Association, Perspectives in Biology and Medicine*, and the *Annals of Internal Medicine*.

5. The computer program was produced by InterActive Software of Knoxville, Tennessee. Its existence was acknowledged humorously in the July–August 1991 issue of the *Hastings Center Report* (Vol. 21, p. 45), and seriously in the Spring 1991 newsletter of the American Association for the Advancement of Science's Committee on Scientific Freedom & Responsibility and Professional Society Ethics Group (Vol. 4, p. 6).

6. In this connection, the Spring 1992 national meeting of the Society for Health and Human Values, held on April 30–May 3 in Tampa, Florida, was organized around the theme "Medicine and Its Stories." Among the major questions it addressed were: "What can medicine learn from narrative fiction and narrative theory? How are medical ethical issues portrayed in literature? What kind of story is the medical case history? What is the role of storytelling in medicine?"

At this time, too, the Society was exploring the question of a change in its name — either to the Society for Medical Humanities, or the Society for Medical Humanities and Bioethics. In its March 1992 *Bulletin*, David Bernard, the then-president of the Society, explained that this was to "identify more accurately the professional and intellectual orientation" of the organization, and to "articulate more clearly [its] place in the landscape of organizations with related interests and agendas."

7. Personal communication from Jeremiah A. Barondess, 10 February 1992.

8. "Choosing Death in America: The Challenge to Religious Beliefs and Practice," draft of a project proposal, Park Ridge Center, Chicago, Illinois, 25 March 1992.

9. The Park Ridge Center is an exception to this pattern. It is explicitly concerned with the challenges that "the cultural shift in American attitudes toward assisted suicide and active euthanasia... presents to religious communities," especially to their "traditional bulwarks against the acceptance of these practices." (Personal communication from Ron P. Hamel and Edwin R. DuBose, 3 April 1992.)

10. Jurist/bioethicist Alexander M. Capron has pointed out that since 1974, in many statutes and court decisions, as well as in medical guidelines, the con-

cept of "futility" has been invoked. He cites as examples the use of the term in connection with medical standards for cardiopulmonary resuscitation; the guidelines accompanying the current "Baby Doe" regulations in the neonatal care nursery; and the 1983 decision of a California court of appeals (in *Barber v. Superior Court*), where the concept was invoked to support the conclusion that the physician had no duty to continue treatment "once it has become futile in the opinion of qualified medical personnel." However, he agrees it was not until the beginning of the 1990s — triggered by certain cases, like *Wanglie,* that "secured a lasting niche in bioethics lore" — that the notion of medical futility became "front-page news" (Capron 1991:26–27).

11. Statement by Arthur Caplan, director of the Center for Biomedical Ethics at the University of Minnesota (cited in Kolata 1992b).

12. For example, in 1990, two such court cases elicited bioethical commentary. The first case, *Davis v. Davis* (1990 Tenn. App. LEXIS 642 [13 September 1990]), concerned the status and disposition of seven frozen embryos conceived by in vitro fertilization, whose custody was contested in a divorce action. The second case, *Johnson v. Calvert and Calvert* (Cal. Super. Ct., Orange Co. Dept 11, No. X633190 [22 October 1990]), involved the custody of a baby conceived by in vitro fertilization from the egg of a woman who had had a hysterectomy and the sperm of her husband and carried to term by another woman who, at the end of the pregnancy, expressed unwillingness to relinquish the baby to his genetic parents.

13. The conference took place on September 23–24, 1991, at the Transplant and Health Policy Center in Ann Arbor, Michigan, a statewide center administered by the University of Michigan.

14. There is at least one other issue associated with AIDS to which more than passing bioethical attention has been paid in the early 1990s: whether, in the name of compassion and urgency, new and experimental drugs that may be able to delay the advance of the HIV virus should immediately be made available rather than first being tested for safety and efficacy via randomized clinical trials as the usual Food and Drug Administration federal regulations require. See, for example, Annas 1990b:35–37; and Petricciani 1991:43–44.

15. Also see the article by Pinit Ratanakul in this volume.

16. The limited involvement of social science and scientists in U.S. bioethics is not solely attributable to the rather unwelcoming ambivalence with which the shapers and gatekeepers of the field view them. The ethos of the social sciences also contributes to the minor role they have played in bioethics, in ways that we will not develop here, but have analyzed elsewhere. See Fox 1989:237–38.

17. "The 1990s will...be a time of fundamental decisions for the environment, both within the United States and on a global scale." See the Hastings Center brochure, "Medical Ethics and Environmental Ethics," announcing the theme of its 1992 General Meeting.

18. Historian of medicine George Weisz has played an especially important role in trying to bring about more collaboration between the social sciences and bioethics. His contribution is acknowledged here, rather than in the body of the text, because he is based in the Canadian-American academic world (at McGill University) rather than in the U.S.A. See Weisz 1990.

19. Several of these physicians, notably Joel Frader and Stuart Youngner, also have social science training. A number of them — for example, Robert Arnold, Joel Frader, and Bernard Lo — are former Robert Wood Johnson Clinical Scholars. Their articles are being published in a cluster of journals that include: the *Journal of the American Medical Association*, the *New England Journal of Medicine*, the *Annals of Internal Medicine*, the *Archives of Internal Medicine*, the *Journal of General Internal Medicine*, the *Journal of Epidemiology*, *Theoretical Medicine*, the *Journal of Medical Philosophy*, and the *Journal of Medical Ethics*. The kind of "social circle" or "visible college" that these "physician/ethicist/clinical epidemiologists" constitute is a development worthy of study in and of itself.

20. The one exception may be Canada, where the development of bioethics has not "lagged behind" the evolution of U.S. bioethics to the same extent. The fact that both are North American societies, with closely linked, though not identical, cultures is probably relevant here.

21. *Fundamentos de Bioética*, by Diego Gracia, professor of the history of medicine at the University of Madrid in Spain.

22. Personal communication from Patricia A. Marshall, 22 April 1992.

23. Personal communication from Laurence J. O'Connell, 27 April 1992.

24. It is still too early to ascertain whether President Clinton's effort to reform the U.S. health care system, and the fact that he included an ethics group in the task force he summoned to Washington, D.C., for this purpose, will affect the outlook of U.S. bioethics or its influence on the national scene. The ethics group's work seems to have been largely confined to drafting a preamble to the larger report. Despite its overall sympathy for the general goals of health care reform, the group is alleged to have been rent by conflicts and disputes. This suggests that the role played by ethicists was minor compared to that of economists, public policy experts, and lawyers.

REFERENCES

Angell, Marcia. 1990. "New Ways to Get Pregnant" (Editorial). *New England Journal of Medicine* 323 (25 October): 1200–1202.

Annas, George J. 1987. "From Canada with Love: Anencephalic Newborns as Organ Donors." *Hastings Center Report* 17:36–38.

———. 1989a. "The Supreme Court, Privacy, and Abortion" (Occasional Notes). *New England Journal of Medicine* 321 (26 October): 1200–1203.

———. 1989b. "A French Homunculus in a Tennessee Court" (At Law). *Hastings Center Report* 21 (January–February): 35–38.

———. 1990a. "Nancy Cruzan and the Right to Die." *New England Journal of Medicine* (6 September): 670–73.

———. 1990b. "FDA's Compassion for Desperate Drug Companies." *Hastings Center Report* 20 (January–February): 35–37.

———. 1991. "Crazy Making: Embryos and Gestational Mothers" (At Law). *Hastings Center Report* 21 (January–February): 35–38.

Annas, George J., Bob Arnold, Mila Aroskar, et al. 1990. "Bioethicists' Statement on the U.S. Supreme Court's *Cruzan* Decision." *New England Journal of Medicine* 323 (6 September): 670–73.

Association of American Medical Colleges. 1988. "Professional Responsibility in Treating AIDS Patients" (Statement). *Journal of Medical Education* 63 (July): 587–90.

Baker, Russell. 1990. "Ethicizationism" (Observer). *New York Times* (27 October): 23A.

———. 1992. "Going to the Dogs" (Observer). *New York Times* (28 March): 23A.

Battin, Margaret Pabst, and Daniel Wikler. 1992. "All Together, Now." *Hastings Center Report* 22 (January–February): 3–4.

Beauchamp, Tom L., and James F. Childress. 1979. *Principles of Biomedical Ethics*. 1st ed. New York: Oxford University Press.

———. 1983. *Principles of Biomedical Ethics*. 2d ed. New York: Oxford University Press.

———. 1989. *Principles of Biomedical Ethics*. 3d ed. New York: Oxford University Press.

———. 1993. *Principles of Biomedical Ethics*. 4th ed. New York: Oxford University Press.

Bellah, Robert N., Richard Madsen, William M. Sullivan, Ann Swidler, and Steven M. Tipton. 1985. *Habits of the Heart: Individualism and Commitment in American Life*. Berkeley and Los Angeles: University of California Press.

Blake, David C. 1992. "The Hospital Ethics Committee: Health Care's Moral Conscience or White Elephant?" *Hastings Center Report* 22 (January–February): 6–11.

Bosk, Charles L., and Joel E. Frader. 1991. "AIDS and Its Impact on Medical Work: The Culture and Politics of the Shop Floor." In *A Disease of Society: Cultural and Institutional Responses to AIDS,* ed. Dorothy Nelkin, David P. Willis, and Scott V. Parris, 150–71. New York: Cambridge University Press.

Bouton, Katherine. 1990. "Painful Decisions." *New York Times Magazine,* 5 August, 6, 22.

Callahan, Daniel. 1989. *What Kind of Life: The Limits of Medical Progress*. New York: Simon and Schuster.

———. 1990a. "Modernizing Mortality: Medical Progress and the Good Society." *Hastings Center Report* 20 (January–February): 28–32.

———. 1990b. "Rationing Medical Progress: The Way to Affordable Medical Care." *New England Journal of Medicine* 322 (21 June): 1810–13.

———. 1990c. "Religion and the Secularization of Bioethics." In Callahan and Campbell 1990:18–20.

———. 1991. "Medical Futility, Medical Necessity: The Problem-Without-a-Name." *Hastings Center Report* 21 (July–August): 30–35.

———. 1992. "When Self-Determination Runs Amok." *Hastings Center Report* 22 (March–April): 52–55.

Callahan, Daniel, and Courtney S. Campbell, eds. 1990. "Theology, Religious Traditions, and Bioethics." *Hastings Center Report* (A Special Supplement) 20 (July–August): 1–24.

Campbell, Courtney S. 1989. "On James F. Childress: Answering Every Person." *Second Opinion* 11 (July): 118–44.

———. 1990. "Religion and Moral Meaning in Bioethics." In Callahan and Campbell 1990:4–7.

Capps, Walter H. 1990. "Putting the Issue in Perspective: Some Statistics." In *Abortion, Religion, and the State Legislator after* Webster: *A Guide for the 1990s* (Report of the Park Ridge Center), 6–7. Chicago: Park Ridge Center.

Capron, Alexander Morgan. 1991. "In Re Helga Wanglie." *Hastings Center Report* 21 (September–October): 26–28.

Cefalo, R. C., and H. Tristram Engelhardt, Jr. 1989. "The Use of Fetal and Anencephalic Tissue for Transplantation." *Journal of Medicine and Philosophy* 14:25–43.

Charo, R. Alta. 1991. "A Political History of RU-486." In *Biomedical Politics,* ed. Kathi E. Hanna, 43–93. Washington, D.C.: National Academy Press.

Childress, James F. 1989. "Ethical Criteria for Procuring and Distributing Organs for Transplantation." In *Organ Transplantation Policy: Issues and Prospects,* ed. James F. Blumstein and Frank A. Sloan, 87–113. Durham, North Carolina: Duke University Press.

———. 1992. "Some Reflections on Joseph Fletcher's Work." *Hastings Center Report* 22 (January–February): 12.

Christakis, Nicholas A. 1988. "The Ethical Design of an AIDS Vaccine Trial in Africa." *Hastings Center Report* 18 (June): 31–37.

Churchill, Larry R., and Rosa B. Lynn Pinkus. 1990. "The Use of Anencephalic Organs: Historical and Ethical Dimensions." *Milbank Quarterly* 68:147–69.

Clouser, K. Danner, and Bernard Gert. 1990. "A Critique of Principlism." *Journal of Medicine and Philosophy* 15 (April): 219–36.

Cooke, Molly, and Merle A. Sande. 1989. "The HIV Epidemic and Training in Internal Medicine: Challenges and Recommendations" (Sounding Board). *New England Journal of Medicine* 321 (9 November): 1334–38.

Crigger, Bette-Jane. 1992. "At the Center." *Hastings Center Report* 22 (January–February): inside front cover.

Daniels, Norman. 1991. "Duty to Treat or Right to Refuse?" *Hastings Center Report* 21 (March–April): 36–46.

Davis, Dena. 1991. "Rich Cases: The Ethics of Thick Description." *Hastings Center Report* 21 (July–August): 12–17.

Dickens, Bernard M., Larry Gostin, and Robert J. Levine, eds. 1991. *Research on Human Populations: National and International Guidelines* (Special issue of *Law, Medicine & Health Care*) 19 (Fall-Winter): 157–295.

Dreyfuss, Rochelle Cooper, and Dorothy Nelkin. 1992. "The Jurisprudence of Genetics." *Vanderbilt Law Review* 45 (March): 313–48.

Elias, Sherman, and George J. Annas. 1986. "Social Policy Considerations in Noncoital Reproduction." *Journal of the American Medical Association* 255 (3 January): 62–68.

Emanuel, Ezekiel J. 1988. "Do Physicians Have an Obligation to Treat Patients with AIDS?" *New England Journal of Medicine* 318 (23 June): 1686–90.

Evans, Roger W. 1990. "Anencephalic Infants as Organ Donors" (Letter to the Editor). *New England Journal of Medicine* 322 (1 February): 332.

Fayerweather, William E., John Higginson, and Tom L. Beauchamp, eds. 1991. *Ethics in Epidemiology* (Special issue of the *Journal of Clinical Epidemiology*) 44 (Supplement I): V-169S.

"*Final Exit:* Euthanasia Guide Sells Out" (unsigned editorial). 1991. *Nature* 352 (15 August): 553.

Fox, Renée C. 1974. "Ethical and Existential Developments in Contemporaneous American Medicine: Their Implications for Culture and Society." *Milbank Memorial Fund Quarterly/Health and Society* 52 (Fall): 445–83.

———. 1988. "The Human Condition of Health Professionals." In Renée C. Fox, *Essays in Medical Sociology: Journeys into the Field,* 572–87. New Brunswick, N.J.: Transaction Books.

———. 1989. "The Sociology of Bioethics." In Renée C. Fox, *The Sociology of Medicine: A Participant Observer's View,* 224–76 (Chapter 7). Englewood Cliffs, N.J.: Prentice-Hall.

Fox, Renée C., and Judith P. Swazey. 1984. "Medical Morality Is Not Bioethics — Medical Ethics in China and the United States." *Perspectives in Biology and Medicine* 27 (Spring): 336–60.

Fox, Renée C., and Judith P. Swazey (with the assistance of Judith C. Watkins). 1992. *Spare Parts: Organ Replacement in American Society.* New York: Oxford University Press.

Frader, Joel, and Robert Arnold. 1993. "Standards for Clinical Ethics Consultation." *Newsletter of the Society for Bioethics Consultation* (Winter): 2–3.

Friedman, Emily. 1989. "The Torturer's Horse." *Journal of the American Medical Association* 261 (10 March): 1481–82.

Geertz, Clifford. 1973. "Thick Description: Toward an Interpretive Theory of Culture." In Clifford Geertz, *The Interpretation of Cultures: Selected Essays by Clifford Geertz,* 3–30 (Chapter 1). New York: Basic Books.

———. 1983. "The Way We Think Now: Toward an Ethnography of Modern Thought." In Clifford Geertz, *Local Knowledge: Further Essays in Interpretive Anthropology,* 147–63 (Chapter 7). New York: Basic Books.

Glass, Richard M. 1992. "AAAS Conference Explores Ethical Aspects of Large Pedigree Genetic Research." *Journal of the American Medical Association* 267 (22/29 April): 2158.

Greenhouse, Linda. 1992. "High Court, 5–4, Affirms Right to Abortion but Allows Most of Pennsylvania's Limits." *New York Times* (30 June): A1, A15.

Gustafson, James M. 1990. "Moral Discourse about Medicine: A Variety of Forms." *Journal of Medicine and Philosophy* 15: 125–42.

———. 1991. "Ethics: An American Growth Industry." *Key Reporter* (of Phi Beta Kappa) 56 (Spring): 1–5.

Hamel, Ronald P. 1991. "Overcoming the Suicide Option." *Philadelphia Inquirer* (9 September): 11A.

————. 1993. "Speaking of God: Must Theology Remain Silent in Bioethics and Public Debate?" *Second Opinion* 18 (January): 83–88.

Hauerwas, Stanley. 1986. *Suffering Presence: Theological Reflections on Medicine, the Mentally Handicapped, and the Church*. Notre Dame, Ind.: University of Notre Dame Press.

————. 1992. "Commentary: The Eyes Have It." *Second Opinion* 17 (April): 41–43.

Heagarty, Margaret C., and Elaine J. Abrams. 1992. "Caring for HIV-Infected Women and Children." *New England Journal of Medicine* 326 (26 March): 887–88.

Hoffmaster, Barry. 1991. "The Theory and Practice of Applied Ethics." *Dialogue* 30:213–34.

Humphry, Derek. 1991. *Final Exit: The Practicalities of Self-Deliverance and Assisted Suicide for the Dying*. Eugene, Oreg.: Hemlock Society.

Ijsselmuiden, Carel B., and Ruth R. Faden. 1992. "Research and Informed Consent in Africa — Another Look." *New England Journal of Medicine* 326 (19 March): 830–34.

"It's Over, Debbie." (A Piece of My Mind). 1988. *Journal of the American Medical Association* 258:272.

Jecker, Nancy S., and Robert A. Pearlman. 1992. "Medical Futility: Who Decides." (Commentary). *Archives of Internal Medicine* 152 (June): 1140–44.

Jecker, Nancy S., and Lawrence J. Schneiderman. 1992. "Futility and Rationing." *American Journal of Medicine* 92 (February): 189–96.

Kass, Leon R. 1985. *Toward a More Natural Science: Biology and Human Affairs*. New York: Basic Books.

————. "Practicing Ethics: Where's the Action?" *Hastings Center Report* 20 (January–February): 6–7.

————. 1992. "Organs for Sale? Propriety, Property, and the Price of Progress." *Public Interest* (Spring): 67–86.

Kaye, Howard L. 1992. "Are We the Sum of Our Genes?" *Wilson Quarterly* 16 (Spring): 77–84.

Kearney, Warren, and Arthur L. Caplan. 1992. "Parity for the Donation of Bone Marrow." In *Emerging Issues in Biomedical Policy: An Annual Review* (Volume I), ed. Robert H. Blank and Andrea L. Bonnicksen, 262–85 (Chapter 19). New York: Columbia University Press.

Kevles, Daniel J. 1992. "Controlling the Genetic Arsenal." *Wilson Quarterly* 16 (Spring): 68–76.

Kolata, Gina. 1992a. "Ethicists Debate New Definition of Death." *New York Times* (29 April): C13.

————. 1992b. "Nomadic Group of Anti-Abortionists Uses New Tactics to Make Its Mark." *New York Times* (24 March): A12.

LaPuma, John, and David L. Schiedermayer. 1991. "Ethics Consultation: Skills, Roles, and Training." *Annals of Internal Medicine* 114 (January 15): 155–60.

Lebacqz, Karen. 1991. "Feminism and Bioethics: An Overview." *Second Opinion* 17 (October): 11–25.

Levine, Robert J. 1986. "Research That Could Yield Marketable Products from Human Materials: The Problem of Informed Consent." *IRB: A Review of Human Subjects Research* 8 (January–February): 6–7.

Lichtenberg, Judith. 1990. "Is There a Middle Ground?" In *Report from the Institute for Philosophy and Public Policy* (Issue on "The Abortion Dilemma") 10 (Spring): 11–13.

Lieban, Richard W. 1990. "Medical Anthropology and the Comparative Study of Medical Ethics." In *Social Science Perspectives on Medical Ethics* (*Culture, Illness, and Healing,* Vol. 16), ed. George Weisz, 221–39. Dordrecht and Boston: Kluwer Academic Publishers.

"A Life-Saving Sibling Helps Once More." 1992. *New York Times* (6 June): 27A.

Lo, Bernard, and Robert Steinbrook. 1992. "Health Care Workers Infected with the Human Immunodeficiency Virus: The Next Steps" (Special Communication). *Journal of the American Medical Association* 267 (26 February): 1100–1105.

Loewy, Erich H. 1992. "An Open Letter." *Bulletin of the Society for Health and Human Values* 22 (March): 3, 8.

Macklin, Ruth. 1991. "Artificial Means of Reproduction and Our Understanding of the Family." *Hastings Center Report* 21 (January–February): 5–11.

Marshall, Patricia A. 1992. "Anthropology and Bioethics." *Medical Anthropology Quarterly* 6:49–73.

Marty, Martin E. 1992a. "Initial Comment: If Only . . . " *Second Opinion* 17 (April): 8–9.

———. 1992b. "Medical Ethics and Theology: The Accounting of the Generations." *Second Opinion* 17 (April): 70–82.

Murray, Thomas. 1987. "On the Human Body as Property: The Meaning of Embodiment, Markets, and the Meaning of Strangers." *Journal of Law Reform* 20 (Summer): 1055–88.

Nau, Jean-Yves. 1991. "Codifier la bioéthique." *Le Monde* (12 June): 1, 15.

Nelkin, Dorothy, David P. Willis, and Scott W. Parris, eds. 1991. "Introduction." *A Disease of Society: Cultural and Institutional Responses to AIDS,* 1–14. New York: Cambridge University Press.

O'Connell, Laurence J. 1987. "The Preferential Option for the Poor and Health Care in the United States." In *Medical Ethics: A Guide for Health Professionals,* ed. David Thomasma and John Monagle, 306–13 (Chapter 26). Rockville, Maryland: Aspen.

———. 1991. "Preface." In *Choosing Death: Active Euthanasia, Religion, and the Public Debate,* ed. Ron Hamel, vi. Philadelphia: Trinity Press.

Paris, John J., Robert K. Crone, and Frank Reardon. 1990. "Physicians' Refusal of Requested Treatment: The Case of Baby L" (Occasional Notes). *New England Journal of Medicine* 332 (5 April): 1012–15.

Park Ridge Center. 1990. *Abortion, Religion, and the State Legislator after Webster: A Guide for the 1990s* (A Report). Chicago: Park Ridge Center.

Peabody, Joyce L., Janet R. Emery, and Stephen Ashwal. 1989. "Experiences with Anencephalic Infants as Prospective Organ Donors." *Journal of the American Medical Association* 321 (10 August): 344–50.

Pellegrino, Edmund D. 1991. "Ethics." *Journal of the American Medical Association* 265:3118–19.

Petricciani, John C. 1991. "AIDS, Compassion, and Drugs" (Letter in reply to Annas' article; "FDA Compassion for Desperate Drug Companies," [January-February 1990]). *Hastings Center Report* 21 (January–February): 43–44.

Phalon, Richard. 1992. "Questions with Human Beings Attached." *National Jesuit News* 21 (April): 1, 5.

Pollak, Otto. 1980. "The Shadow of Death over Aging." In *The Social Meaning of Death,* ed. Renée C. Fox. Special Issue of *Annals of the American Academy of Political and Social Science* 441 (January): 71–77.

Quill, Timothy E. 1991. "Death and Dignity — A Case of Individualized Decision Making." *New England Journal of Medicine* 324:691–94.

Quindlen, Anna. 1991. "The Heart's Reasons," *New York Times* (6 June): A25.

Ratanakul, Pinit. 1991. "An Asian Perspective on U.S. Bioethics." Unpublished Working Paper.

Rosenblatt, Roger. 1992. "How to End the Abortion War." *New York Times Magazine* (19 January): 26–27, 41–42, 50, 56.

Rothman, David J. 1991. *Strangers at the Bedside: A History of How Law and Bioethics Transformed Medical Decision Making.* New York: Basic Books.

Schöne-Seifert, Bettina, and Klaus-Peter Rippe. 1991. "Silencing the Singer: Antibioethics in Germany." *Hastings Center Report* 21 (November–December): 20–27.

Shenkin, Henry A. 1992. "Medical Ethics in Review" (Letter to the Editor). *Journal of the American Medical Association* 267 (12 February): 806.

Shewmon, D. Alan, Alexander M. Capron, Warwick J. Peacock, and Barbara L. Schulman. 1989. "The Use of Anencephalic Infants as Organ Sources: A Critique." *Journal of the American Medical Association* 261 (24/31 March): 1773–81.

Siegler, Mark. 1992. "A Medicine of Strangers or a Medicine of Intimates: The Two Legacies of Karen Ann Quinlan." *Second Opinion* 17 (April): 64–69.

"A Sister Is Saved." 1992. *Time* (23 March): 73.

Spinsanti, Sandro (with the editorial assistance of Jacquelyn Slomka). 1992. "A Handbook of Mediterranean Bioethics." *Medical Humanities Review* 6 (January): 73–75.

Truog, Robert D., and John C. Fletcher. 1989. "Anencephalic Newborns: Can Organs Be Transplanted before Brain Death?" (Sounding Board). *New England Journal of Medicine* 321 (10 August): 388–91.

———. 1990. "Anencephalic Infants as Organ Donors" (Letter to the Editor). *New England Journal of Medicine* 322 (1 February): 333.

Truog, Robert D., Allan S. Brett, and Joel Frader. 1992. "The Problem with Futility" (Sounding Board). *New England Journal of Medicine* 326 (1 June): 1560–64.

Verhey, Allen D. 1990. "Talking of God — But with Whom?" In Callahan and Campbell 1990:21–24.

Walters, LeRoy, and Joy Kahn Tamar, eds. 1991. *Bibliography of Bioethics* (Vol. 17). Washington, D.C.: Kennedy Institute of Ethics, Georgetown University.

Weed, Douglas J. 1991. "The Merger of Bioethics and Epidemiology." *Journal of Clinical Epidemiology* 33 (Supplement I): 15S–22S.

Weisz, George. ed. 1990. *Social Science Perspectives on Medical Ethics,* Vol. 16. Dordrecht and Boston: Kluwer Academic Publishers.

Wikler, Daniel. 1991. "What Has Bioethics to Offer Health Policy?" *Milbank Quarterly* 69:233–51.

Wind, James F. 1990. "What Can Religion Offer Bioethics?" In Callahan and Campbell 1990:18–20.

Wolf, Susan M. 1992. "*Final Exit:* The End of Argument." *Hastings Center Report* 22 (January–February): 30–33.

Zaner, Richard M. 1989. "Anencephalics as Organ Donors." *Journal of Medicine and Philosophy* 14:61–78.

Zylke, Jody W. 1992. "Examining Life's (Genomic) Code Means Reexamining Society's Long-Held Codes" (Medical News and Perspectives). *Journal of the American Medical Association* 267 (1 April): 1715–16.

~ 2 ~

PRINCIPLES-ORIENTED BIOETHICS
AN ANALYSIS AND ASSESSMENT FROM WITHIN

James F. Childress

Which ethical perspective or framework can most helpfully illuminate and direct biomedical ethics? For many years, according to some commentators, a principles-oriented perspective has dominated the field. However, for at least a decade the criticisms of that perspective have been widespread and profound. In view of these criticisms, I recently asked Daniel Callahan about the warrant for his claim that a principles-oriented perspective (about which he has serious reservations) remains the dominant paradigm in bioethics. He responded by noting the preponderance of articles within this paradigm submitted to the *Hastings Center Report.*

As a defender of one principles-oriented framework, especially in several editions of *Principles of Biomedical Ethics* (hereafter *PBE*),[1] which I co-authored with Tom L. Beauchamp, I have been impressed by the number and strength of the criticisms. Even though Beauchamp and I have not been persuaded to abandon our framework of principles, the successive editions of *PBE* reflect the impact of several of these criticisms, particularly in the ways we have clarified, elaborated, and altered the framework. Despite the major changes reflected in the forthcoming fourth edition of *PBE,* the framework is still recognizably principles-oriented, but it is, we believe, considerably enriched by our increased attention to method, emotions, virtues, care, relationships, all in response to major challenges to principles-oriented approaches to bioethics.

In this essay I will sketch some principles-oriented approaches to bioethics. Critics often overlook the great variety of principles-oriented approaches, wrongly supposing that a successful assault on one variety damages all. I will argue that some principles-oriented approaches are much closer to critical perspectives, such as casuistry, than is recognized in some typologies of major approaches to bioethics. Furthermore, some principles-oriented approaches can be revised to accommodate important criticisms from other perspectives. Even though I will often explicate and even defend some features of the principles-oriented approach I have taken elsewhere, I am here mainly interested in the contours of the debate.

I will use as shorthand the term *principlism* to refer to various principles-oriented approaches. However, some qualifications are in order. Critics first applied this term, and for many it is thus a pejorative label. I use it, however, as a descriptive label. Furthermore, according to many who deny that theory and rules, as well as principles, are central in bioethics, the very critics who affixed the label of principlism are themselves principlists, engaged in what appears to be a mere family quarrel (Clouser and Gert 1990; Green 1990).

Whether principlism actually dominates in bioethics depends on how this approach is delineated. No single approach can be called *the* principles approach. Nor is it clear that the formal statement of a principlist approach in *PBE* would be universally accepted: These principles "are intended to provide a framework of moral theory for the identification, analysis, and resolution of moral problems in medicine" (*PBE*, 1989:16). However, at the very least, to be a principlist one must view general moral norms as central in biomedical ethics, without necessarily denying other features that are central in other frameworks. Some of these general moral norms may be viewed as principles, others as rules. Both principles and rules are "general action guides specifying that some type of action is prohibited, required, or permitted in certain circumstances" (Solomon 1978:408). In this essay I will use the term *principles* to encompass both principles and rules, unless otherwise indicated. When they are distinguished, as is important to do in some contexts, principles are often conceived as more general and sometimes as sources or foundations of rules, while rules specify more concretely the type of prohibited, required, or permitted action. In addition to principles and rules, it is useful to note two other levels or tiers of moral discourse identified in *PBE:* theory and particular judgments. Ranked according to their level of generality we have: (1) theory, (2) principles, (3) rules, and (4) particular judgments. Part of the debate about principlism focuses on the relation between the four levels of ethical theory and, especially, how the first three lead to particular judgments in cases.

Justification of Principlist Approaches

The language of principles often appears to reflect a strictly rationalist and foundationalist approach to ethics that dispenses fairly quickly with history, convention, community, tradition, and so on. Thus it might be supposed that *PBE*, Robert Veatch's *Theory of Medical Ethics* (1981), and H. Tristram Engelhardt, Jr.'s *Foundations of Bioethics* (1986) all represent rationalistic, foundationalist theories.[2] The views expressed in these books, however, are complex and are not all strictly foundationalist. Among different interpretations of ethical theory, the most rationalistic, foundationalist version requires, as Stanley Clarke and Evan Simpson note, a "set of normative principles governing all rational beings and providing a dependable procedure for reaching definite moral judgments and decisions." But another version of ethical theory, which uses the method of reflective equilibrium, "construes ethical inquiry as a matter of reflective testing of ethical beliefs against others or against particular ethical conceptions presented for exploration" (Clarke and Simpson 1989:4). The first version tends to be deductivist, the second tends to be coherentist. In the second version of ethical theory, debates about the acceptability or superiority of any framework hinge on such obvious, formal criteria as coherence, consistency, simplicity, and comprehensiveness, and more controversially, on such substantive criteria as the framework's capacity to account for, illuminate, and direct moral experience (see *PBE*, chap. 1; these criteria are considerably expanded in the fourth edition).

How can various principles be justified? Here Beauchamp and I in *PBE* have taken a more clearly historicist turn rather than a turn to strong conceptions of theory (of the sort defended by Clouser and Gert). For instance, the third edition of *PBE* accepts historicism and rejects "foundationalism in moral justification, in the sense of holding that moral theories are rooted in some ahistorical domain rather than in history and tradition." Nevertheless, principles can still "transcend the insights and beliefs of many particular groups and traditions, and...are often useful for critically examining and restructuring past moral thinking and present moral perplexity" (*PBE*, 1989:24, n. 20). Our first edition in 1979 was probably still under the sway of a strong conception of ethical theory, even when many of our arguments took a somewhat different direction. And in the fourth edition we still discuss various theories, at least schematically. However, we do not really press justification to ultimate foundations of our principles; instead, we rely on convergence between different theories on a set of prima facie principles and rules. Now the Rawlsian language of "overlapping consensus" is attractive.

Furthermore, we recognize that ethical reflection usually occurs within a community (or communities), and within a tradition (or traditions), and this reflection does not involve an ahistorical theory as much as the discernment of principles that are embedded in laws, policies, and practices. This mode of reflection is not inconsistent with the language of principles. While principles are sometimes viewed as ultimately foundational, rationalistically established, ahistorical norms from which other norms or judgments are deduced, that is not our conception of principles. Instead of deriving principles or rules from moral theory, *PBE* involves a dialectic between theory, principles, rules, and particular judgments (case judgments), with a reflective equilibrium operating at each level as well as between the levels.

Those who accept the rationalistic, foundationalistic version of ethical theory — such as Gert, Clouser, and Green — criticize the lack of "rigor" in some historicist versions of ethical theory. I believe, however, that *PBE's* principlism provides as much theoretical rigor as morality permits, for morality itself is not a rigid system. Furthermore, the distinction between theoretical and applied, or practical, ethics needs rethinking and perhaps even abandoning (Beauchamp 1984). And even where there is no comprehensive, rationalistic, foundationalist ethical theory, there may still be important theoretical distinctions in bioethics (e.g., the distinction between obligatory and ideal beneficence). Principlist bioethics may thus be a work *in* moral theory, even if not a work *of* moral theory in the comprehensive, rationalistic, foundationalist sense.

Which Principles and Rules?

The literature in biomedical ethics in the last twenty years or so has identified several moral principles, often but not always the same ones. For example, the National Commission for the Protection of Human Subjects of Biomedical and Behavioral Research (1978) justified its recommendations for policies by appealing to three major principles: respect for persons, beneficence (which includes what some have called nonmaleficence), and justice. Whatever the principles in biomedical ethics are called, they represent the following sorts of general moral considerations: obligations to respect the wishes of competent persons (respect for persons or autonomy); obligations not to harm others, including not killing them or treating them cruelly (nonmaleficence); obligations to benefit others (beneficence); obligations to produce a net balance of benefits over harms (utility); obligations to distribute benefits and harms fairly (justice); obligations to keep promises and contracts (fidelity); obligations of truthfulness; obligations to disclose information; and obligations to respect privacy and protect confidential information (confidentiality).

Sometimes these obligations are stated as principles; sometimes as rules. Some obligations are viewed as primary and fundamental; others as secondary and derivative. For example, *PBE* recognizes respect for autonomy, nonmaleficence, beneficence (including utility), and justice as primary principles, and veracity, fidelity, privacy, and confidentiality as derivative principles or rules. Veatch's list of primary principles overlaps in important respects but differs in others: beneficence, contract keeping, autonomy, honesty, avoiding killing, and justice. He also recognizes several moral rules or intermediate moral formulations, such as informed consent. In a much shorter list, Engelhardt accepts only the principles of autonomy and beneficence, reducing justice to these two considerations, but he then recognizes several derivative obligations. Thus one major difference among principlists is how they sort out obligations. Some principlist frameworks may encompass several obligations under a few general headings, while others may view them as distinct and even separable obligations.

Some critics connect principlism closely with rights talk. However, principlists do not necessarily favor the language of rights over the language of obligation or duty. Indeed, *PBE* includes only a brief section on "rights," and throughout the text the language of rights is clearly subordinated to the language of obligation (which is used interchangeably with duty). Nevertheless, *PBE* recognizes a rough correlation between rights and obligations; thus it does not matter too much which term is used. The terms may have different rhetorical force, however, and in a society shaped by liberal individualism, the language of rights may have stronger rhetorical force. In the end, our principlism, just as that of many others, can be stated in the language of either rights or obligations.

Critics of principlism often associate it not only with rights language but also with the dominance of one particular right: autonomy. But here again variety is evident; the principle of autonomy does not play the same role in all principlist frameworks. For example, *PBE* simply includes respect for autonomy as one basic principle among others, and it is only prima facie binding, as are all other principles. It may often triumph, but it does not have *a priori* superiority over other principles. Furthermore, I have argued sharply against overextending and overweighing the principle of respect for autonomy in relation to other general moral considerations (Childress 1990). But other principlists have different emphases. For example, Engelhardt does assign priority to autonomy as a side constraint, while Veatch holds that nonconsequentialist principles of autonomy and justice outweigh consequentialist ones, but that when autonomy and justice conflict, justice takes priority. This variety is best explicated in the context of debates about the meaning and weights of various moral principles.

Meaning and Weights of Principles and Rules

Even proponents of the same principles and rules diverge widely about what those principles and rules imply for particular cases because of disputes about their meaning and their weights. It is important to consider meaning and weight together. For example, consider the case of the father who is reluctant to donate a kidney to try to save his dying daughter (Levine et al. 1977). He asks the physician to tell the other members of the family that he is not histocompatible when in fact the tests that he underwent establish him as histocompatible. The father's request is based on his fear that full disclosure would wreck the family because his wife and others would accuse him of allowing his daughter to die. The physician is not comfortable with this request but finally agrees to say that for "medical reasons" the father should not donate a kidney. The physician might have held that the rule of confidentiality outweighed the rule of truthfulness or that the avoidance of bad consequences (wrecking the family) outweighed the rule of truthfulness. However, there are different interpretations of the meaning of the rules of confidentiality and truthfulness, as well as of their weight and stringency. Consider the following two possibilities.

First, if lying is defined as making an intentionally deceptive statement, it might be held that the physician told a lie when he said that for "medical reasons" the father should not donate a kidney. After all, he made an intentionally deceptive statement, designed to conceal the full truth from the family. In view of this definition, the moral debate would focus on whether the rule against lying could be overridden by another rule (the rule of confidentiality) or by the consequences (avoiding the destruction of the family). Whatever is held about this particular case, few if any ethical theories consistently hold that lying so defined is absolutely wrong.

Second, if lying is defined as intentionally withholding information from or deceiving someone who has a right to the truth, the moral debate about this case would focus on whether the physician actually lied and, ultimately, on whether the man's wife had a right to the information that had emerged in the relationship between her husband and the nephrologist. If this second definition of lying is accepted, it would be possible to hold that the rule against lying is absolute, for all of the difficult moral questions would be answered by determining who has a right to the truth.

The necessity of considering the meaning and the weight of a rule together is evident in a recent study of physicians' attitudes toward using deception to resolve difficult ethical problems. Dennis Novak and his colleagues conducted research on physicians' attitudes by means of a questionnaire with hypothetical cases, including the case of Mrs. Lewis, a fifty-two-year-old patient who is undergoing her annual examination (Novak et al. 1989). "You tell her that everything looks normal and that you are going to order routine blood tests and her annual screening mammography, which you feel is important for women of her age. She is against the mammography, saying that the last time you ordered it, she had to pay for it herself. You know she is of modest means and cannot easily afford it. You are surprised that her health insurance did not cover it. Upon asking your secretary, you learn that the insurance covers the cost of mammography only if there is a breast mass or objective clinical evidence of the possibility of cancer. The secretary tells you that the way to get around this is to put down 'rule out cancer' instead of 'screening mammography' on the form." The physicians were asked what they would do, and their responses were most interesting. Close to 70 percent said they would write "rule out cancer," but 85 percent of those said that they would not be deceiving the insurance company by doing so. They could have conceded that they were deceiving the insurance company but then argued that their deception was justified in order to help the patient. But many simply denied that the act would be one of deception. And thus they could also consistently view deception as absolutely wrong, while putting "rule out cancer" on the form.

There are three major interpretations of the weight or stringency of moral principles and rules. They may be viewed as absolute, as prima facie, or as relative maxims or rules of thumb. At one extreme are the legalists who appeal to absolute principles and rules. They define these principles and rules, however, in such a way as to eliminate irresolvable moral dilemmas, often because of philosophical or theological views about harmony in the moral universe. To take one example, Paul Ramsey (1967) is widely viewed as an absolutist in many areas of biomedical ethics, and he handled hard cases of moral conflict not by overriding significant rules but rather by deepening their meaning. Thus, rather than justifying lying, he probed and deepened the meaning of the rule against lying. By contrast, Joseph Fletcher (1966) offered his method of "situation ethics" as a way to avoid both legalism and its extreme opposite (antinomianism). He insisted that there is only one absolute principle — neighbor-love, or utility — and that all other principles and rules are relative maxims or rules of thumb, parallel to baseball's "don't bunt on the third strike." These other principles and rules suggest actions that people have found to produce or subvert good consequences. They only illuminate courses of action; they do not prescribe what ought to be done. Reducing all principles and rules to mere maxims regarding utility, Fletcher came perilously close to antinomianism. His position failed to recognize that principles and rules can be prescriptive without being absolute. They can be prima facie binding (i.e., binding, other things being equal). As prima facie binding, they direct courses of action, but other prima facie principles and rules can override or outweigh them when they come into conflict in a situation.

In *PBE,* Beauchamp and I argue that the principles we identify — respect for autonomy, nonmaleficence, beneficence (including utility or proportionality), and justice, along with such derivative principles or rules as veracity, fidelity, privacy, and confidentiality — are only prima facie binding. None can be considered absolute. And these principles and rules have to be weighed and balanced in situations of decision. This perspective might appear to be very close to Fletcher's maxims or rules of thumb, and even to revived casuistry, which will be considered below, but there is an important difference. For *PBE,* the principles and rules are prima facie binding and thus prescriptive, whereas for Fletcher they only illuminate the application of the one ultimate principle of neighbor-love (or utility). Hence, for *PBE,* the moral agent has to justify departures from principles by showing that in the situation some other principles have more weight. However, the assignment of weight or priority depends on the situation rather than on an abstract, a priori ranking. This approach suffers from the limitations of any pluralistic approach that does not assign weights or priorities to various principles in advance. A great deal rests on what has been variously called prudence, practical moral reasoning, or discernment in the situation within the framework of prima facie principles.

A rule utilitarian (i.e., one who justifies all other principles and rules by the ultimate principle of utility) may be able to appeal to the ultimate principle of utility that justifies various other principles and rules in order to adjudicate conflicts among them. Some rule deontologists (i.e., those who recognize various independent principles and rules of intrinsically right and wrong action) have explored priority rules, for example, contending that the principle of autonomy always trumps or overrides the principle of beneficence, when the only beneficiary is the competent person whose wishes, choices, or actions are overridden.

A major effort to find a lexical or serial ordering of principles appears in Veatch's *Theory of Medical Ethics*, where all the deontological or nonconsequentialist principles "are given lexical priority over the principle of beneficence." In cases of conflict, however, the deontological or nonconsequentialist principles are themselves balanced against each other in what Veatch labels a "balancing strategy." Veatch thus finds "a solution to the inevitable unacceptable tension between Hippocratic individualism and the utilitarian drive toward aggregate net benefit." This solution "comes from the articulation of other nonconsequentialist principles that will necessarily have a bearing on medical ethical decisions: contract keeping, autonomy, honesty, avoiding killing, and justice" and from assigning them collective priority over the production of good consequences for individuals (Hippocratic individualism) or society (utilitarianism). Nonconsequentialist principles are thus given "coequal ranking" in relation to each other and "lexical ranking" over the principle of beneficence. Similarly Engelhardt gives the principle of autonomy priority over the principle of beneficence. Some of the problems of interpreting the meaning and weights of principles and rules can best be explored by considering different ways principlists seek to move from general principles to particular case judgments.

Decision Procedures:
The Movement from Principles to Cases

Using principles-oriented ethics to arrive at concrete, particular judgments requires interpretation. Suppose a family considers whether to terminate artificial nutrition and hydration for an elderly, incompetent patient. They may be uncertain whether their case falls under a principle that prohibits harming the patient or a principle that requires benefiting the patient. The same principle may point in different directions — for example, the principle of benefiting the patient may offer ambiguous directions. In addition, a relevant principle may conflict with other principles, such as respecting the patient's prior express wishes. Some of these conflicts may be apparent rather than real and dissolve upon closer inspection, but others may persist. Finally, different parties involved may have moral conflicts with each other about the appropriateness of withdrawing artificial nutrition and hydration.

In contrast to some criticisms, principlists do not all have the same decision-making procedure. Principlists connect principles to cases in one or more of several possible ways, often combining them. These different decision-making procedures also reflect different views of the interpretation of principles, particularly regarding whether conflicts between principles can be resolved by further elaborating the principles or only by balancing them. Indeed, according to Henry Richardson's helpful analysis, there are three main models of connection between principles and cases: (1) application, which involves the deductive application of principles and rules; (2) balancing, which depends on intuitive weighing of conflicting principles; and (3) specification, which proceeds by "qualitatively tailoring our norms to cases" (1990).

Although *PBE* has used the metaphor of *application*, as in *applied ethics*, this was a mistake that misled some readers, as did its charts that sometimes appeared to indicate a top-down approach through a process of justification. Very few principlists actually take a mechanical view of application, as in a limited model of engineering. Even though there may sometimes be genuine application of principles, the terms applied or application cannot cover all significant relations between principles and cases. In other words, not all connections between principles and particular judgments in cases involve rational deduction. Furthermore, this model suggests a top-down approach, with all the movement from principles and rules to case judgments. (I return to this matter below when I discuss casuistry.) Although absolutist interpreters of principles often attempt this model of application, in practice, as noted above, they frequently incorporate some exceptional cases through deepening the meaning of the principles or rules, a process that is very close to specification.

Balancing is closer to what the first three editions of *PBE* attempted to do, and it fits best with a conception of principles as prima facie binding but potentially in conflict in particular cases. The third edition of *PBE* attempted to reduce the intuitive assignment of weights to conflicting principles in a situation by a more formal procedure for resolving conflicts among principles. Specifically, if two prima facie principles come into conflict, several conditions need to be met before one can override the other. Thus it is not simply a matter of their weights as intuited in the situations. Take, for example, the cases mentioned earlier: the physician who in order to protect confidentiality or to avoid wrecking the family said the father should not donate a kidney for "medical reasons" and the physician who wrote "rule out cancer" on the form so that the insurance company would pay for his patient's screening mammography. If we assume that these are deceptive acts, the rule against deception can be justifiably breached only if the competing principle is weightier or stronger in these circumstances; if the deceptive act could realistically achieve its objective of protecting the competing principle, including avoiding bad consequences; if the deceptive act is necessary in the circumstances in the sense of a lack of morally acceptable alternatives; and if the deceptive act infringes the moral rule against deception to the smallest extent possible, commensurate with achieving the primary goal (*PBE*, 1989:53). These conditions reduce but do not eliminate intuition in the decision-making procedure of balancing.

Specification is Richardson's preferred method for connecting principles and cases. Even though *PBE* did not explicitly identify and develop specification as an approach to principles, specification was involved throughout in determining the meaning, scope, and range of principles such as respect for autonomy, and in indicating how principles can take shape in rules (such as rules requiring voluntary informed consent). Specification also appears in our discussion of the meaning of lying (*PBE*, 1989:49–50). Specification should be expected in principlism, for as R. M. Hare notes, "any attempt to give content to a principle involves specifying the cases that are to fall under it.... Any principle, then, which has content goes some way down the path of specificity" (1989:54).

Even though elements of all three models appear in *PBE*, we were not as clear as we might have been in our theoretical statements or our practical applications. The work of Richardson and of David DeGrazia proposed what they call "specified principlism"; this has helped us see these matters more clearly (DeGrazia 1992). The forthcoming fourth edition proposes that specification be tried first, in an effort to tailor norms so that they can guide actions in concrete situations before balancing occurs. I am not convinced, however, that specification can serve as the exclusive model for relating principles and particular judgments. My main reason for skepticism is my belief that moral conflict is inevitable, not only between people but also within the moral universe. Hence, I think we will still have to engage in some balancing because we cannot specify principles fully enough to avoid all moral conflicts. Furthermore, we may find specification to be as arbitrary as balancing, especially if we have no controls over the interpretation of meaning of the key moral categories. An example appears in our earlier discussion of the moral category of lying in physicians' willingness to put "rule out cancer" on the insurance form because the company would not pay for annual screening mammographies. Without adequate controls on how lying is defined, agents may deceive themselves by supposing that the statement "rule out cancer" requires no moral justification because it infringes no moral rule in that particular context, when in fact it deceives the insurance company about the actual reason for the mammography.

For example, we would first need to define lying in the case presented earlier about mammography to rule out cancer.

Thus, instead of viewing application, balancing, and specification as three alternative models, it is better, I believe, to recognize the importance of all three approaches. Sometimes a principle or rule can be directly applied; sometimes potentially conflicting principles and rules are illuminated through specification; at still other times a conflict requires resolution by balancing, within the constraints and direction of the decision procedure I identified. It is a substantive, and not simply a formal, moral debate about which approach works where. Perhaps the most appropriate general category for what is involved is that of interpretation, as long as it includes both the meaning and weights or strengths of different principles, with attention to the particularities of real situations.

The Primacy of Particular Case Judgments: Casuistry's Challenge to Principlism

So far, in connecting principles to cases, I have discussed how principlists can move from their principles to particular judgments. Casuists charge that principlists fail to give independent and sufficient attention to particular judgments about cases because principlism neglects the primacy of particular judgments about cases over general moral judgments expressed in principles.

Before exploring this charge, I want to consider how some casuists characterize the principlism they attack and also how some casuists explicitly recognize a modest role for principles and incorporate more principles than they explicitly recognize. To take one example, Albert Jonsen and Stephen Toulmin's excellent and important book *The Abuse of Casuistry* (1988) vigorously opposes "the tyranny of principles" (a formulation that appeared earlier in Toulmin's article by the same title).[3] Nevertheless, a careful reading of their book reveals that their target, despite their language, is not the inevitable tyranny of principles as such, but rather the tyranny of some conceptions of principles, particularly "eternal, invariable principles, the practical implications of which can be free of exceptions or qualifications" (Jonsen and Toulmin 1988:2). Such principles lead to problems, particularly deadlocks and fruitless standoffs. And yet, as we have seen, most principlist approaches in biomedical ethics, in contrast to popular debate, recognize few if any absolute principles. In short, this casuistry-based attack on tyrannical principlism focuses on its absolutist versions rather than on versions that

view principles and rules as prima facie binding and require balancing
and other modes of interpretation in situations of decision.

Moreover Jonsen and Toulmin themselves recognize principles. At
one point, they state that their aim is to argue for "good casuistry," that
is, casuistry "which applies general rules to particular cases with discernment [in contrast to] bad casuistry, which does the same thing sloppily"
(Jonsen and Toulmin 1988:16). And elsewhere Toulmin concedes that
principles have special relevance in relations between strangers rather
than intimates (a matter to which I return below) (Toulmin 1981).
Furthermore, in addition to their explicit concessions, casuists often
have principles and rules that they do not appear to recognize clearly.
When casuist Jonsen distinguishes ethically wrong, permissible, and
obligatory actions, he focuses on relevant similarities and differences between paradigm cases and current cases, and in the process, implicitly
or indirectly appeals to what may be viewed as principles. For example, in identifying the features and conditions that distinguish justified
autopsy from unjustified vivisection of criminals, Jonsen focuses on the
fact that autopsy does not involve harm or pain (because the subject is
dead), coercion, or unfairness, even if the prospect of benefit is limited
(Jonsen 1988). All four of the major principles in *PBE* are implicit in
Jonsen's argument: the noninfliction of pain expresses the principle of
nonmaleficence; avoidance of coercion expresses the principle of respect
for autonomy; and avoidance of unfairness expresses the principle of
justice. In addition, the interest in autopsy stems from the principle of
beneficence: producing good. Principlists contend that it is better first to
recognize that general moral considerations, which can be called principles, function broadly in our judgments and then to examine them
directly for their adequacy rather than to allow them to enter covertly.

Similar points can be made about the casuistical categories of medical indications, patient preferences, quality of life, and socioeconomic
factors, featured in the book *Clinical Ethics,* which Jonsen co-authored
with Mark Siegler and William Winslade (1986). These four factors correlate closely with what others call moral principles — e.g., attention to
medical indications and quality of life involves principles of beneficence
and nonmaleficence; respect for patient preferences involves respect for
persons and their autonomy; and the external factors, which focus on
the impact of actions on others including family and society, involve
considerations of utility and justice. In fact, these ethical factors or considerations function in their argument about clinical ethics in roughly
the way that similar principles and rules function for some other theories
of biomedical ethics. They are prima facie or presumptive rather than
absolute, but they are more than maxims. Fear of the tyranny of prin-

ciples that are absolute or simplistic does not provide sufficient reason to discard the language of principles altogether, especially when these ethical considerations function as principles.

Central to Jonsen and Toulmin's argument for casuistry over (absolutist) principlism is their interpretation of the work of the National Commission for the Protection of Human Subjects of Biomedical and Behavioral Research. (Jonsen was a commissioner and Toulmin a staff philosopher.) According to Jonsen and Toulmin, "the locus of certitude in the commissioner's discussions did not lie in an agreed set of intrinsically convincing general rules or principles, as they shared no commitment to any such body of agreed principles. Rather, it lay in a shared perception of what was specifically at stake in particular kinds of human situations" (Jonsen and Toulmin 1988:18). Nevertheless, the commissioners did issue the *Belmont Report,* which, as noted above, articulates three fundamental principles: beneficence (which includes what Beauchamp and I call nonmaleficence), respect for persons (which includes what Beauchamp and I call respect for autonomy), and justice. To be sure, this report came late in the National Commission's deliberations, after much of the work on problem areas had been completed (Jonsen and Toulmin 1988:356, fn. 14), and it may have been motivated in part by the legislative mandate to identify the ethical principles that should govern research involving human subjects. But another plausible interpretation is that these general principles were already embedded in the Commission's agreements about problem areas, such as research involving children and prisoners, and that the *Belmont Report* simply articulated these principles with greater clarity. A clear articulation of these underlying principles could both illuminate the particular recommendations and provide a basis for testing consistency and adequacy.

Furthermore, the National Commission's analysis of types of cases in research involving human subjects occurred within a general consensus about a paradigm case (the Nazi experiments on unconsenting human subjects) and also about the relevant moral principles and rules (the Nuremberg Code, which embodies virtually all the principles and rules that would now be taken to govern research involving human subjects). For purposes of moral education and enforcement, it was important to formulate the Nuremberg Code. Even though the Nuremberg Code itself emerged after moral revulsion to the Nazi experiments (a case judgment), it would be a gross oversimplification to suppose that historically it was only after a negative judgment about the Nazi experiments that moral principles and rules emerged for judging such experiments. The relations between particular judgments, principles, and rules are more complex. Because of consensus about the principles and rules embodied in the Nuremberg Code, the National Commission could more easily deal with new or ambiguous cases not captured by the paradigm case.

So far my discussion of casuistry has focused on the unclear target of some major casuists and on their acknowledged and unacknowledged incorporation of principles in their case analyses. The heart of the casuists' positive claim, as stated in *The Abuse of Casuistry* (1988:330), is that (1) "casuistry is unavoidable," (2) "moral knowledge is essentially particular, so that sound resolutions of moral problems must always be rooted in a concrete understanding of specific cases and circumstances," and (3) moral reasoning proceeds by paradigm cases and analogies. I agree with much in these statements, but I would argue that moral knowledge is general as well as particular, that the locus of certitude is not limited to particular cases, and that forms of principlist reasoning are compatible with the use of paradigm cases and analogies.

What does it mean to affirm the primacy or priority of particular judgments? First, it might mean that particular judgments chronologically come first. But then the question is for whom. Each individual participates in communities, many of which involve traditions of moral reflection. These traditions include both general principles and judgments about cases. Even if the particular judgments came first historically (a claim that is difficult to establish), we do not encounter the moral wisdom of our communities and their traditions only through their particular judgments, for these communities and traditions usually present general principles and rules too. Indeed, it is hard to imagine moral education proceeding without general principles and rules as well as paradigm cases. Hence, the Jonsen-Toulmin view and critique of principles as "top-down" holds only if we are thinking in terms of theoretical derivation; it does not fit with a historical, communal interpretation of morality.

Second, the primacy of particular judgments might suggest normative priority. Here the language of dialectic is the most illuminating. Where particular judgments appear to conflict with general principles, adjustments are required, but it is not possible to say that either should always take priority.

Third, the primacy of particular judgments might mean logical priority. However, it is not clear that logical priority can be assigned to either principles or case judgments; the relation between them is better viewed as dialectical, with neither one fully and completely derived from the other but each potentially modifying the other.

It is also important to ask what is implied when we make a judgment that an action in a particular set of circumstances is wrong. R. M. Hare argues that "if we, as a result of reflection on something that has happened, have made a certain moral judgment, we have acquired a precept or principle which has application in all similar cases. We have, in some sense of that word, learnt something." If we learn something useful from reflection on a particular case, Hare claims, the principle we gain must be somewhat general rather than having unlimited specificity. Since no two real cases are exactly alike, we have results of reflection that can be useful in the future only if we "have isolated certain broad features of the cases we were thinking about — features which may recur in other cases" (Hare 1989:54). Hare's argument presupposes the principle of universalizability, which Beauchamp and I also take to be a condition of moral judgments (*PBE*, 1989:18–20). Acceptance of the principle of universalizability does not distinguish principlism from casuistry, for this formal principle is also presupposed by the Jonsen-Toulmin approach to casuistry. The focus on paradigm cases and analogical reasoning depends on identifying relevant similarities and differences between cases, and its force derives from the requirement of the principle of universalizability to treat relevantly similar cases in a similar way. This principle also appears in the common law doctrine of precedent, which serves as a model for casuistry.

Beauchamp and I have not always stated our (current) view of the relation between principles and cases clearly. (I include the qualifier "current" because our position may have become clearer to us as we worked on it over time, but I would argue that even the first edition of *PBE* in 1979 was richer on this point than is sometimes recognized.) In particular, as I noted above, problems in interpreting our principlism could easily arise because of our continued use of the metaphor of "application," along with such metaphors as hierarchical tiers, foundation, basis, and ground, and the use of diagrams that sketch the relations between theories, principles, rules, and particular judgments in ways that seem to deny or diminish the certitude in casuistical judgments other than by way of application of general principles and rules. We have stressed, however, that particular moral judgments have relative independence and can lead to a modification or reformulation of general principles; for example, we note that it is a mistake to say that ethical theory and principles are "not *drawn* from cases but only *applied* to cases" (*PBE,* 1989:16). And throughout our editions we have viewed the relation between principles and rules, on the one hand, and particular judgments about cases, on the other, as *dialectical,* with each potentially modifying the other.[4]

We admit that one cannot determine meaning and weights of principles in total abstraction from situations, or at least types of situations;

so, then, what terribly important differences exist between our principlism and casuistry? In practice, Jonsen and Toulmin do not reject principles (but only those with certain characteristics or qualities, such as absoluteness, invariability, and exceptionlessness) and concede that casuistry involves the discerning application of principles; meanwhile, Beauchamp and I recognize a more complex relation of principles and cases than some of our language and diagrams of principlism suggest. Thus our approaches may share more than is sometimes recognized. Beauchamp and I do not claim that principles are indispensable for every particular judgment and moral decision, but we do claim that principles play an important role in many moral judgments and decisions, in moral education, and in moral justification in a communal setting (e.g., regarding public policy). At the very least, Jonsen and Toulmin's casuistry and our principlism share an important similarity in spirit.

Responses of Principlists to Other Selected Criticisms

In this section, I briefly highlight some other (but by no means all) important criticisms of principlist bioethics and indicate in passing how well they succeed, with attention to whether they hit their identified target, whether all principlist approaches are equally susceptible to the charges, and whether revision is possible to salvage principlism.

Bioethics for intimates or strangers. One criticism of principles and rules in biomedical ethics holds that they are appropriate in interactions among strangers but not among friends and intimates, a point Toulmin makes in his article. Hence, a fundamental question is whether in our society patients and physicians or other health care professionals interact as friends or as strangers.

Major changes in health care have rendered problematic a conception of medicine in terms of friendship. Pluralism in values; the decline of close, intimate contact over time between professionals and patients; the rise of specialists who treat only part of the whole person; and the growth of large, impersonal, and bureaucratic institutions of health care have all contributed to the loss of intimacy and community. Trust among strangers cannot presuppose knowledge of each others' traits of character or values. In the absence of community, then, principles, rules, and procedures become increasingly important. As reconceived in a pluralistic setting, trust may amount to confidence in and reliance upon health care professionals to adhere to such principles as autonomy and truthfulness which do not presuppose knowledge of the professionals' interpretation of benefits and burdens or harms. Thus, rights within health care, as distinct from rights to health care, may limit and constrain the professional's actions even when they are putatively directed at the patient's welfare. Trust may also be expressed as confidence in and reliance upon others to adhere to moral limits that derive from respect for persons, justice, and so on, rather than from beneficence. In short, principles and rules may provide the basis for interaction among "friendly strangers." They are not friends, but they are not estranged and hostile. Even though they do not have (or at least do not know if they have) shared conceptions of the good life, including balances of benefits and harms, they can trust each other to respect common principles and rules. As Alasdair MacIntyre has noted,

> When a community of moral and metaphysical beliefs is lacking, trust between strangers becomes much more questionable than when we can safely assume such a community. Nobody can rely on anyone else's judgments on his or her behalf until he or she knows what the other person believes. It follows that nobody can accept the moral authority of another in virtue simply of his professional position. We are thrust back into a form of moral autonomy. (1977)

Our social situation thus supports claims not only about the importance of moral principles and rules for interaction among strangers but also about the importance of some moral principles and rules over others. Developing bioethics for secular, pluralistic societies, Engelhardt has argued that physicians "must come to terms with the moral commitments and views of individuals from various moral communities while preserving the moral fabric of a peaceable, secular, pluralist society" (1986).

Preference for liberal individualism over communitarianism. Because principlism is often viewed as rights-oriented and as giving primacy to rights of autonomy, privacy, and liberty of the individual, it is also viewed as a form of liberal individualism rather than communitarianism. Perhaps no recent discussion has been beset with as many unclarities as the one centered on communitarianism. It is important to distinguish at least two forms of communitarianism: methodological and normative.[5] Methodologically, I have argued that some principlist approaches (including the one I find defensible) can be viewed as communitarian in that they ground principles in communal life rather than in a foundationalist theory and use a coherentist rather than a deductivist procedure.

As a normative approach, communitarianism may view community as identifying desirable human relationships and may assign communal values priority over other values. Nothing in the approach of principlism itself dictates a conclusion about the relative weights of the individual and the community in cases of conflict, even if many principlists have been liberal individualists in part because of their views about the fragmentation of contemporary society. Principlists need not neglect special and particular communal relations, but they will also note that principles of justice are often necessary to set priorities among conflicting communal relations and to limit the undue claims of particular communities. Moreover, principlists can assign a variety of weights to the claims of individuals and the claims of communities. For example, a principlist who holds that several moral principles are prima facie binding and that they must be balanced in particular circumstances may sometimes give community priority over individuals and vice versa. There is no a priori ranking. And even if presumptions exist that favor individual rights of autonomy, liberty, and privacy, those presumptions are rebuttable and can sometimes be overridden in the name of community. Consider the debate about selective mandatory HIV screening and testing. A principlist who is a "liberal communitarian" may favor respect for autonomy and derivative rules such as liberty, privacy, and confidentiality but also identify conditions that must and in some cases could override the "liberal" principles (and thus, support mandatory screening under some circumstances) (Childress 1991).

Principlism as regulatory bioethics. Principlists are often viewed as undertaking regulatory bioethics for the society rather than offering prophetic judgments, perhaps based on particular religious traditions.[6] James Gustafson distinguishes four varieties of moral discourse: ethical, prophetic, narrative, and policy (Gustafson 1988). Ethical discourse uses concepts and categories from moral philosophy and theology to decide how one ought to act in particular circumstances. By contrast, prophetic discourse tends to offer more general indictments or utopian visions, and narrative discourse invokes the values and visions of communities as shaped by their stories. Policy discourse tends to ask what is possible. Gustafson argues that we neglect morally significant issues if we employ only one form of moral discourse. Principlists, to be sure, have concentrated on ethical analysis and argument and have often participated in trying to shape public policy in a liberal, democratic society. With the casuists and others, however, they have used a variety of narratives. And despite claims of some critics, principlists have often been prophetic in denouncing various aspects of health care and its social setting — examples include the criticism of professional paternalism and the unequal distribution of health care. It is true that some principlists (as well as some casuists and theorists) have sought to work out acceptable policies in such areas as human fetal tissue transplantation research.[7] But which position is prophetic — one that supports the ban on federal funds for human fetal tissue transplantation research because the tissue comes from deliberately aborted fetuses and is alleged to create the risk of additional abortions, or one that opposes the ban because of the possible benefits of the research compared with the improbable increase in abortions?

Nothing about the framework of principlism itself, in contrast to casuistry, makes it less prophetic and more regulatory. In the kind of principlism I find most satisfactory, principles are discerned in social practices rather than established by a unified theory. They can still serve a critical function, perhaps more readily than the taxonomic approach of a pure casuistry that attempts to operate without principles. Even if one could locate the historical origins of principles in case judgments, general principles operate in communities' and traditions' moral discourse and education and provide ways to criticize practices that are not available in case-to-case analysis. Building on some suggestions by John Arras (1991), I would note that in moving from actual case to actual case, the ethicist (casuist) may be limited to what practitioners and others present for analysis and assessment as *felt* problems or dilemmas. General principles may help identify other cases that should be on the moral agenda, and they may direct our attention to *real* problems and dilemmas that practitioners have not yet experienced as such.

Sometimes this charge of regulatory bioethics focuses on principlism's alleged neglect of particular religious traditions and other particular communities in its effort to articulate principles that can guide and direct actions and policies in a secular, pluralistic society. Principlists do tend to concentrate on principles that can operate across the society rather than within one particular tradition in the society. But while some principlists identify an explicitly secular bioethics, others relate their principles, however loosely, to shared themes in religious traditions.[8] And principlists generally do not deny an important role for religious traditions in moral discourse about bioethics, even if they concentrate on the larger social framework. The issues raised by principlism also emerge within particular religious traditions — for example, the recent debate in Catholic moral theology about proportionalism and the earlier debate in Protestant ethics about norm versus context (see Gustafson 1965; Outka and Ramsey 1967; Hoose 1987).

Mechanical application. Several critics of principlism lament the "tiresome invocation of the applied ethics mantra (i.e., the principles of respect for autonomy, beneficence, and justice)" (Arras 1991:48–49). They oppose what they view as ritualistic incantation of the mantra and mechanical application of principles along the lines of a narrow engineering model. Clouser and Gert's graphic description is noteworthy:

> Throughout the land, arising from the throngs of converts to bio-ethics awareness, there can be heard a mantra "...beneficence... autonomy...justice...." It is this ritual incantation in the face of biomedical dilemmas that beckons our inquiry....Brandishing these several principles, adherents to the "principle approach" go forth to confront the quandaries of biomedical ethics. (1990:219; see also Wikler 1991)

This criticism sometimes suggests that principlism has distorted bio-ethics, and scholarship in bioethics, by offering some relatively abstract, philosophical categories (especially autonomy, beneficence, and non-maleficence) that have tempted some newcomers to philosophical or theological ethics to suppose that they have been initiated into a mysterious realm, and thus have become experts in ethics because they can chant the mantra. Then these newcomers mechanically apply the principles. It is sufficient to note in response that there is good and bad scholarship in bioethics, whatever the approach (Brody 1990). After all, as Jonsen and Toulmin concede, casuistry fell into disfavor because it developed into a form of self-serving logic-chopping (or at least the critics so charged). While some works in biomedical ethics offer unsophisticated interpretations and mechanical applications of principles, others present careless casuistry or sermonic renditions of the virtues. Thus critics must compare the best scholarly presentations of each approach, as well as note deficient versions.

Obsession with quandaries. One common criticism of principlism is that it fosters a conception of bioethics as quandary ethics, always focused on moral dilemmas and problems, which then have to be resolved. That is a misconception of principlism. Even if principlists concentrate on quandaries that face various parties who affirm these moral principles, they do not suppose that the moral life simply consists of various disconnected moral problems. They can recognize that much of the moral life is a matter of doing what one recognizes to be right, good, obligatory, and so on without any direct appeal to principles. For example, moral agents recognize that they ought to act as "Good Samaritans" because of a neighbor's need, without reflection based on principles. Only when novel situations and moral conflicts, both intrapersonal and interpersonal, arise, must principles be invoked. However rare, quandaries do have to be faced when they arise. Preventing them is desirable, but preventive ethics, just as preventive health care, is not uniformly successful, and then critical cases have to be faced and resolved. Thus, to concentrate on dilemmas in biomedical ethics because of their importance and difficulty is not to suppose that dilemmas as shaped and resolved by principles exhaust biomedical ethics.

The neglect of character and virtue. A related criticism of principles and rules comes from proponents of the primacy of character and virtues. In a framework of character and virtues, actions are assessed according to what they express about the agent and his or her motives and traits or character. According to character or virtue ethics, many putatively different frameworks (e.g., principlists and casuists, deontologists and utilitarians) have more in common than is usually recognized, for each focuses on "What ought I do?" in the context of moral dilemmas, quandaries, and problems that must be approached either through principles or through analogical reasoning. By contrast, proponents of the primacy of virtue — though by no means a uniform group — address the question "What ought I to be?" and hold (1) that a virtuous professional can *discern* the right course of action in the situation without reliance on principles and rules, and/or (2) that a virtuous person will *desire* to do what is right and avoid what is wrong. The first approach is often combined with situation ethics, and it downplays rules and principles in moral decision making. Leon Kass articulates this viewpoint: "I increasingly believe that the attempt to replace the often inarticulate yet prudent judgments of discerning physicians with explicit rules or procedures will not lead to better decisions" (1980:1811). Principlists respond that if we do try to determine which approach will lead to "better decisions," we must appeal to principles and rules to identify courses of action that are right, obligatory, wrong, or permitted. And when agents have to justify their conduct, they cannot simply appeal to their "discernment" or "prudence" or "conscience" without reference to principles and rules. There is simply no assurance that good people will discern what is right. The second approach to virtues concentrates on the agent's motivation to do what is right, assuming that what is right is clear in most situations and that the major problem is the lack of motivation to do what is right. When moral requirements and self-interest conflict, the problem may be one not of knowledge but of motivation, and virtues dispose people to act in morally appropriate ways from morally appropriate motives. For example, according to Gregory Pence, "the ultimate argument" for discussing biomedical ethics "in the framework of the virtues" is that researchers, physicians, and other professionals can subvert rules such as informed consent if they desire (Pence 1980:177). Thus it is important to create a climate in which professionals have the right kind of desires. Pence is certainly correct to emphasize the role of virtues in disposing people to right actions, but it is necessary to have an independent assessment of acts in light of moral principles. Virtues include certain motivations to perform right actions but are not themselves sufficient to determine which actions are right. In many cases it is simply not clear what a virtuous physician would do. Would such a physician, for example, breach confidentiality in order to warn a person that his or her lover has AIDS or order an involuntary hospitalization for a patient contemplating suicide? And finally, in much (but by no means all) of the moral life, principles of action help to determine which virtues should be developed. Many virtues are correlated with principles and rules (e.g., benevolence with beneficence, truthfulness with veracity), and many other virtues (e.g., conscientiousness and courage) are important for morality as a whole.

Care in relationships. A final criticism of principles and rules in biomedical ethics could be built on the arguments offered by Carol Gilligan (1982) about male and female moralities. Noting that both Piaget and Kohlberg omitted girls and women from their studies of moral development, Gilligan contends that women are not morally retarded, as Kohlberg's tests suggest, but rather speak in a different moral voice, which is not adequately recorded by the tests developed on male models. In particular, Gilligan notes that women tend to concentrate on narrative, context, and relationships, in which they express care and caring, rather than on tiers of moral principles and rules with their logic of hierarchical justification, as in male perspectives on morality. She argues that women see and resolve moral problems differently. This is a very important argument, but it needs further clarification and elaboration. Gilligan emphasizes that what is involved is not gender but socialization, and she insists that what is needed is a recognition of the complementarity of the two moralities of care and justice, including rights.

While this complementarity is possible within an individual's life over time, it is not yet clear what it would imply for some social roles, like those in medicine. Consider again the case of the father who did not want to donate a kidney to his dying daughter and asked the physician to lie. Would a physician with a caring perspective come to a conclusion different from one reached by a physician with a principlist perspective, which, as we have suggested, could itself lead to several different conclusions? It is hard to predict with confidence whether these perspectives would produce significant differences in this case, not only because the socialization process in medicine may inculcate "male" morality, but because the major question is the *moral significance* of the nephrologist's relationships with the father and with the other members of the family. Hence the physician in that case would have to determine, at least in part through principles and rules, how much weight each relationship should have.

It is plausible to hold that some moral principles and rules as well as some modes of moral reasoning will be more important in one setting than in another, whether females or males occupy the social roles. Within research, medicine, and health care, which, as I have stressed, often involve relations among strangers, the appeal to principles and rules may be important and even indispensable, whether the strangers are male or female. Furthermore, principles of respect for autonomy and justice, particularly in the form of equality, are often invoked to argue for women's rights. And some feminists, who take seriously the social context of oppression of women under patriarchy, wonder whether female caring is to a great extent a product of this oppressive social system (Sherwin 1992). Nevertheless, the moral perspective of care in relationships does identify a major limitation of some principlist approaches. Methodologically, as Alisa Carse stresses, " 'care' reasoning is concrete and contextual rather than abstract; it is sometimes principle-guided, rather than always principle-driven, and it involves sympathy and compassion rather than dispassion" (Carse 1991). Although casuistical and care perspectives overlap, the latter properly stresses emotional qualities and character traits sometimes neglected by both casuists and principlists.

Finally, then, it does not appear to this principlist that the various critics have dislodged principles from a central place in the structure of biomedical ethics. At least some principlist approaches, with appropriate modification and revision, appear to withstand the most important challenges. The fundamental question is not whether to invoke principles and rules in the identification, interpretation, and resolution of moral problems — and there are such problems in contemporary science, medicine, and health care, as well as in public policies regarding them. The legitimate and perplexing questions surround which principles and rules should be adopted, how they can be justified, how they should be interpreted and specified in particular cases, how they should be modified in light of particular cases, how much weight and strength they should have, which should have priority if they conflict in particular circumstances, and what significance they have in various contexts and relations, such as those between strangers and those between intimates.

Answers to these questions are not easy, or uncontroversial, but seeking the answers in the context of science, medicine, and health care remains a fundamental responsibility in biomedical ethics. Thus the critics of principlism need to attend more carefully to what different approaches, loosely labeled principlist, actually hold about principles and their function and interpretation. But principlists also need to attend more carefully and thoughtfully to the critical challenges and to revise their frameworks as appropriate in light of those criticisms. For, as Carse suggests, being principle-guided is different from being principle-driven. And the most defensible principlist frameworks entail only principle-guidance.

NOTES

1. We are now (in late 1993) preparing the fourth edition for publication.

2. When Veatch's and Engelhardt's names appear in the text without a reference or note, these volumes are the sources for the information. Also for Veatch, see his essay "The Principles for Medical Ethics," in *The Patient-Physician Relation: The Patient as Partner*, Part 2 (Bloomington: Indiana University Press, 1991), chap. 6.2.

3. Hereafter page references to this work will be given in the text. See also Stephen Toulmin, "The Tyranny of Principles," *Hastings Center Report* 11 (December 1981):31–39.

4. 1st ed., p. 13; 2d ed., p. 13; 3d ed., p. 16.

5. I am using these terms in a sense somewhat different from that in the source from which I have drawn them. See Shlomo Avineri and Avner de-Shalit, eds., *Communitarianism and Individualism* (New York: Oxford University Press, 1992).

6. In discussions at the Hastings Center, Daniel Callahan has used the label "regulatory" bioethics to characterize much of contemporary bioethics.

7. See statements by James Childress and K. Danner Clouser in National Institutes of Health, *Human Fetal Tissue Transplantation Research* (1988), as well as Jonsen 1988.

8. Contrast Engelhardt with Robert Veatch, *The Foundations of Justice* (New York: Oxford University Press, 1986).

REFERENCES

Arras, John. 1991. "Getting Down to Cases: The Revival of Casuistry in Bioethics." *Journal of Medicine and Philosophy* 16:29–51.

Avineri, Shlomo, and Avner de-Shalit, eds. 1992. Introduction. *Communitarianism and Individualism.* New York: Oxford University Press.

Beauchamp, Tom L. 1984. "On Eliminating the Distinction Between Applied Ethics and Ethical Theory." *Monist* 67:515–531.

Beauchamp, Tom L., and James F. Childress. 1989. *Principles of Biomedical Ethics,* 3d ed. New York: Oxford University Press.

Brody, Baruch. 1990. "Quality of Scholarship in Bioethics." *Journal of Medicine and Philosophy* 15:161–178.

Carse, Alisa L. 1991. "The 'Voice of Care': Implications for Bioethical Education." *Journal of Medicine and Philosophy* 16:5–28.

Childress, James F. 1991. "Mandatory Screening and Testing." In *AIDS and Ethics*, ed. Frederic Reamer. New York: Columbia University Press.

———. 1990. "The Place of Autonomy in Bioethics." *Hastings Center Report* 20 (January/February): 12–17.

Clarke, Stanley G., and Evan Simpson, eds. 1989. *Anti-Theory in Ethics and Moral Conservatism*. Albany: State University of New York.

Clouser, K. Danner, and Bernard Gert. 1990. "A Critique of Principlism." *Journal of Medicine and Philosophy* 15:219–36.

DeGrazia, David. 1992. "Moving Forward in Bioethical Theory: Theories, Cases, and Specified Principlism." *Journal of Medicine and Philosophy* 17 (October): 511–39.

Engelhardt, H. Tristram, Jr. 1986. *Foundations of Bioethics*. New York: Oxford University Press.

Fletcher, Joseph. 1966. *Situation Ethics: The New Morality*. Philadelphia: Westminster Press.

Gilligan, Carol. 1982. *In a Different Voice*. Cambridge: Harvard University Press.

Green, Ronald. 1990. "Method in Bioethics: A Troubled Assessment." *Journal of Medicine and Philosophy* 15:179–197.

Gustafson, James M. 1988. *Varieties of Moral Discourse: Prophetic, Narrative, Ethical, and Policy*. (Stob Lectures of Calvin College and Seminary, 1987–1988.) Grand Rapids, Mich.: Calvin College and Seminary.

———. 1965. "Context versus Principles: A Misplaced Debate in Christian Ethics." *Harvard Theological Review* 58:171–202.

Hare, R. M. 1989. "Principles." *Essays in Ethical Theory*. Oxford: Clarendon Press.

Hoose, Bernard. 1987. *Proportionalism: The American Debate and Its European Roots*. Washington, D.C.: Georgetown University Press.

Jonsen, Albert R. 1988. "Transplantation of Fetal Tissue: An Ethicist's Viewpoint." *Clinical Research* 36:215–19.

Jonsen, Albert R., Mark Siegler, and William J. Winslade. 1986. *Clinical Ethics*, 2d ed. New York: Macmillan.

Jonsen, Albert R., and Stephen Toulmin. 1988. *The Abuse of Casuistry*. Berkeley: University of California Press.

Kass, Leon. 1980. "Ethical Dilemmas in the Care of the Ill." *Journal of the American Medical Association* 244 (17 October): 1811.

Levine, Melvin D., Lee Scott, and William J. Curran. 1977. "Ethics Rounds in a Children's Medical Center: Evaluation of a Hospital-Based Program for Continuing Education in Medical Ethics." *Pediatrics* 60 (August): 205, reprinted in Beauchamp and Childress, *PBE*, 404–5.

MacIntyre, Alasdair. 1977. "Patients as Agents." In *Philosophical Medical Ethics: Its Nature and Significance,* ed. Stuart F. Spicker and H. Tristram Engelhardt, Jr. 197–212. Boston: D. Reidel Publishing Co.

National Commission for the Protection of Human Subjects of Biomedical and Behavioral Research. 1978. *The Belmont Report: Ethical Guidelines for the Protection of Human Subjects of Research*, DHEW Publication No. (OS) 78–00. Washington, D.C.: Department of Health, Education, and Welfare.

National Institutes of Health, Report of the Advisory Committee to the Director. 1988. *Human Fetal Tissue Transplantation Research*. Bethesda, Md.: National Institutes of Health, C7–C8, and C17–C18.

Novak, Dennis H., Barbara J. Detering, Robert Arnold, et al. 1989. "Physicians' Attitudes Toward Using Deception to Resolve Difficult Ethical Questions." *Journal of the American Medical Association* 261 (26 May): 2980–85.

Outka, Gene, and Paul Ramsey, eds. 1967. *Norm and Context in Christian Ethics*. New York: Charles Scribner's

Pence, Gregory. 1980. *Ethical Options in Medicine*. Oradell, N.J.: Medical Economics Co., Book Division.

Ramsey, Paul. 1967. *Deeds and Rules in Christian Ethics*. New York: Charles Scribner's.

Richardson, Henry S. 1990. "Specifying Norms as a Way to Resolve Concrete Ethical Problems." *Philosophy and Public Affairs* 19:279–320.

Sherwin, Susan. 1992. *No Longer Patient: Feminist Ethics and Health Care*. Philadelphia: Temple University Press.

Solomon, William David. 1978. "Rules and Principles." In *Encyclopedia of Bioethics*, vol. 1, ed. Warren T. Reich. New York: Macmillan and Free Press.

Toulmin, Stephen. 1981. "The Tyranny of Principles." *Hastings Center Report* 11 (December): 31–39.

Veatch, Robert. 1991. "The Principles for Medical Ethics." In *The Patient-Physician Relation: The Patient as Partner*, part 2, chap. 6. Bloomington: Indiana University Press.

———. 1986. *The Foundations of Justice*. New York: Oxford University Press.

———. 1981. *A Theory of Medical Ethics*. New York: Basic Books.

Wikler, Daniel. 1991. "What Has Bioethics to Offer Health Policy?" *Milbank Quarterly* 69:233–51.

Part Two

Principlism
and
Its Critics

~ 3 ~

PRINCIPLISM
A WESTERN EUROPEAN APPRAISAL

Henk ten Have

Introduction: Transformation of Medical Ethics

Interest in the moral problems of medicine and health care has burgeoned over the last three decades, in the U.S. as well as in the majority of European countries. Although medical practice has always been the subject of ethical critique, two recent developments in particular have transformed the traditional notion of medical ethics: (1) advances in medicine and health care due to the influence of biotechnology and technology-oriented medicine, and (2) the rapidly changing sociocultural context in Western countries, marked by an increased plurality of values, especially those values that bear on the provision of health care.

Since the middle of the nineteenth century, medicine and health care have advanced significantly, and previously life-threatening diseases are now met with effective therapeutic interventions. However, advances in biotechnology and biomedicine have also stimulated the realization that the medical enterprise is in need of reappraisal (Greaves 1979). Not only have advances in medical technology become disvalued as impersonal and inhumane, but increasingly, the goals, direction, and effectiveness of technology-oriented medicine have come into question.

The sociocultural context of medical practice has changed in many respects as well. During the last three decades, the influence of religious values in the resolution of moral problems in medicine has diminished, whereas a nonreligious, secularly grounded view of human life has become more influential. This view emphasizes personal autonomy and each patient's right to make his or her own health care decisions. At the same time, the writings of Zola, Illich, and Foucault focused on the power of health care professionals in present-day society, as well as on the so-called medicalization of postmodern culture. Such critiques have resulted in a changed attitude toward health care professionals and an increasing demand by patients to participate in medical decision making at virtually every level — not only in the physician-patient encounter but also within the health care system.

The social status of physicians has been affected significantly by these factors. Traditionally, medical ethics referred to the deontology of the medical profession, to codes of conduct which consist partly of ordinary moral rules, partly of rules of etiquette, and partly of rules of professional conduct (Downie 1974). Inasmuch as it shares these concerns, traditional medical ethics had the following characteristics:

First, it was essentially a set of problems that focused on the internal morality of medicine — those values, norms, and rules intrinsic to the actual practice of health care. Medicine is not considered a merely technical enterprise that can be morally evaluated from some exogenous standpoint. On the contrary, the professional practice of medicine always presumes and implies a moral perspective or point of view; therefore, what is judged to be sound medical practice is determined by the shared rules and standard procedures of the practice.

Second, it was related to the professionalization of medicine. The historical process of professionalization merged an appeal to the self-interest of the members with emphasis on the common good. Social recognition could only be gained on the basis of a strong internal organization and self-imposed standards of behavior. Self-regulation by physicians and a special style of life, structured by high ideals, duties, and virtues, could promote the physician's image, and thus the power and prestige of each member of the medical profession.

Third, because they were primarily concerned with explicating norms and formulating standards of professional conduct, medical ethics and etiquette have been segregated for a long time from general intellectual history (Fox 1979). Moreover, before the 1960s, medical ethics was not a subject frequently discussed in public forums and the extant literature. Apparently, there was a consensus concerning the moral commitments of those who provided medical care, and the explication or codification of these commitments was regarded as the principal concern of medical professionals.

Since the 1960s, professional medical ethics has gradually detached from its traditional deontology (ten Have and van der Arend 1985), although there are important phase differences between the U.S. and European countries, especially in southern European countries where the emphasis in medical ethics is still on medical deontology. In northwestern European countries and in the U.S., professional medical ethics more and more is subsumed under *health care ethics* or *bioethics*. These new terms indicate that the discipline of ethics includes not only problems that arise in the physician-patient relationship but also moral problems posed by other health care professionals, moral issues created by the health care system, and public policy issues engendered by biomedical advances and the results of research. This trend is further illustrated by the dramatic increase in publications on moral problems in medicine and health care authored by nonphysicians. Consequently, the range of problems properly subsumed under the rubric *medical ethics* is considerably enlarged; there are ever new and more complex moral issues, and new participants emerge to engage in an intensified set of medico-ethical debates.

The gradual transformation of medical ethics has had two results. It has produced a new professional — the health care ethicist, or bioethicist, who possesses a specific body of knowledge and particular cognitive skills; publishes in specialized journals; participates in newly formed societies; and teaches in newly established centers, institutes, and departments. It has produced a new sociocultural interest in medico-moral matters of significant public concerns — particularly in those countries where advanced biomedical technology permeates public as well as private life. Bioethics is a way of publicly addressing, explicating, and debating problems generated by science and technology.

The outcome of the above-mentioned transformation is more salient in the U.S. than in most European countries. In U.S. bioethics moral problems in health care are generally approached more analytically and from more of an applied perspective than is usually the case in many Continental approaches.

The first part of the following discussion identifies and critiques the dominant conception of bioethics that seems to prevail in the U.S. Such critique at the same time, however, calls into question the specific characteristics of European approaches to moral problems in health care. The second part describes significant ideas and developments in European medical ethics. Therefore, a European appraisal of U.S. bioethics (i.e., principlism) results in a clarification of the European dimension of medical ethics.

A European Criticism of U.S. Bioethics

Today we see growing dissatisfaction with the results of this transformation in medical ethics. As noted, professionalization and institutionalization of medical ethics received an enormous stimulus because both the adequacy and the relevance of medicine's internal morality were called into question. In response, professional ethicists have placed more and more emphasis on the role of external morality: the principles, norms, and rules operative in society that may bear on medicine and are frequently codified in law. Thus for some ethicists, medicine and health care have become nothing more than interesting intellectual phenomena with respect to which general ethical theories, principles, and rules may be applied. This shift to an external morality and to a predominant interpretation of medical ethics as applied ethics encouraged physicians to criticize present-day bioethics for its lack of attention to the practical vicissitudes of health care, for its theoretical biases, and for its conceptual alienation from clinical reality ("Medical Ethics" 1990; Vandenbroucke 1990).

Many observers claim that the conceptual ground of bioethics is too limited and even reductive when seen from the perspective of the tradition of philosophical ethics itself. Must medical ethics be conceptualized as applied theory rather than as reflective practice (Baier 1985; Kass 1990)?

In addition, a serious discrepancy may exist between the public's attention to moral questions, the actual impact of ethical analysis on the routine practices of medicine, and the current direction of medicine's development. Moral issues tend to appear every day, but how successfully do bioethicists address these novel issues? To be sure, the media reflect a constant fascination with the myriad of moral problems in health care, but what concrete effect do these debates have on physicians' decisions in daily clinical medicine, on nursing practice, and on public health policies? Arguably, such "discrepancies" result from the very conception of medical ethics in our time (ten Have and Kimsma 1990).

The Dominant Conception of Bioethics

During the last thirty years, a new and unique view of medical ethics as a discipline somewhat disconnected from philosophy as well as medicine has emerged. In this disconnectedness lie both its strength and its weakness.

The mainstream of scholarly literature conceives of bioethics as applied ethics. In Beauchamp and Childress's well-known textbook, bio-medical ethics is defined as "the application of general ethical theories, principles, and rules to problems of therapeutic practice, health care delivery, and medical and biological research" (1983:ix–x).

This conception implies the following set of interdependent presup-positions (ten Have 1990b):

1. Bioethics is application of ethical theory and ethical principles.

2. There is a body of available ethical theories, principles, and rules to be applied to a variety of practical, biomedical problems.

3. Professional ethicists have a special expertise in applying ethi-cal theories and principles, whereas non-ethicists (for example, physicians) merely provide moral problems for applied ethics.

4. Bioethics is general ethics applied to medicine. That is, the context in which these problems arise is not unique: it is not characterized by specific values that generate special problems. Indeed, the med-ical context is viewed as a practice ground for a new profession of biomedical ethicists.

5. The aim of bioethics is to proffer practical recommendations and prescriptions based on or deduced from ethical theories and principles.

This set of presuppositions to some degree clarifies why many perceive bioethics as an independent discipline. For example, some hold to the view that ethics should perform four tasks: to clarify concepts, ana-lyze and structure arguments, weigh alternatives, and advise a preferable course of action (deBeaufort and Dupuis 1988:19–20). The central con-tribution of bioethics is therefore restricted. It does not necessarily result in judgments regarding what we should do. The bioethicist only pro-vides the topography of arguments and objectifies the options. He or she acts as a disinterested and neutral observer of medical practice, who is in the best position to weigh moral alternatives.

The Dominant Conception: Critique and Alternatives

Only recently have the presuppositions underlying the prevailing con-ception of bioethics and applied ethics been critically questioned. Con-sider the following three arguments:

First, in daily medical practice, *bioethics focuses on mid-level prin-ciples* — respect for autonomy, beneficence, nonmaleficence, and justice.

Bioethicists apply these principles to dilemmas, cases, and problems encountered in the practice of health care. From a specific principle, the bioethicist derives guidelines or recommendations in order to resolve various problems. Yet no single rational criterion exists to decide which principle is overriding; no definitive scheme orders principles and guides the choice between them. As long as the principles of applied medical ethics are not integrated into some broader theoretical framework, they lead to conflicting judgments about which actions and social policies one ought to carry out.

Even if one proceeds from some articulated moral theory (for example, consequentialism or contractarianism), one cannot evade the chaos of conflicting moral judgments (B. Brody 1988). Confronting physicians and medical students with a variety of conflicting but plausible theories, applied medical ethics may give no moral guidance but, instead, reinforce the belief that whatever one does in problematic situations, some moral theory will condone it, another will condemn it (Baier 1985). Thus, the primacy of applied ethics and the deductivist model of applying general moral theories and intermediate principles can only lead to an inadequate way of conceiving the relation of ethics to medicine (Jonsen 1990). Because the dominant conception of medical ethics focuses on the application of principles, norms, and rules, it is rather loosely embedded in philosophy and lacks a more encompassing critical, theoretical perspective on its own practical activities.

Second, *the dominant conception of bioethics has developed within a particular cultural context.* The fundamental ethos of applied bioethics, its analytical framework, methodology, and language, its concerns and emphases, and its very institutionalization have been shaped by beliefs, values, and modes of thinking grounded in specific social and cultural traditions. Nowadays, the bioethics literature serves as one of the most powerful means by which to express and articulate these traditions. This literature, however, only rarely attends to or reflects upon the sociocultural value system within and through which it operates. Scholars usually assume that its principles, theories, and moral views are transcultural.

H. Tristram Engelhardt, Jr. (1986), for example, distinguishes between *two* levels of culture: that of secularized pluralistic society and that of the many particular moral communities with competing visions of the good life. Bioethics, in his opinion, should focus on the first, or societal, level, speaking across gulfs of moral discourse: it has a common neutral language, a secular moral grammar, guaranteeing a peaceable society. In fact, the most interesting task of ethics is on the first level: promoting and defending, in the context of health care, the general secular moral language of mutual respect. Critics agree that this is an important task, but it flows from a rather thin or minimalist conception of ethics (Callahan 1981). Ethics is conceptualized as procedural; it regulates social relations through peaceable negotiation. In order to speak the language of mutual respect, all other moral languages must be pacified.

But why should we abstain from our particular moral language in favor of a neutral common language? This question points to an important problem: how neutral is the common neutral language? Is Engelhardt's language itself not the specific moral language of a specific moral community? Is this language itself not the expression of a commitment to a certain "hypergood" (Taylor 1989), in particular, that demands universal and equal respect and self-determining freedom — primal values in the liberal tradition? Such questions assume that the value of mutual respect and rights to privacy are not decontextualized standards but are themselves expressions of community-bound agreements.

Only recently have we come to see that we must critically examine the sociocultural context if we are better to understand the strengths and weaknesses of this currently dominant conception of bioethics. Renée Fox (1989), for example, has shown how the political norms of liberalism and individualism characterize North American bioethics. By stressing the autonomy and rights of individuals, other significant considerations (for example, community and the common good, duties and responsibilities) have been neglected, as have critical philosophical questions concerning the value of medical progress and personal and public health in communal life. Although the philosophy of medicine in Europe seems to emphasize the social aspects of medicine and the common good over individual autonomy, the dominating conception of bioethics in the Netherlands seems quite similar to that in the U.S., where liberalism and personal autonomy are stressed.

Third, *the dominant conception of bioethics is inattentive to the particularities of the practical setting.* Moral theories and principles are necessarily abstract and therefore not relevant to the particular circumstances of actual cases, the concrete reality of clinical work, and the specific responsibilities of health care professionals. By appealing to principles, norms, or rules, applied ethics may fail to realize the importance of the concretely lived experience of health care professionals and patients. The moral agent is taken to have an abstract existence. Contemporary philosophers elaborate this point.

Ethics, according to Bernard Williams (1988), for example, does not respect the personal integrity of the concrete moral subject. It requires that the subject give up a personal point of view and exchange it for a universal and *impartial* point of view. This is, Williams argues, an absurd requirement, because the moral subject is requested to give up the very thing that constitutes his or her personal identity and integrity. The idea that knowledge of normative theories and principles can be applied to medical practice simply ignores the fact that moral concerns tend to emerge from experiences in medical settings themselves. Charles Taylor raises a similar issue in his recent work when he considers morality and identity as two sides of the same coin (Taylor 1989). To know who we are is to know to which moral sources we should appeal. The community, the particular social group to which we belong, is usually at the center of our moral experience. Even our use of ethical language depends on a shared form of life. The Wittgensteinian notion that our understanding of language is a matter of picking up practices and being inducted into a particular form of life is germane here.

In short, bioethicists should come to appreciate the actual experiences of practitioners and attend to the context in which physicians, nurses, patients, and others experience their moral lives: the roles they play, the relationships in which they participate, the expectations they have, and the values they cherish (Zaner 1988). The physician-patient relationship is not ahistorical or acultural; nor is it an abstract rational notion; persons are always persons-in-relation, members of communities immersed in a tradition, and participants in a particular culture.

From these criticisms of bioethics two conclusions may be drawn (ten Have and Kimsma 1990). One, morality is something we all participate in, and bioethics in particular is not the result of esoteric knowledge; anyone involved in the medical setting is *ipso facto* a moral participant and "expert" at least with regard to moral experience and intuitive knowledge. Two, the moral experience inherent in health care practices must be taken into account — more than the conformity of these practices with pre-existing ethical theories. From the perspective of applied medical ethics, abstracting from the reality of practices and appealing to moral principles and rules outside these practices are necessary conditions to criticizing health care practices. The problem, however, is not only how such a standpoint external to concrete practices is possible, but also whether appeals to external morality are made in vain without intimate knowledge of the morality internal to the practices in question (Jensen 1989).

Given the criticisms noted above, an alternative conception of bioethics is clearly needed — a conception that provides a more comprehensive understanding of the nature, scope, method, and application of ethics in the contemporary health care context. In other words, bioethics must reconnect with both a general philosophical standpoint and the concrete practice of medicine. Such reconnection is being explored in several promising new perspectives.

In response to the theoretical and methodological weaknesses of applied ethics, phenomenological ethics (Zaner 1988), hermeneutic ethics (Carson 1990), and narrative ethics (H. Brody 1987; Hunter 1988) have emerged. Furthermore, traditional conceptions have been revitalized, notably the new casuistry, drawing from the classical casuistic mode of moral reasoning (Jonsen and Toulmin 1988), and the virtue approach, emphasizing qualities of character in both individuals and communities (Drane 1988). These approaches are examined in this volume.

The recently appreciated relevance of the *social and cultural matrix* in which bioethics operates has generated still other approaches. For example, Callahan (1990) has argued that the ethical problems generated by the need for health care resource allocation and for the formation of new health policy have forced us to explore the goals and ideals of medicine as well as the meaning of health in modern society. Nevertheless, thoughtful empirical research into the value systems relevant to the formation of moral issues in health care is relatively rare. For example, data acquired from sociological value research as well as the methodological approaches of social scientists (for example, Halman et al., 1987; Inglehart 1990) are virtually unknown and therefore ignored in U.S. bioethics. The rigid distinction between descriptive and normative ethics could, in part, account for the absence of empirical value studies in bioethics. Only recently, however, are there signs that a more positive interaction between bioethics and the social sciences can be achieved (Weisz 1990).

A recent conception of bioethics (especially in the United States) is *clinical ethics*, though it is not influential in the Netherlands. It has emerged in response to the criticism that applied ethics is too far removed from the realities of medical practice. Clinical ethics aims to reorient medical ethics within the daily health care setting (Jonsen, Siegler, and Winslade 1986). It differs from the prevailing conception of applied ethics in the following ways:

First, at the basis of clinical ethics is the interdependence of technical and normative dimensions of medical judgment. This interdependence is repeatedly underlined by recent work in philosophy of medicine. Clinical medicine, the argument goes, is intrinsically a moral enterprise because it presumes a healing relationship between physician and patient. Since value judgments pervade clinical decisions, moral concerns are inseparable from certain technical concerns, for example, the correct diagnosis and the most effective treatment.

Second, clinical ethics relies on an insider perspective. The ethical problems that arise in the practice of surgery, this argument goes, are not identical to those that arise in pediatrics, obstetrics, or gynecology. Moreover, they are not of the same nature "medically," because they differ with respect to risks and benefits. Only insiders, then, can determine whether risks, in routine investigations, are low, or whether they are substantial with questionable benefits. Thus the insider can frame the ethical questions that arise in clinical encounters and can acquire empirical data relating to these questions: How do patients and physicians actually make decisions? What moral options are involved? What are the effects of personal and professional values in reaching clinical decisions?

Third, clinical ethics uses the method of induction. Instead of applying general theories and principles to practical moral dilemmas, some assert, bioethicists should begin with a careful analysis of specific empirical conditions (the inductive method). This view partly accounts for the renewed interest in classical casuistry (Jonsen and Toulmin 1988). The casuistical method includes the search for paradigm cases in which a particular moral maxim for right action is clearly applicable. Analogies are then proposed regarding cases in which, because of different circumstances, other moral maxims appear less suitable. The casuist explores a range of cases and scenarios and forms a series of plausible arguments. Thus the factual circumstances of a case are extremely relevant: as one modifies them, one gains new insights. The casuist's task is to determine the degree to which relevant moral maxims "fit" the particular circumstances. Even more: the casuist seeks to determine which factors, personal preferences, and social conditions and values are relevant enough to be judged as significant "moral facts."

In sum, clinical ethics is an inherent function of medicine itself. When physicians consider ethics as intrinsic to their craft, then the ethical analyses of medical decisions cannot proceed from an externally imposed system but are an inherent, second-order function of clinical medicine itself.

A limited conception of ethics presently dominates U.S. bioethics — the *application* of moral theories and principles to cases. This conception depreciates the fundamental internal morality of the professional practice of medicine by stressing external morality. This conception also reveals a lack of interest in the empirical realities of clinical medicine and neglects the sociocultural value-contexts in which medical care is provided. Clearly, a broader philosophical framework is needed.

European Approaches to Medical Ethics

It is problematic to identify typically European perspectives to medical ethics. Heterogeneous philosophical ideas and theories rule the Continent (postmodernism, hermeneutics, critical theory, to name a few) without any major dominating school. The same is true for ethics. Although in some European countries — for example, the Netherlands — the principles approach is influential, the range of approaches to medical ethics in Europe seems broader than in the U.S. In many countries, ethics is very much under the influence of philosophical and theological traditions and is not dominated by analytical philosophy. Only in a very few countries, such as the United Kingdom, the Netherlands, and the Nordic countries, is medical ethics the specialized enterprise of a new profession; most often it is the recognized business of medical practitioners, who therefore dominate public debate. This is, presumably, one of the reasons that the term *bioethics* is not as frequently used in Europe as is *medical ethics* or *health care ethics*.

In Europe, *bioethics* often is identified not with a discipline of moral philosophy but with a specific approach to moral problems. Sometimes the label carries negative connotations, as when bioethicists (not medical ethicists) have been accused of facilitating medical technologies that soften moral resistance to biomedical and biotechnological innovations. For example, one can argue that moral intuitions about the intrinsic dignity of human embryos do not in general favor the instrumental use of embryos for research; in order to undermine intuitive opposition to embryo research, bioethicists have introduced, according to this argument, the new terminology of "pre-embryo" and new conceptions of personhood, thus connecting moral status and human development. These arguments must be evaluated against the background of recent events in Germany. In 1988 and 1989, Peter Singer was invited to lecture on the subject of euthanasia for severely disabled newborn infants in Germany, but the invitation was canceled. When Singer was trying to lecture at another university, protesters made it impossible for him to speak. A broad coalition of left- and right-wing groups did not want issues like euthanasia and the right to life of handicapped people to be discussed in Germany (Singer 1990). Since then, other activities against bioethics have taken place, for example, the canceling of the annual conference of the European Society for Philosophy of Medicine and Health Care in Bochum in 1990 and the International Wittgenstein Symposium in Kirchberg in 1991, and the disruption of courses on practical ethics in several German universities. For the protesters, bioethics is an imported product that supports the U.S. medical-industrial complex.

Other European countries have not generated such a radical opposition to bioethics. But one does notice a growing awareness that the dominant conception of U.S. bioethics, though in a sense very effective in education and public debate, is lacking in certain fundamental aspects. If a difference exists between the medical ethics literature of Europe and North America, it is that European authors put more emphasis on (1) the historical perspective on ethical issues, (2) the sociocultural context, (3) substantive normative viewpoints, and (4) a philosophical approach to moral problems.

The Historical Perspective

Present-day European interest in medical ethics is the latest phase in a tradition of theoretical reflection upon medicine. In the thematic development of a European philosophy of medicine over the last hundred years, three phases can be distinguished: epistemological, anthropological, and ethical (ten Have 1990c). It is remarkable that from 1870 a rapid growth of medico-philosophical literature has occurred, particularly in Germany, France, and Poland. Initially, the identity of modern medicine was described in epistemological terms: medicine was characterized as a natural science. In this scientific conception of medicine, the artistic element, the art of medicine, was eliminated. At the same time, the unity and coherence of medicine were endangered through the successes of the scientific approach. In the philosophical literature, two epistemological problems were identified: first, medical knowledge was fragmented and medical practice one-sided because of specialization; second, the patient as the object of medicine was no longer adequately addressed because the conceptual tools of medicine are insufficient and too simple. Solutions to these problems have been sought by proposing more rigorous methodologies, by synthesizing medical knowledge in grand theories, and by re-interpreting medicine as an art.

The interpretation of medicine as an art evolved into a new conception of medicine as anthropological science, influential from 1930 until 1960, particularly in Germany and the Netherlands. This interpretation criticized the tendency of natural medical science to objectify the doctor-patient relationship. According to the anthropological point of view, the subject should be reintroduced into medicine: the implied acknowledgment of the subjectivity of the knowing and acting subject (the physician) also should extend to the patient. Medicine, then, is considered a unique profession in systematically and methodically attending to the patient as an irreducible person.

Since the 1960s, this anthropological orientation has been rapidly superseded by a growing interest in medical ethics. A marked continuity exists, however, between these two phases of philosophy of medicine. Through concentrating on the subjectivity of the patient, anthropological medicine paved the way for the subsequent ethical phase. It opened the moral dimension of medicine for public reflection, because it argued that medicine itself is a normative science of life.

The current preoccupation with ethical problems is, in this view, not discontinuous with earlier efforts to philosophize about medicine. In a certain way, it shares the same commitments and fundamental problems as earlier phases, although with different concepts and vocabulary. Medical ethics, therefore, is part of a long tradition of philosophical reflection in health care. What is new is the current tendency to phrase fundamental problems in the language of good or bad, right or wrong, acceptable or unacceptable. Furthermore, within the traditional philosophical view, medical ethics is not focused so much on solving problems but on clarifying their value-context, analyzing, for example, the goals of medical practice and the subjectivity or personhood of the patient. Anthropological medicine paved the way for the subsequent ethical phase.

The Sociocultural Context

Europeans tend to analyze medical ethical problems in relation to the structure and organization of the health care system in a particular country as well as in the framework of social values in which the problems present themselves. For example, moral problems concerning neonatology are related to the rise of neonatology as an independent discipline, the use of increasingly sophisticated technology, and the development of a specific ethos in its practitioners. The sociocultural context is also considered important for both the perception and the management of moral issues in medicine. In the euthanasia debate in the Netherlands, for instance, it is important not only to analyze the moral arguments for and against euthanasia but also to examine the changing attitudes toward a good death, the rapid secularization of an extensively religion-based and religiously organized society, as well as the fact that many patients have a long-standing relationship with a general practitioner who can "manage mortality" at home. Contextualism also implies that the role of individual actors is related to sociocultural conditions (and explained in reference to them). For example, although much discussion is heard about the welfare state, the basic notions of solidarity and state protection of the vulnerable are not really disputed (ten Have and Keasberry 1992). Introducing libertarian and free-market thinking into health care has in many European countries only resulted in some degree of strongly regulated competition for, in most instances, marginal services. Two examples from the Dutch context can illustrate this point. When the government announced that it wanted to introduce competitive elements in health care financing, many insurance companies merged; from initially over 200 companies, only a few dozen remain that now have divided the potential market among themselves without much competitive risk. Another example are governmental proposals to restrict the pharmaceutical budget. It was announced that only a restricted number of medicines would be fully reimbursed through health insurance. The response of the pharmaceutical industry almost annulled the effect of such proposals. (Although in the Netherlands the use of medicines is almost the lowest in Western Europe [8 units per capita in 1989, compared to 49 units in France and 27 in Italy], the consumer price per unit is the highest [162 per unit, compared to 90 in Italy and 62 in France] [*Kiezen en delen* 1991].)

Substantive Ethical Issues

Although European nations are in principle as pluralistic as the U.S., an ethics that emphasizes procedures (principlism) seems less pervasive as the privileged solution to moral controversies. At least in politics, many countries have strong social-democratic and Christian-democratic traditions and share substantive normative ideas on communal relations, labor, social welfare, health care. Value research has shown that in postmodern societies there is de facto a lot of agreement and overlapping consensus concerning moral values (like tolerance, equality, solidarity) (Halman et al. 1987).

Moreover, for the most pressing problems in medical ethics, a procedural approach typical of U.S. bioethics is insufficient. How can scarce resources in health care be allocated without substantial ideas on essential or adequate care? And how can such ideas be developed without a philosophy of the kind of society we want, without a substantive conception of health and human life, without a politics of the good? An ethics of principles is too much focused on cure and technology. Such a thin conception of ethics is unsatisfactory, and a broader conception is needed, for example an ethics of care concerned with meaningful life and filial morality.

Philosophical Ethics

The dominant U.S. conception of medical ethics is loosely embedded in philosophy, thereby lacking a more encompassing critical, theoretical perspective on its own practical activities. The success of this conception flows from its applicability to practical problems (for example, in vitro fertilization, organ transplantation, or the forgoing of life-sustaining treatment) and its pragmatic concentration on elucidating and resolving these problems. Doing so, U.S. bioethics itself has been transformed into a techno-ethics, or technethics. This is a paradoxical result. Moral issues arise from an almost exclusive technological orientation to the world and a predominant scientific conceptualization of human life; we try to address these issues with a conception of ethics, itself impregnated with scientific-technical rationality. The dominant conception of medical ethics still seems very much under the spell of the Marxist formula that philosophy should change the world, not interpret it. Unfortunately, through its emphasis on pragmatism and applicability, it cannot change the world of medical science and technology, because it is too much part of it.

Connecting Internal and External Morality

The body of European literature on medical ethics seems to have a common denominator: a focus on the connection between the internal and external morality of medicine, without reducing one set of norms and values to another. It is heuristically assumed on the one hand that there are specific values, norms, and rules intrinsic to the actual practice of medical care (the "internal morality"), and on the other hand, values, norms, and rules prevailing in social, cultural, and religious traditions that function as external determinants of medicine (the "external morality"). The dominant U.S. conception of bioethics proceeds from a too strong distinction between these two sets of values, norms, and rules, as well as an overestimation of the relevancy and importance of the external morality. In order to obtain a better understanding of the interaction of both moralities, it is necessary to establish a theoretical framework that adequately takes account of the norms and values inherent in the practice of medicine but at the same time has sufficient detachment to provide a critical normative perspective on medical practice.

But how can one develop a theoretical perspective on medical ethical issues that connects philosophical reflection with the everyday realities of medical practice?

Such a perspective aims not only at elucidating specific bioethical problems but at critically examining various conceptions of bioethics that purport to deal with such problems. It should also make clear why and how such bioethical problems appear, reappear, and even disappear in medical discourse; why certain problems emerge in various health care practices and others do not; and how such problems can be discussed and even resolved during daily interactions among physicians, nurses, patients, hospital administrators, and others.

In order better to achieve the ideal relationships between the internal and external morality of medicine, at least four steps should be considered:

1. The methods of clinical ethics in different health care contexts should be examined so that the *internal morality* of these practices can be better understood. This will require both empirical research and philosophical investigations. A new theoretical perspective on bioethics can be developed only if we take certain fundamental notions of clinical ethics seriously (for example, that certain internal standards and norms govern professional medical practice) (ten Have 1990a). The reconnection of practice-internal and practice-external moralities depends on the careful examination of daily health care practices. Surely clinical ethics requires such a reorientation; yet for many practitioners, *clinical ethics* denotes only the application of ethical rules and principles to cases. That is, to them, clinical ethics simply means doing ethics in the clinical setting and thus is simply a special case of applied ethics. The disadvantages of this approach can be overcome, however, if one introduces ethical discourse directly into the clinic, thereby retaining the values and norms internal to medical practice. Clinical ethics then becomes a radically different interpretation of ethics because it takes place within the medical clinic. It is possible, therefore, to benefit from clinical ethics without reducing clinical ethics to applied ethics.

2. The *external morality* governing health care practices should be analyzed and interpreted. Making use of the results of recent social research and specific empirical investigations, this step requires the study of values, norms, and attitudes concerning medical ethical issues. To date, value studies have only occasionally examined patients' values regarding health, disease, dysfunction, disability, dying, illness prevention, and health care. These values in society need to be explored if we are to understand more fully the value context in which current bioethical debates occur.

An example of this approach would be a research project that focuses on values regarding health, disease, dying, illness prevention, and health care that are explicit or implicit in public policy documents concerning care for the chronically ill. What norms and values are reflected in public policy documents as well as actual public policy decisions for the chronically ill? Important values in this context are, for example, solidarity and justice. In the Dutch health care system, solidarity seems to imply not only that the community will take care of the ill and helpless but also that the weak will limit their claims to care when there is no longer any prospect of a meaningful life for them. The value of justice is significant as well because we seem to lack a guiding vision of how a just and good society should accommodate the special needs of its chronically ill members. In view of the growing prevalence of chronic illnesses, traditional concepts of solidarity and justice will become more problematic. The question will be how much society wants to afford to care for the chronically ill, but the issue is also how chronic suffering is valued in a particular society. Before we can gain a better understanding of the current bioethical problems in chronic health care practices, we need to explore the normative context of such practices (in social debate, in public policy decisions, and in policy documents).

3. *New theoretical perspectives* on health care practices should be created. History of medicine as well as philosophy of medicine share a growing interest in the empirical realities of medicine. The so-called empirical shift in philosophy of science some decades ago has led to new approaches, e.g., several kinds of social constructivism (ten Have and Spicker 1990). From this point of view, diagnoses, diseases, medical knowledge, and health care institutions are considered social constructions, which can be understood only in their *empirical* social and cultural context.

Philosophy, ethics, and history of medicine may thus find common ground in creating new theoretical perspectives on health care practices. Philosophy of medicine analyzes the cognitive components of health care practices: concepts, methods, and ideas. Medical ethics examines the activities and action-guides embodied in health care practices as well as the values embedded in such practices. History of medicine studies the construction and transformation of practices. In any practice (for example, surgery or psychiatry), a complex set of activities guided by shared rules, cognition, action, and normativity are inextricably linked. Focusing on the notion of *practice* as the common theoretical starting point, the interdependence of the disciplines as well as the specificity of their expertise will become apparent.

A critical evaluation of theories of medical practice is therefore necessary. The work of the Danish philosopher Uffe Juul Jensen (1987) gives a useful and interesting example of a philosophical theory of medical practice. Jensen's theory is a conceptual framework as well as a

heuristic instrument for studying the problems of modern health care —
such as those arising in the care of chronic patients — from moral, philosophical, and historical perspectives. Jensen specifically distinguishes
three kinds of practice — orientations that are woven together in the
modern health care system: the disease-oriented practice, the situation-
oriented practice, and the community-oriented practice. Obviously, a
critical analysis of Jensen's viewpoints is necessary; however, the focus
of his model for the interrelationship of knowing, acting, and valuing
in health care practices is a promising starting point for analyzing and
elucidating present-day moral problems in chronic health care.

4. A *new conception of bioethics* that illuminates and clarifies the
complex interaction between the internal and external moralities of
health care practices should be developed. As a particular domain of
philosophy, ethics proceeds from empirical knowledge, namely, moral
experience. The moral dimension of the world is first and foremost experienced. Moral experience is humanity's way of understanding itself
in moral terms (Tongeren 1988). Ethics is therefore the interpretation
and explanation of this primordial understanding. Before acting morally
we must already know, at least to some extent, what is morally desirable or right. Otherwise, we would not recognize what is appealing in a
moral sense. On the other hand, what we recognize in our experience is
typically unclear and in need of further elucidation and interpretation.

In short, we all approach the moral dimension of the world from
a set of prior understandings; they form the basis of our interest in
what at first seems odd and strange to us, requiring us continuously to
reconstruct the moral meaning of our lives. Such an interpretive perspective will help integrate the experiences disclosed in the clinical-ethical
studies, as well as utilize the insights gained from describing the value
contexts of health care practices. Additional research questions include
these: How can we clarify and interpret the meaning of the internal and
external moralities relevant to today's bioethical quandaries? How can
we better understand the interaction (or lack of interaction) between the
internal and external moralities that govern health care practices? Which
conception of bioethics most comprehensively takes this interaction into
account? To answer these questions, fundamental philosophical research
is necessary.

The data, insights, and theoretical notions obtained and analyzed in
the previous steps require integration through developing a theory of
medical practice (with emphasis on its ethical dimensions) that can illuminate and clarify the complex interaction between the internal and
external moralities of various health care practices. Criticism of principlism can help to articulate what kind of theory is needed and which

conception of bioethics is most adequate for understanding medical practice.

REFERENCES

Baier, Annette. 1985. *Postures of the Mind: Essays on Mind and Morals.* London: Methuen.

Beauchamp, Tom L., and James F. Childress. 1983. *Principles of Biomedical Ethics,* 2d ed. New York and Oxford: Oxford University Press.

Brody, Baruch A., ed. 1988. *Moral Theory and Moral Judgments in Medical Ethics.* Dordrecht: Kluwer Academic Publishers.

Brody, Howard. 1987. *Stories of Sickness.* New Haven and London: Yale University Press.

Callahan, Daniel. 1981. "Minimalist Ethics: On the Pacification of Morality." In *Ethics in Hard Times,* ed. A. L. Caplan and Daniel Callahan, 261–81. New York: Plenum Press.

———. 1990. *What Kind of Life: The Limits of Medical Progress.* New York: Simon and Schuster.

Carson, Ronald A. 1990. "Interpretive Bioethics: The Way of Discernment." *Theoretical Medicine* 11 (5):1–9.

deBeaufort, I. D., and H. M. Dupuis. 1988. *Handboek Gezondheidsethiek.* Assen/Maastricht: Van Gorcum.

Downie, Robert Silcock. 1974. *Roles and Values: An Introduction to Social Ethics.* London: Methuen.

Drane, James F. 1988. *Becoming a Good Doctor: The Place of Virtue and Character in Medical Ethics.* Kansas City: Sheed and Ward.

Engelhardt, Hugo Tristram, Jr. 1986. *The Foundations of Bioethics.* New York: Oxford University Press.

Fox, Daniel M. 1979. "The Segregation of Medical Ethics: A Problem in Modern Intellectual History." *Journal of Medicine and Philosophy* 4:81–97.

Fox, Renée C. 1989. *The Sociology of Medicine: A Participant Observer's View.* Englewood Cliffs, N.J.: Prentice-Hall.

Greaves, D. 1979. "What Is Medicine? Towards a Philosophical Approach." *Journal of Medical Ethics* 5:29–32.

Halman, L., Frank Heunks, R. de Moor, and H. Zanders. 1987. *Traditie, secularisatie en individualisering Een studie naar de waarden van de Nederlanders in een Europese context.* Tilburg: University Press.

Have, Henk ten. 1990a. *Ethiek tussen alliantie en dissidentie.* Inaugural lecture, Maastricht: University of Limburg.

———. 1990b. *Een hippocratische erfenis: ethiek in de medische praktijk.* Lochem: De Tijdstroom.

———. 1990c. "Verleden en toekomst van medische filosofie." *Scripta Medicophilosophica,* Schrift 7:5–18.

Have, H. ten, and A. van der Arend. 1985. "Philosophy of Medicine in the Netherlands." *Theoretical Medicine* 6:1–42.

Have, H. ten, and H. Keasberry. 1992. "Equity and Solidarity: The Context of Health Care Allocation in the Netherlands." *Journal of Medicine and Philosophy* 17:467–81.

Have, H. ten, and Gerrit K. Kimsma. 1990. "Changing Conceptions of Medical Ethics." In *Changing Values in Medical and Health Care Decision Making,* ed. U. J. Jensen and G. Mooney, 33–51. Chichester: John Wiley and Sons.

Have, H. ten, and Stuart F. Spicker. 1990. "Introduction." In *The Growth of Medical Knowledge,* ed. Henk ten Have, G. Kimsma, and S. F. Spicker, 1–11. Dordrecht: Kluwer Academic Publishers.

Hunter, Kathryn Montgomery. 1988. "Making a Case." *Literature and Medicine* 7:66–79.

Inglehart, Ronald. 1990. *Culture Shift in Advanced Industrial Society.* Princeton, N.J.: Princeton University Press:

Jensen, Uffe Juul. 1987. *Practice and Progress: A Theory for the Modern Health-Care System.* Oxford: Blackwell Scientific Publications.

———. 1989. "From Good Medical Practice to Best Medical Practice." *International Journal of Health Planning and Management* 4:167–80.

Jonsen, Albert R. 1990. "Practice Versus Theory." *Hastings Center Report* 20:32–34.

Jonsen, Albert R., Mark Siegler, and William J. Winslade. 1986. *Clinical Ethics: A Practical Approach to Ethical Decisions in Clinical Medicine.* 2d ed. New York: Macmillan Publishing Company.

Jonsen, Albert R., and Stephen Toulmin. 1988. *The Abuse of Casuistry.* Berkeley: University of California Press.

Kass, Leon R. 1990. "Practicing Ethics: Where's the Action?" *Hastings Center Report* 20:5–12.

Kiezen en delen. 1991. Rapport van de Commissie Keuzen in de Zorg. Den Haag.

"Medical Ethics: Should Medicine Turn the Other Cheek?" 1990. Editorial. *Lancet* (6 October): 846–47.

Singer, P. 1990. "Bioethics and Academic Freedom." *Bioethics* 4 (no. 1): 33–44.

Taylor, Charles. 1989. *Sources of the Self: The Making of Modern Identity.* Cambridge: Cambridge University Press.

Tongeren, P. van. 1988. "Ethiek en praktijk." *Filosofie & Praktijk* 9:113–27.

Vandenbroucke, J. P. 1990. "Medische ethiek en gezondheidsrecht; hinderpalen voor de verdere toename van kennis in de geneeskunde?" *Nederlands Tijdschrift voor Geneeskunde* 134:5–6.

Weisz, George, ed. 1990. *Social Science Perspectives on Medical Ethics.* Dordrecht/Boston/London: Kluwer Academic Publishers.

Williams, Bernard A. 1988. "Consequentialism and Integrity." In *Consequentialism and Its Critics,* ed. S. Scheffler, 20–50. Oxford.

Zaner, Richard M. 1988. *Ethics and the Clinical Encounter.* Englewood Cliffs, N.J.: Prentice-Hall.

~ 4 ~

COMMUNITY AND COMPASSION
A THERAVADA BUDDHIST LOOK AT PRINCIPLISM

Pinit Ratanakul

Theravada Buddhist Ethics and Moral Precepts

Theravada Buddhism, also known under the name *Hinayana*, prevails in such countries as Sri Lanka, Thailand, Burma, Cambodia, and Laos.[1] In its teaching of *nibbana*, the supreme goal of human existence, Theravada Buddhism stresses purity of the heart and other related virtues. At the same time, with its doctrine of *kamma,* the law of cause and effect, Buddhism is concerned very much with the precepts of right actions, or moral principles for dealing with what actions are right (*kusala,* or what we ought to do) and what are wrong (*akusala,* or what we ought not to do).

This mixed ethics is formulated to accommodate people who desire and have the potential to attain *nibbana* as well as those who are concerned only with good *kamma* (right actions) and who seek guidance toward the conduct most likely to produce good *kamma*. The precepts protect them as well from generating bad *kamma*, for which they would have to suffer in the future. These people are not saints (*arahan*) and do not aspire to be perfectly right (*parama kusala*). They are creatures of mixed motivations, combinations of personal strengths and weaknesses. For them, purity of heart and of motivation are moral ideals. But if doing what is right, what they ought to do in relationship to others, fully depended on the presence in them of such moral purity, few or none of their acts could ever be considered right. The precepts, then, help them distinguish right from wrong actions and guide them toward conduct most favorable to the production of good *kamma* and away from conduct that generates bad *kamma*.

In the context of *kamma*, people are considered good in the first place if they do right actions by observing the precepts, even though their motives are mixed and their hearts are not pure. Buddhism does not want us to wait until our hearts are pure to do good. Purity of heart is the Buddhist moral ideal for those who want to attain *nibbana*, to cut the bonds that tie them to the endless life cycles (*samsara*). The path to *nibbana* is the most arduous path, and only few can tread it to the end.

Thus, while teaching the heart to cleanse itself from all defilements (*kilesa*), Buddhism lays down moral precepts for deciding on right actions. Hence it is not difficult to see that Buddhism is sympathetic with principlism and its formulation of moral principles as guidelines for moral decision making in the practice of medicine. Doctors and nurses need these principles to determine right action with regard to their patients or to society in given situations.

The virtues or traits of character that seem essential to and implied by the practice of medicine (e.g., caring, compassion, sensitivity to the needs of others) either are assumed to be present in doctors and nurses to some degree or are held before them in their training as composing the model of the "good" doctor or the "good" nurse. Individuals who possess few or none of these qualities probably ought not be permitted to enter medicine in the first place, but unfortunately, there are few character tests given for admission; high scores in the hard sciences distinguish the applicants who are accepted to medical training. This may be one of the problems of modern medicine — that more emphasis is placed on scientific and technological ability and knowledge than on the human qualities of those who possess them.

These highly skilled doctors and nurses, then, need the help of structured principles and a method for decision making to determine what their concrete obligations are and what they or others ought or ought not to do in specific sets of circumstances. Even "good" doctors, those who have morally good attitudes, dispositions, motives, and overall character, do not know intuitively how to decide complex moral questions. Rational structures help people of good will come to wise decisions and reach consensus. We usually expect that doctors and nurses who are conscientious, compassionate, and trustworthy will perceive what is morally right to do and do it. But this is often not the case. From experience we know that good people sometimes fail to perceive what is right to do in a given situation, and they are often the first to recognize that they face a moral dilemma, a conflict in which they do not know what to do. To have standards and principles that help decide right actions remains therefore indispensable to doctors and nurses whether they are "good" or not.

Moral Principles and Virtuous Life

Though Buddhists have some reservations about principlism, which I discuss below, they agree with the central place given to principles or rules of conduct. Buddhists recognize the recent concern for cultivating virtues in doctors, nurses, and members of other professions. But they also realize that virtues cannot be commanded. They are acquired from childhood on, as a matter of learning, encouragement, and habit formation, and through the observation of admired and respected adults. Religion can also motivate one to possess them. But virtues cannot be taught as an academic discipline. In an academic setting, one can only hold up the qualities that are considered admirable as personal ideals to encourage individuals to nurture and cultivate them in themselves in order to become better people and therefore better doctors and nurses.

From a Buddhist viewpoint, the concern with moral principles is an initial step toward the cultivation of virtues in doctors and nurses. For there is a correlation among virtues, duties, and the observance of these principles. Doctors and nurses, for example, have a duty to observe the principle of veracity in their relationships to patients. This principle recognizes the moral value of honesty and the virtue of trustworthiness, so we can ask doctors and nurses to cultivate these qualities and have the strength of character to manifest them. The Buddhists thus agree with Beauchamp and Childress (1979:235) that "specifically, for medical practice, the important virtues are correlated with the duties and ideals of the profession. Virtues are settled habits and dispositions to do what we ought to do" to fulfill our professional obligations. Doctors and nurses will be valued members of their profession the more they make the effort to observe precepts or moral principles and have the desire to cultivate certain relevant virtues. Regular observance of the precepts will color all their associations with other people and help build a consistently moral character.

Autonomy and Individual Rights

The basis of Theravada Buddhist ethics is the concept of *kamma,* which places responsibility for conduct on the individual. In the Buddhist perspective, the individual is the sum of his or her own *kamma* (cause-effect) and the architect of his or her own life. He reaps what he has already sown. Her destiny is not predetermined but depends on her own decisions and choices. Even in the givens of life, the effects of *kamma* — for example, being born as male or female, of certain parentage, of a particular country, culture, religion, and time in history — the person is free to accept or reject, to give new meanings and values, to what has been given. In the light of *kamma* the individual is both unique and autonomous. Uniqueness derives from one's *kamma*, which differentiates him or her from others in all the givens of life including intellectual ability and moral character.

The autonomy of the individual, in Buddhist thought, consists mainly of the ability to make one's own decision, to plan one's life according to one's own perception of what is good and right. Buddhism recognizes the value and the importance of social life, but it also points out that in the end, we all have to strive individually and reach the goal individually. Beyond a certain point, no one can help us. Even the Buddha can only show the Way — he cannot tread it for us. As a result, Theravada Buddhist ethics expresses a strong faith in the individual and a high regard for individual differences.

In this respect also, then, Buddhists would be in sympathy with principlism for the importance it places on the autonomy of the individual. They, however, have strong objection to the way principlism isolates the individual from the social context. Such separation, they believe, reflects the dominant American cultural mentality of individualism. This cultural commitment is philosophically and historically based on the assumption that inalienable "rights," possessed by all individuals from birth, exist antecedent to the establishment of any social organization. Within this cultural orientation, "good" is a matter more of personal than of collective concern. Even the collective good might have to be compromised to protect and preserve individual rights. This strong cultural commitment to individual autonomy has influenced not only biomedical ethics in the United States but also other aspects and institutions of American culture (see Ward 1974).

By firmly embedding in itself this cultural value of individualism, principlism has oriented U.S. biomedical ethics to the well-being and welfare of the individual at the cost of the welfare of others, or the public good. In such ethics, moral issues are discussed primarily in relation to the individual and his or her rights. The right to health care, for example, is individualistically understood as one of private "entitlement" and claimed without due attention to the social context, communal need, and the common good of society as a whole. Such orientation, in the Buddhist perspective, is unhealthy because it has put U.S. biomedical ethics in danger of slipping into egoism.[2]

The Individual and Conditionality

Theravada Buddhist ethics is individualistic, because its final aim is the perfection of the individual. But it is not an egoistic ethics, for such perfection, which consists in perfect beauty, perfect wisdom, perfect goodness, and perfect freedom, is used as a means of serving others. True morality demands not only that we consecrate ourselves to others but also that we fully develop our own power for the benefit of such consecration. Selfishness does not consist in elevating the intrinsic and social worth of oneself but in ignoring or denying the rights, claims, and worth of others. Although the Buddhist goal is an individual one, not a collective one, it is permeated with selflessness, for to have attained perfection means to have destroyed selfhood and egoism. Besides, while endeavoring to tread the path to *nibbana*, one perfects oneself by the observance of precepts and by the practice of compassion. Without compassion and altruism, the perfection of *nibbana* is inaccessible.

Theravada Buddhist ethics therefore is not preoccupied with egoism or individual rights but is concerned very much with virtues and precepts of right action. The concept of the inalienable "right" or "rights" that originated in the liberal democratic reformist philosophies of the West is absent from Buddhist ethical thinking and moral codes. For Buddhists, the medical ethics of principlism would be less egoistic if its concept of the autonomy of the individual were modified by the Buddhist concept of conditionality (*paticca-samuppada*) (see Mahathera 1986). This concept affirms interrelational existence, or the connectedness of all phenomena at both the macrocosmic and individual levels. Within this concept, the individual consists of the physical and psychological elements that are intimately linked to form the overall human system and personhood, which should not be segmented into separate parts. This personal identity is also linked to social relations. In other words, the individual does not exist in isolation; rather, one exists in social contexts and interrelationships — for example, as a member of a family, a society, or a religious group with its own particular values, customs, traditions, and religious life. One's worth as an individual is partially tied to the relationship one has with others. In such relationships, duties and obligations are appreciated more than individual rights.

The emphasis on the conditionality of the individual does not mean that the Buddhists would want U.S. principlism to give up its concept of the autonomy of the unique individual by replacing it with the Marxist conception of the collective self or with the ideology of authoritarianism. Theravada Buddhist ethics itself is individualistic in its affirmation of the autonomy and integrity of the individual, but this ethics is also social-istic. It does not emphasize the importance and value of the individual at the cost of a concern for the common good. Through its concept of conditionality, Buddhism places the individual in relation to others and the community as well as the whole social and cultural environment.

To prevent biomedical ethics from making the ego-assertive instinct grandiose, a Buddhist would say, principlism must tone down its indi-vidualistic elements, for example, by adopting the Buddhist concept of conditionality to curtail individual rights and to address moral issues more in terms of social relations. Such values as human rights and in-formed consent, for example, should be interpreted in a much larger context involving the community or the public. The public as a whole, not merely isolated as individuals, has the right to be informed about issues relevant to its own welfare. Similarly, informed consent should be enlarged from the setting of two individuals meeting face-to-face; it needs to become an interaction between the profession and the pub-lic. The public has the right to know about biomedical research, about what the scientists are doing in their laboratories. Such information is necessary for its consent. Because the concept of the autonomy of the individual is firmly rooted in American culture, however, it remains to be seen how much this value can be modified. Such modification, if it does occur, will have far-ranging effects on U.S. biomedical ethics and the health care delivery system.

Buddhism and principlism do not conflict on the values of nonmalef-icence, beneficence, and justice in dealing with complex ethical issues in medicine. Buddhism, however, points out that all these moral values are superseded by compassion, which embraces and transcends them. What the Buddhists call compassion is neither a sentiment nor an emotion, neither an emotional identification with the suffering of others nor the agonized, vicarious bearing of the world's suffering in one's own self. Rather, it radiates from the mind as a result of knowledge — the real-ization of the selflessness of all beings and the consequent, fundamental equality of all beings with one another.

All beings are vulnerable to pains and sufferings and desire likewise to avoid them to attain happiness. Compassion means, in the first place, our desire to enhance the health of individual patients and alleviate their suffering as best we can, not because they are this or that kind of per-son but simply because they are human and therefore vulnerable to pain and suffering. Compassion implies not only an amount of self-sacrifice but also a feeling of gladness arising from helping those in need. With such recognition of the human condition we can provide loving care to patients effortlessly and in a way that acknowledges them as whole persons with emotional, psychological, mental, and spiritual, as well as physical, dimensions. This loving care also involves protecting them and preventing harm to them.

The moral ideal of compassion should be given a central place in biomedical ethics for two reasons. First, compassion is the motive most frequently given for entering medicine, for becoming a doctor or a nurse. This motive involves a special concern for the evident suffering of fellow human beings — the suffering and pain of illness, disability, and defect that can lead to death — and a desire to cure people and relieve their suffering. Second, human compassion is most called for where people are the most vulnerable to pain and suffering — in infancy, in early childhood, in sickness, in disability, and near death. In these conditions, people are least able to act for themselves. They rely on, are dependent upon, are really at the mercy of other human beings to help them and care for them. Without the active concern and efforts of others, people so vulnerable cannot survive or can live only a minimal existence. Compassion, then, has a special application in the field of medicine. Without those who have compassion, without those who hold this moral ideal before them as the motive of their professional activity, the most vulnerable of our human brothers and sisters are threatened even more.

Buddhists agree that the principle of justice is a valuable moral principle in medicine. Justice, for Buddhists, means to render to each what is his or her due. It obligates us to treat individual patients as fellow human beings, as full persons on the basis of their common humanity. Buddhists commend principlism for its concern with distributive justice, a principle that would enable all people to have a fair share in the health care resources provided by society. This equal access and opportunity are worth striving for, particularly to reduce the gap between the "haves" and the "have-nots" in the community. From the Buddhist viewpoint, the effort to eradicate this gap is good because it represents a good volition that will bear fruit in the future, not because of any possibility of its succeeding completely. But this socioeconomic gap reflects the selfishness of human nature, and it will disappear only when that nature is transformed. All improvement must come from within, for we are the creators of our world. Even the conditioning it imposes is ultimately traceable to us. If the wealth of the world were to be equally distributed one morning, there would be the rich and the poor by that evening. We will have equality only when all *kamma* — that is, the past and present thoughts and deeds of all — are equal. And when can that be? Being in such a state would obligate us to treat individual patients as fellow human beings, as full persons on the basis of their common humanity.

The principle of justice, therefore, should be superseded by the principle of compassion, which embraces and goes beyond it, and therefore beyond equality and human rights. Compassion is self-giving and self-denial — the voluntary sacrifice of one's rights beyond what is socially obligated. Compassion demands that we give up claims to which we have an unquestionable right so that we will not cause harm to others. Compassion also requires us to overlook our personal injuries and refrain from taking revenge when such opportunity is present. When a patient voluntarily refuses medical treatment or gives up his or her right to health care — even if such sacrifice may lead to death — so that another can be treated or so that his or her family does not suffer, this is an act of compassion. When a doctor or nurse stays with a patient who needs him or her night and day, forgoing rest and family, this also is an act of compassion. If a doctor or a nurse chooses to work among the rural poor, forgoing her or his high income and social status to spend her or his life with those in dire need, voluntarily and without reward, this is an act of compassion. In each case, the person assumes a burden that she or he is not socially obligated to take. To pursue the principle of compassion is to transcend the language of justice and individual rights. It is to be unconcerned for whether one is getting what one deserves, being treated fairly, or securing one's rightful claims on others.

As we face the challenges of high-tech medicine and the unwholesome tendencies of dehumanization in medical care, we see an urgent need for a shift in the paradigm of biomedical ethics: compassion must become an ethical imperative. In the words of the Metta Sutta:

Sabbe Satta Sukhita Hontu (May all living beings be happy.)

Sabbe Satta Avera Hontu (May all living beings be free from enmity.)

Sabbe Satta Abyapajjha Hontu (May all living beings be free from affliction.)

Sabbe Satta Anigha Hontu (May all living beings be free from trouble.)

Sabbe Satta Sukhi Attanam Pariharantu (May all living beings care for themselves with ease.)

NOTES

1. Around 110 years after the Buddha's death, a second Buddhist meeting, known as the Second Council, took place, and resulted in the schism of the Order into two factions — the Theravada, or "Teaching of the Elders," and the Mahasanghika, or "Member of the Great Order."

2. Sociologist Robert N. Bellah and his colleagues call this affirmation of self-centeredness in the name of individual rights "rampant individual utilitarianism" (Bellah et al. 1985). See also Callahan 1981.

REFERENCES

Beauchamp, Tom L., and James F. Childress. 1979. *Principles of Biomedical Ethics*. New York and Oxford: Oxford University Press.

Bellah, Robert N., et al. 1985. *Habits of the Heart*. New York: Harper and Row.

Callahan, Daniel. 1981. "Minimalist Ethics: On the Pacification of Morality." In *Ethics in Hard Times*, ed. Arthur L. Caplan and Daniel Callahan, 261–81. New York: Plenum Press.

Mahathera, Ledi Sayadaw. 1986. *The Buddhist Philosophy of Relations*. Kandy: Buddhist Publication Society.

Ward, John William. 1974. "Individualism: Ideology or Utopia?" *Hastings Center Studies* 2, no. 3 (September): 11–22.

~ 5 ~

Bioethics in a Liberationist Key

Márcio Fabri dos Anjos

By and large, bioethics in the United States is concerned with the problems raised by high-cost and high-tech medicine and experimentation. Other issues, however, await the attention of bioethics, issues that affect a vast proportion of the world's population who live and die far from the resources of sophisticated medical techniques. Against this backdrop, I want to introduce the question of the poor: what chance do poor people have of seeing their problems dealt with by bioethics? Once raised, this question immediately takes on a methodological coloring: how does one go about doing bioethics immersed in the world as it is lived in and perceived by the poor? How does one at least include on the agenda a treatment of their problems? Are these problems of interest to bioethics?

My intention is to offer a Latin American perspective on these questions. The enormous contrasts between rich and poor undoubtedly provoke the development of such a perspective. It is necessary to recognize, however, that a treatment of bioethics in a liberationist key, in Latin America, is as yet but sketchy. Broad methodological principles can be found that apply to bioethics, but it is much more difficult to locate studies that take this broad approach systematically. Thus the embryonic state of bioethical reflection in Latin America leads me to be cautious in treating the theme at hand.

Still, we can describe the general shape of a bioethics elaborated in a liberation key. One characteristic of the liberationist methodology is its propensity to bring into close relationship theory and practice. In that spirit, I have taken lived experience in Latin America as the backdrop for my reflection, a move that should not be construed as a desire to project our problems uncritically into the North American bio-ethical scene. Rather, it should be seen as a demonstration of an applied methodology that may help, at least indirectly, in the rethinking of U.S. bioethics.

Furthermore, I am working within the context of an effort in Latin America to develop a particular Christian, theological vision. The relevance of theology's contribution to bioethics, I believe, goes beyond any sectarian interest. At the same time, I recognize the legitimacy of other convictions and the richness that dialogue with them brings.

Basic Inspiration

A suitable starting point for outlining a vision of bioethics in a liberationist key is its basic inspiration. Inspiration? For a long time, the sciences have assumed principles without considering themselves obliged to prove them. Currently, many authors alert us to the nonneutrality of the sciences and point to the world of convictions that constitute the *credo* presiding over every one of them.[1] It is what lies behind these convictions that we refer to as *inspiration*.

Bioethics finds its fundamental inspiration in seeking answers to some of the basic questions about human life and its end, the deeper meaning of suffering and death, and the rationality of human relationships in these circumstances. The answers that one gives to these questions determine the various models of bioethical practice. Therefore, not just religious interests are at stake. Facing the question of the fundamental inspiration of bioethics carries a requirement for safeguarding its academic seriousness. These remarks not only indicate areas in which theology can legitimately contribute to bioethics, but also make clear the wealth of cultural and scientific dialogue to be explored in the attempt to answer these basic questions.

Let us first consider several ideas that have inspired a liberationist bioethics and then look at some practical consequences that can be drawn from them.

Life as a Gift

The affirmation that human life is a gift rings ironic when one considers the bitter experience of death and the various forms in which life is denied in Latin America. It is not even necessary to have recourse to history, recalling the genocide of indigenous peoples and the violence of slavery, to illustrate this. Even today, in many places in Latin America life expectancy barely reaches the fifty-year mark, and the mortality rate for children between the ages of one and five is above 10 percent per year.[2] The drama of this experience of death is heightened when we see it legitimized by some as being *the will of God*.

Christian theology nonetheless affirms that God is the God of life and not of death. Life is a *gift* that we receive and is intended to be shared and developed responsibly. We receive life from God, and by God's power we transmit it. Implicit in this clearly religious affirmation is the recognition that we do not wish to suffer and die.

Another statement, which complements the previous one, is that God is Father and that makes all of us brothers and sisters. This affirmation commits us, on the one hand, to affirm the basic equality of all human life as a foundational ethical principle, and, on the other, to recognize a responsibility that unites us in a mutual promotion and defense of life, without appeal to privileges or discrimination against individuals or groups. In practical terms, statements about God are, in this context, ethical proposals for the governance of our vital relationships: be committed to one another in the search for life and in the overcoming of death; because we have God as a common "father," we should treat each other as brother and sister; and because we experience "God as the God of Life," this should impel us to overcome the processes that generate death (Gutiérrez 1989).

The Reality of Death

It would be naive to attempt a reflection on life without any reference to death. The harsh reality of violent death immediately shatters any such romanticism. Within the Christian perspective, life and death are not to be understood as two single-sense, mutually exclusive concepts. The notion of the transcendence of justice, for example, permeates the concept of life. If this were not so, death in any form, but particularly the death of the poor person who has suffered injustice, would be unredeemably absurd. By means of the concept of transcendence, death is transposed into an ethical key. It is total death only for the one who produces it unjustly.[3]

For the Christian, death and suffering negate life to the extent that they proceed from injustice, which is understood as any violation of the fundamental rule that the other is brother or sister. Grounded in such a rule, liberationist bioethics presupposes a critical reading of sickness, of suffering, and of death; it examines not only their *biological* but also their *ethical* roots. Expressions of this injustice are the *lack of commitment* that ignores or excludes people; *violence* that inflicts suffering and death; *dominion* that simply uses human beings, exploiting the life-force within them. The principal enemy faced by bioethics is thus not simply death but *premature death* and *suffering* as the *fruits of injustice.*

In a certain sense death has its own place on the horizon of life, as have also sickness and suffering. First, inasmuch as we all suffer and die, we can feel the solidarity with others by which human life is woven. Second, in death and suffering we are pointed to the places where human life reaches its limits. In the first case, the end of one person's life generates life for another. In the second case, the end of a life forces us to confront that critical moment in which we must re-elaborate the sense of our own lives. These moments allow us to comprehend pain and death as profound experiences of life and not simply as evils to be avoided at all costs. Such a broadened horizon of meaning raises pointed questions for a bioethics that confines itself to the challenges of killing pain and keeping death at bay.

A Consciousness of the "Other"

A consciousness of the "other" is a third notion that inspires bioethics in a liberationist key. The "other," leaving aside for the moment the question of the transcendence of God, is our fellow human being, and the faith dimension allows us to perceive the other as brother or sister. Solidarity with those who suffer, who are sick or close to death follows. By means of this first step, one breaks with the individualism that allows one to act as if one's own interests were the only interests. We make ourselves capable of seeing the other with the eyes of the heart.

This faith dimension of consciousness is complemented by a *critical* dimension of consciousness of the other. In this critical dimension, consciousness awakens, in the most scientific way possible, to the situation in which the other is found; one is aware of how that other is being treated and of what needs must be met if he or she is to be treated truly as brother or sister. This double consciousness constantly returns to concrete experience as a starting point for the elaboration of ethics. It also frees ethical reflection from the temptation of making faith a hiding place for lack of commitment or a pretext for exploiting one's fellow.

Gratitude

From a Christian perspective, an ethical consciousness would be incomplete and even incorrect if gratitude were lacking. In our very existence we carry the marks of gratuity: no one is born or grows up without the intervention of others. Thus life is affirmed not merely as a gift from God to the individual to do with as he or she would wish. Life is also a gift that one weaves in solidarity with others in a circulating gratitude that builds life, even if, in the process, one passes through suffering and death. This perception lies behind the great synthesis made by the Christian faith in its passage through the violent death and resurrection of Jesus.

Derived from this perception is a concept of justice that is important for a liberationist bioethics. We are used to understanding justice as *distributive equity*, and that is undoubtedly one of its fundamental meanings. But experience of the God of life, the Father of all, shows that "justice alone does not have the last word" (Gutiérrez 1987:142). The fundamental discovery is the gratuity that we learn from the very affirmation of life as a gift of God. To exclude gratuity would be to undermine the ground on which we walk.[4]

This perspective opens up an alternative path for bioethics, precisely when society in general seems to be accepting competitiveness as the rule of the game of life, leaving behind the "vanquished." It questions not only the legitimacy of lack of commitment to the life of the other but also the mentality of those who are content with strictly legal relationships.

A Vision of Liberation

Because the vision that coheres around the concepts of justice, solidarity, and gratuity seems unrealizable, many of the poor and marginalized abandon their hopes, pragmatically bending before the demands of individualism. One aspiration, therefore, is important in any discussion of bioethics in a liberationist key. It is the aspiration to *liberate bioethics* itself,[5] so that it may avoid being merely a legitimizer of practices that fail to promote commitment between people and avoid being a bioethics that serves the currently dominant social system, without any capacity for criticizing it.

Bioethics inspired by the desire for liberation takes as its task not only the eminently practical challenge of discerning ethical norms for action in the medical field, but also a more theoretical reflection on the general values that are the basis for human solidarity. Such reflection involves a serious critique of human relationships as they exist and the development of new forms of human relationship capable of transforming the exploitation, discrimination, and individualism. Without this reflection and transformation, the poor and excluded are not likely to find their place in bioethical reflection, and what is produced is not likely to be a liberationist bioethics.

The Challenges that Practice Poses for Theoretical Reflection

A close relationship between theory and practice characterizes the method used by those who share in the liberationist vision, and reflection on experience is a critical and obligatory moment in the reflective process. The concepts described above point bioethics in a direction that is unsettling on both the theoretical and the practical level.

It is important to study the implications of these concepts for the methodology of bioethics. First, though, I wish to focus on the practices that challenge bioethics as theory elaborated from a liberationist perspective: from what, and starting from where, does one liberate?

The Challenge of Concrete Practices

The way we treat human life in practice is the basic point of departure and the raw material for our reflection. When we do bioethics, the vantage point from which we initiate reflection affects the quality of our reflection. It is one thing to do bioethics in the tranquility and relative isolation of a university study; it is quite another to elaborate one's thoughts within earshot of the cries of the suffering sick in a Rio de Janeiro *favela*.

For a liberationist bioethics, our *locus, our vantage point*, is not simply a matter of geography. It has to do with our network of social relationships, the people to whom we attribute importance, the necessities or problems to which we give priority. It signifies at once the point from which we gaze and the perspective with which we "read" and interpret our experience and project possible lines of action.

The perspective adopted normally points toward a community that nourishes our options and our practices. For example, a Latin American liberationist is rooted in a community of persons who develop a preferential solidarity with those who are impoverished and marginalized by society. Hearing cries of suffering in the midst of sickness and death, the listener is led to consider, in terms pertinent to bioethics, the root causes of the suffering and death of the poor and marginalized.

What topics emerge when we consider bioethics from a point of view that corresponds to that of the poor within our society?

1. *The degradation of life.* Despite the sophistication of medical technology, the devaluation and degradation of life is a tangible fact among those in Latin America. It is evident — to give only a few examples — in the high levels of infant mortality, in the low levels of life expectancy for adults, in the number of diseases that are endemic, in the number of accidents in the workplace. And these facts are but the tip of the iceberg. They show that the path leading to the doctor and the hospital, in our context, passes first through an acute social degeneracy. Sickness and death have their social roots in hunger, in unhealthy living conditions, in the lack of sewage systems and running water, in precarious working conditions, in the lack of education about basic health precautions, and in the lack of economic resources to put them into practice.

A few statistics help to summarize this situation. For example, the percentage of the population (urban and rural) that subsists below the level of absolute poverty is 46 and 83 percent in Peru; 40 and 65 percent in Ecuador; 32 and 70 percent in Colombia.[6] These figures send one back to the economic realities behind health policy options. Sickness and premature death bear all the marks of hunger and unhealthy conditions, which themselves can be linked with subemployment and low wages.[7] The social and economic policies of a nation, in their turn, depend on international political and economic systems. The sickness and premature death of the poor person in Latin America are therefore closely linked with both the foreign and domestic debt of his or her country.

The logic of the degradation of life that appears in this macrosocial scheme of things shows itself equally in the ecological problems that we face today. There is a growing conviction that these problems cannot be dealt with without concerted action from society as a whole. This complexity of social relationships within which sickness and death occur challenges bioethics to face up to one fact: the majority of viruses that the doctor scrutinizes under the microscope not only feed and develop on the biological body of the patient, but also nurture themselves in the body politic.

2. *The discrediting of folk medicine.* It is illuminating to consider the relationship between technological advances in medicine and health care and the culture of the poor. Poor people in Latin America have developed their own ways of interpreting, resisting, and facing sickness and death. Certainly exaggerated claims for their results should not be

made. On the other hand, advanced technology, while demonstrating to the poor a high level of efficiency in the medical and pharmaceutical fields, ends up discrediting the health care interpretations and resources of their culture. That in itself would not be a serious problem. The difficulty arises when, having deprived the poor of the resources provided by their folk medicine, the health care system also denies them access to the more technologically advanced forms of medicine. The poor are made culturally dependent in the area of health care, and then they are distanced and even excluded from access to its technologies by means of economic filters.

3. *The preference for curative medicine over preventive medicine.* Social health policies, on a large scale, give preferential treatment to curative medicine at the expense of preventive medicine. This is not an innocent preference. Behind it lies a string of interrelated interests. For example, hospital systems and pharmaceutical and health insurance companies, while undoubtedly providing social services, are also highly lucrative ventures. Clearly, sickness must exist so that profit can be made from it. The search for health is organized according to the demands of the market economy; paradoxically, health needs disease so it can offer itself as a "product" (Macedo 1981).

These economic realities help to explain the general lack of interest in seeking out the socially rooted causes of disease. Measures of public health more frequently indicate the lack of disease rather than the presence of health (Dallari 1987:18). More serious, however, is the fact that a lack of concern for the close relationship between health and quality of life leads to a falsification of the statistics, which fail to portray the true state of the health of the population: a pile of percentages obscures the huge inequalities in quality of life and health (Laurentie 1985). Even worse is the Malthusian cynicism that says, "Only disease and hunger are capable of controlling the South's mad demographical situation."[8]

4. *The objectification of the patient.* The most common experience for someone who falls sick is to be treated as an object, as someone to whom things are done. Further, within the hospital complex, the "patient" is isolated from the cultural and affective ties of his or her everyday world. Death in the hospital thus becomes a drama. To the extent that medicine becomes a technique for curing disease and not a science that helps treat people who are sick, those who are incurably ill or who are old become highly problematic.

5. *The dispensability of persons.* The social and interpersonal practices that characterize medicine and health care among the poor add up to a frightening pragmatism. People become dispensable. The macropolitical and economic level reflects this sense as well, where certain

Third World countries are considered "dispensable" in the international economic scheme. Technological advances have reached a point where the rest of the world can do without the labor and even the raw materials from the Third World.[9]

This logic, which is beginning to be called the "logic of dispensability," has in its own way already penetrated the hospital, with the result that the claims of certain people to health care are simply discarded. A text on liver transplants in children crudely illustrates this pragmatism. The words are of a doctor and researcher: "The queue of children waiting for a liver transplant is long, and the criteria used for discarding a candidate are variable. Automatically one eliminates, for example, a child that wouldn't have the minimum sociocultural conditions, who lives in a miserable hovel, in subhuman living conditions.... On his first day home, back in contact with poor quality sanitation, he would quite likely end up with diarrhea, for example, and the operation would have been a waste of time."[10]

The influence of social factors in these cases needs no commentary. What is certain is that ethical reflection cannot afford to ignore these data.

The Challenge of Producing an Adequate Theory of Practice

Bioethical theory is itself a form of practice, expressed concretely in the principles, systematizations, and arguments that bioethics uses and in the proposals that it produces. The question is whether the theory sheds adequate light on concrete procedures and whether it can help in the transformation of the current situation. Before treating the question of method, we should note some of the challenges involved in the liberation of bioethics itself.

Bioethics, as a discipline, has received a great deal of attention lately, especially because of the interdisciplinary way in which its fundamental concepts are treated. Certain questions, however, persist, not the least of which concern the very concept of bioethics. In the Latin American historical context, there is a strong tendency to reduce bioethics to a mere deontology for the doctor, taught as an appendix to forensic medicine and mainly concerned with defending the interests of the medical profession.

In this situation, the scope of bioethical reflection frequently is restricted to the individualist concerns of the doctor or of the patient and rarely escapes beyond the boundaries of the hospital or the laboratory; the problems attended to have their origins in intensive care units or in the use of advanced laboratory techniques. These issues are not without merit, but bioethics should not isolate itself from the real context of life and health, death and disease that goes on in the world outside the hospital walls.

For example, in an article about the tendencies of bioethics in the last twenty years, the author included an item on those who confuse bioethics with social questions (Elizari 1991:103–16). But the current patterns of thinking testify predominantly to a *disassociation* between bioethics and serious social problems. One reason for this, quite possibly, is that bioethical reflections are being elaborated by people who have no experience of these social problems. Another possible reason is the tendency to isolate the context in which one does bioethics from political and economic questions. I have critiqued these tendencies elsewhere: "In the first case we have a bioethics that is inadequate for the Third World. In the second case arises the question of how one could possibly think through a bioethics without reference to politics and economics. On the level of anthropology it would signify neglecting the political, social, and economic dimensions of the body, while on the level of the reality of the social systems in which we live, it would signify ignoring the interplay of political and economic interests which underlie the themes treated by bioethics" (Anjos 1988:219).

Thus we see that one must view bioethics more holistically if one is to avoid the danger of reducing it to an individualist vision of things. Further, it is necessary to attend to two dimensions of this holistic approach. One dimension permits us to understand the human person in the totality that constitutes his or her subjectivity. Consequently, one cannot arrive at an adequate bioethics without taking into account the horizons of meaning of human life, of suffering, of death — the horizons of the motivations and convictions that drive the subject or that may be proposed to him or her.

Second, one cannot possibly avoid the social dimension. A consideration of this dimension would start from a reflection on human solidarity as a necessary condition for the flourishing of the subjective life. In this way, bioethics rediscovers the social commitment that presides over our lives and our potentialities, concurrently being energized so that it does not become a simple legitimizer of selfish and subjective individualism.

A third and final challenge for the practice of bioethical theory arises from reflecting on these questions: For whom does one do bioethics? Who benefits? The theology of liberation alerts us to a vice that frequently occurs in ethical discourse: the tendency to legitimize ethically the status quo, with its dominant social, economic, and political system, forgetting to question whether the presuppositions of the system are anti-ethical.[11] The underlying question is whether and to what extent bioethics is capable of self-criticism so that it does not become a cluster of principles and systematizations at the exclusive service of people powerfully installed in society.

All these considerations converge to reinforce the necessity of an interdisciplinary approach to the doing of bioethics. Obviously, the social sciences which analyze society, its cultural traditions, and its structures, and the sciences of religion play an important role.

Some Methodological Principles

Here I propose some methodological principles for a bioethics conceived within a Latin American theological perspective. Of interest is not so much the religious convictions in themselves but rather their impact on the method used.

See, Judge, Act

The methodological procedure I propose includes three steps, popularly known as "see, judge, and act." This method aims at concretizing a strict relationship between theory and practice, drawing conclusions from the theoretical phase concerning the appropriate action. It seeks, at the same time, to maintain a certain dynamism by means of a circularity: new practices provoke a new way of seeing the world, which in turn provokes a revision of theory, from which derives a revision of one's practical proposals. This methodological circularity works its effect on the level of concrete practices, on the level of the practice of theory and, in our case, on the practice of theory that we call bioethics. Specifically in the case of bioethics, we can note the following.

During the *first moment* in the process, one looks at and analyzes the realities that would be a challenge in the field of bioethics. Specifically, the sciences examine the various dimensions of that reality. On the empirical level, it falls to bioethics to seek the help of the sciences that study the structures and mechanisms of the medical and health care world; on the philosophical level, to seek the aid of sciences that analyze the horizons of meaning of human life. This first moment is, therefore, one of interdisciplinary activity, during which bioethics opens itself to a broad field of concern both in terms of individuality and in terms of society. Obviously, it is not possible to investigate exhaustively all facets of this moment before taking subsequent steps. Precisely because of this limitation, however, we see the importance of the inspiration that presides over bioethics and that generates the options that we necessarily choose as we proceed with our analysis of reality. A Latin American, liberationist vision tends to lead preferentially to a search for the root causes of disease and of the suffering and death of the poor and excluded.

The *second moment*, methodologically speaking, is devoted to ethical and theological discernment. Here one confronts the options chosen during the process of analysis, and the initial conclusions to which one may have come with the criteria of faith. The spiritual faith tradition, enriched especially by biblical hermeneutics, nourishes fundamental convictions about human life in all its dimensions: historical, transcendent, individual, and communitarian. It offers criteria for choosing liberating practices as a response to the reality analyzed during the first phase.

In the *third moment,* one begins to develop practices of liberation that flow from the reflection elaborated during the first two moments. In the case of bioethics, it is a question of developing a new theory of practice that would be at the service of concrete liberating practices in the area of biomedicine.

The Question of Subjects

This liberating characteristic is made clearer if we look at some of its more constant preoccupations. The first of these preoccupations concerns the subjects of bioethics. Here, we cease giving privileged status to the social classes whose interests have tended to predominate until now, while at the same time discovering *new subjects* in the faces of the impoverished and the excluded. These new partners in dialogue even confront the more academic discourse of bioethics, at least to the extent that it (a) considers their problems and health needs, and (b) takes seriously their cultural world and their sentiments. This question concerning the subjects of bioethical discourse is indispensable if we are to liberate bioethics from a possible cynicism and hypocrisy in its choice of whom to exclude from the benefits of its service.

Microsocial, Midisocial, and Macrosocial Levels

The liberationist method is also constantly preoccupied with the extent of its social scope — with the extent and quality of the relationships between the subjects involved in the issues treated by bioethics. At times, these relationships are merely interpersonal, scarcely going beyond the interests of the individual patient or doctor. Three levels of activity are crucial in the doing of bioethics: the microsocial, the midisocial, and the macrosocial levels.

The *microsocial level* extends principally to interpersonal relationships that involve the doctor, the sick person, and his or her family. Case studies and a variety of questions raised by medical ethics frequently treat problems exclusively on this level.

The *midisocial level* refers to relationships that extend to the interests and necessities of groups, as for example, doctors as a social class, or high-risk groups, such as AIDS victims.

The *macrosocial level* focuses attention on the great social systems and political, economic, or cultural structures, with their implications for a huge variety of relationships within the field of bioethics.

I indicated above the importance of these levels when I spoke of the need to consider the impact of macropolitics and macroeconomics in bioethical practice. In general, most bioethicists agree on the importance of reflecting on the subjective and interpersonal dimensions of issues treated. But reflection on the right of a sick person to die with dignity is not the only moving concern of bioethics. Just as significant is reflection on the quality of life and on the right to health for segments of the population who are often denied this right because of their social and economic exclusion. Various types of discrimination, especially in health care, are relevant topics for bioethicists. All these dimensions, however, escape scrutiny if bioethics does not reflect upon them at an appropriate level.

The necessity to bear in mind the social dimensions of our existence leads us finally to a preoccupation with discerning, with regards to human life, the values that are *most important* and *most urgent*. This means a commitment to recognizing a strongly relational character both in health in general and in the life of the individual. The health interests of the individual need to be confronted with the interests of the general public, and vice versa.

Challenges for Bioethics Today

Several important challenges must be recognized before one attempts to elaborate bioethics in a liberationist key. In addition, it may be helpful to locate points of contact between the Latin American way of seeing things and the critical re-reading of bioethics that is under way in the United States.

Our sharp criticism of the technicalization in biomedicine should not be confused with a rejection of scientific and technological advances. Human life and its complexity constantly require some scientific decoding and some technology to give it direction. Liberation does not and cannot signify naiveté in the face of vital processes; the conquests made in the area of medical care should not be despised.

Ethical criticism of technicalization in biomedicine has other sources, however, and it is there that we find the current major challenges for bioethics: to reconsider the subjects of bioethics; to be open to new *horizons of meaning* in the field of bioethics; to recognize the importance of social context for bioethics, and to appreciate the necessity for bioethics to have its own *mystique.*

Reconsideration of New Subjects in Bioethics

The question of the subjects of bioethical discourse arises as a prerequisite for doing bioethics effectively. This question challenges us to make people and not technological casuistry the focus for reflection. It also challenges us to reflect on our situation, which is one of being in relationship with others. This means that we must be prepared to open ourselves to questions about life that come from the poor and the needy; we must overcome, as a response to this questioning, a discriminatory and selective bioethics that merely concerns itself with the problems of a particular class of people who have access to the sophisticated world of well-equipped hospitals and laboratories. Here we identify a further challenge: the need to overcome a narrow view that reduces bioethics to the professional problems of the doctor and that tends to justify the treatment of the sick person as a "patient-object." A final challenge in this context relates to a consciousness of the cultural boundaries within which one develops one's reflections, a factor that leads to respect for forms of bioethics that are found in other cultural contexts.

Facing up to this group of challenges is a complex task. No matter how close our fellow human beings may be physically, it is at times a long haul to perceive truly the other as our fellow and our equal. It is undoubtedly true that in the United States, whole groups of people are excluded from access to health care. Thus one of the challenges for U.S. bioethics is precisely to make evident and unmask the mechanisms of such inequality. As a next step, it could then examine seriously the question, for whose benefit is bioethics being done?

Recognition of the Sociopolitical Dimension

Closely linked with the question of the *subjects* is another: the question of developing a sociopolitical dimension within bioethics. Bioethics would lose its critical sense if it did not consider the wide social context in which its problems and solutions interweave with political and economic problems and options. Even admitting that epistemological objections may make the evolution of bioethics on the level of politics and economics difficult, the necessity of, at the very least, conducting bioethical reflection in dialogue with social ethics persists.

Social ethics today makes strong criticisms of the political and economic systems that currently predominate in the West. In view of this, bioethics, if its field of activity is reduced to the hospital or the laboratory, ends up being a domesticated prisoner, and the risk constantly grows that it will be co-opted by an anti-ethical system. Bioethicists must examine what is going on outside the hospital and be aware of the factors that lead people to need a doctor. The challenge, then, is to introduce into bioethics the questions that have been identified by macrosocial ethics. It is true that some studies have led bioethics to concern itself with the problem of the distribution of health care resources,[12] but the question is much broader than that, and one should look directly at the national and international relations themselves that have an impact on bioethics. Precisely on that point, even in countries like the United States, bioethics must begin to reflect on its national options, bearing in mind the quality of life of all its citizens but also the implications of its international options for the life and health of other peoples and nations.

Openness to New Horizons of Meaning

It is vitally important for bioethics to reconsider the horizon of meaning within which we understand life, suffering, and death itself. For example, in the present horizon of meaning characterizing modern medicine, we see first that technological efficiency increasingly transforms death into a dehumanizing, a lingering, and often, for the people involved, a senseless horror. Second, an emphasis on strong individualism discards the bond of solidarity between people and insists on *individual well-being* as an indispensable prerequisite for meaningful life. Within such a narrow horizon of meaning, bioethics tends to be reduced to an ethics of efficiency applied predominantly on the individual level. This is surely an important limitation to overcome.

The opening up to new horizons of meaning challenges us to recover elements of our humanistic heritage, for example, a sense of the transcendence of life. Such a sense can confer on suffering and on death itself a meaning that embraces a life shared and transformed. Intercultural dialogue can reveal these new horizons with a certain facility, and undoubtedly the same can occur in dialogue with theology. As a science, theology has among its principal tasks precisely that of reflecting on and systematizing the questions and answers concerning the meaning of our lives.

The Challenge of Evolving a Mystique for Bioethics

It may seem strange to a way of thinking marked by pragmatism and the cult of efficiency to suggest that bioethics needs a *mystique*. In a liberationist vision of things, however, there is no way of escaping from this proposal. Bioethics needs a horizon of meaning, no matter how narrow it may be, in order to develop its reflections and its proposals. At the same time, one cannot do bioethics without selecting a series of options within the world of human relationships. That in itself is an indication of the need for some form of *mystique* or set of fundamental meanings that we accept and by means of which we cultivate our idealisms, weave our options, and organize our concrete practices.

It is not possible to define in a few words a liberationist *mystique* for bioethics. It would, however, include a conviction of the transcendence of life that rejects the notion that sickness, suffering, and death are unbearable absolutes. It would also include a perception of the others as partners capable of living in solidarity and of accepting life as a gift. It would witness the central emphasis on individual interests giving way to a willingness to hear the voice of *others,* to hear the cry of the needy and the excluded. It would witness a new willingness to redefine the values, principles, and norms that constitute bioethics. It may even herald the coming of a biomedicine that explicitly accepts being ruled by the demands of human solidarity.

As I present this vision of bioethics, I am of course aware of a much greater complexity to be explored in the terms here used. Moreover, a great deal of idealism is necessary if one is to forge ahead with developing a bioethics that allies itself with so many "losers" and with so many people who are excluded from the onward march of society. At the same time, it is encouraging to know that many people and groups, in different social and cultural contexts, are making enormous efforts to guarantee a life in which all are called to share and participate.

NOTES

1. The theology of liberation exploits extensively this notion of a fundamental *credo* in its assessment of the political and economic sciences, noting in their structure a close analogy with religion. See, for example, Assman and Hinkelammert 1989.

2. UNICEF 1992.

3. There exists an extensive biblical tradition which affirms: "God did not make death, and he does not delight in the death of the living. For he created all things that they might exist, and the generative forces of the world are wholesome, and there is not destructive poison in them; and the dominion of Hades is not on earth. For righteousness is immortal" Wisdom 1:13–15 (RSV).

4. See Moser and Leers 1987:121–26.

5. This notion is borrowed from Segundo 1975.

6. UNICEF 1992:72–73.

7. The average wage of 50 percent of Latin American workers is less than 100 U.S. dollars a month. In Brazil nearly 41 percent of the workers earn between 45 and 135 U.S. dollars for a whole month's work. See Anuário Estatístico do Brasil 1990:104; also UNICEF 1992:72–73.

8. See Rufin 1991.

9. Hinkelammert 1991:1–6. The quotation is from an interview given by J. C. Rufin to *Paris Match* (15 October 1992):40.

10. "Transplante de fígado infantil: 85 percento de êxito. O trabalho do Prof. Maksoud e sua equipe," in *Prática Hospitalar* 6 (1991):9.

11. E. Dussel calls this way of elaborating ethics "intra-systemic morals." Cf. *Etica Comunitaria* 1986:43–44.

12. An early interesting article on the subject is Outka 1976:373–95.

REFERENCES

Anjos, Márcio Fabri dos. 1988. "Bioética a partir do Terceiro Mundo." In *Temas Latino-americanos de ética,* 219. Aparecida: Ed. Santuario.

Aquinas, Thomas. *Summa Theologica* I, q. I, a. 8.

Assman, Hugo, and Franz Joseph Hinkelammert. 1989. *A Idolatria do Mercado. Ensaio sobre Economia e Teologia,* 114–17. São Paulo: Ed. Vozes.

Dallari, Sueli Gandolfi. 1987. *A Saúde do Brasileiro,* 18. São Paulo: Ed. Moderna.

Dussel, Eduardo. 1986. *Etica Comunitaria.* Petropolis: Ed. Vozes.

Elizari, Javier. 1991. "Veinte Años de Bioética." In *Moralia* 13, no. 49: 103–16.

Gutiérrez, Gustavo. 1987. *Falar de Deus a partir do sofrimento do Inocente,* 142. Petropolis: Ed. Vozes.

———. 1989. *El Dios de la Vida.* Lima: CEP.

IBGE. 1990. *Anuario Estatístico do Brasil.*

Hinkelammert, Franz Joseph. 1991. "La crisis del socialismo y el tercer mundo." In *Pasos,* no. 30:1–6.

Laurentie, R. 1985. *Estatísticas de saúde.* São Paulo: EDUSP.

Macedo, Carmen Cinira. 1981. "A produção social de saúde." In *Vida Pastoral* 22:9–12.

Moser, A., and Bernadino Leers. 1987. *Teologia Moral: Impasses e alternativas,* 121–26. Petropolis: Ed. Vozes.

Prática Hospitalar. 1991. 6, no. 5:9.

Outka, Gene. 1976. "Social Justice and Equal Access to Health Care." In *Bioethics,* ed. T. A. Shannon, 373–95. New York: Paulist Press.

Rufin, J. C. 1991. *L'Empire et les nouveaux Barbares.* Paris: J. C. Lattes.

Segundo, Juan Luis. 1975. *Liberación de la teología.* Buenos Aires: Ed. Carlos Lohlé.

UNICEF. 1992. *Situação Mundial de Infância — 1992.*

~ 6 ~

European-American Ethos and Principlism
An African-American Challenge

Cheryl J. Sanders

Introduction

One of the most significant contributions thinkers of European-American descent have made to the field of bioethics is the development of a deductive approach that applies ethical theory and principles to a broad range of problems and cases. The work of Tom Beauchamp and James Childress perhaps represents the best of this line of thought, lifting up such principles as autonomy, nonmaleficence, beneficence, and justice, and rules regarding veracity, confidentiality, fidelity, and the like. Still, notably absent from their *Principles of Biomedical Ethics* (1983) is any discussion of the perspectives, writings, thought, or experience of African-Americans as theorists or participants in the American health care system. Moreover, the authors' apparent marginalization of race or religion as noteworthy factors in the thirty-five cases they cite in their book indicates a devaluation of the community and belief systems characteristic of African-American ethical discourse and social life. As a specific cultural phenomenon, principlism in bioethics seems to fall short in the effort to posit a body of knowledge that is intellectually rigorous and universally applicable cross-culturally.

A version of this essay appeared in Harley E. Flack and Edmund D. Pellegrino, eds., *African-American Perspectives on Biomedical Ethics* (Washington, D.C.: Georgetown University Press, 1992).

In the April 1989 issue of the Kennedy Institute of Ethics *Newsletter*, Harley Flack and Edmund Pellegrino presented an exploratory discussion of the importance of African-American perspectives in biomedical ethics. This brief article (1989) offers insightful reflections on data gathered during a February 1987 conference of African-American scholars, educators, health professionals, and philosophers. It suggests that African-Americans and Anglo-Americans differ significantly in their ideas about morality and ethics. It further offers a credible account of the dominant ideas of the African-American perspective on morals in terms of the greater importance ascribed to community, religion, the ethics of virtue, and personal life experiences in comparison to Western value systems. The authors called for further dialogue on the question of how these two moral systems differ in relation to biomedical ethics.

However, that article made a couple of problematic assertions that have influenced my own critical analysis of the problems and limitations of an African-American perspective on biomedical ethics. First is their explanation of the unique nature of the African-American experience, as manifested in norms such as the dominant value of community, the importance of religion and ethics of virtue, and the weight given to personal life experiences:

> Slavery, segregation, discrimination, poverty and a disadvantaged position with respect to education, health and medical care sensitize African-Americans in specific ways. These experiences evoke a more empathetic response to the social-ethical questions — justice in the distribution of resources, sensitivity to the vulnerability and dependence of the sick person, and a sense of responsibility for the poor and rejected members of society. (Flack and Pellegrino 1989:2)

While their description of the norms of the African-American perspective seems accurate enough, they seek to account for this distinctiveness in terms that seriously understate the issue. In their view, what makes the African-American experience unique is a greater empathy for social-ethical concerns. What they leave unsaid is that the social injustice, insensitivity, and irresponsibility that have created this empathy are direct manifestations of a racist Anglo-American ethos that is itself uniquely indifferent to community, religion, virtue, and personal experience. In other words, it seems absurd to speak of the unique moral context of the African-American experience of suffering without at the same time addressing the cause of this suffering in the broader moral context of European-American racism.[1]

A second problem is the call for dialogue and the parenthetical observation that "so few African-Americans are involved in scholarly work in biomedical ethics and how their number might be increased" (Flack and Pellegrino 1989:2). Again, I take issue not with what they say but rather with what they don't say. Clearly, African-Americans are engaging in biomedical ethical discourse on a daily basis, but not necessarily in ways that European-Americans would regard as scholarly or even noteworthy. Further, it may be that African-Americans have thoughtfully concluded that Western biomedical ethics is not useful or applicable to their dilemmas precisely because their data and input have not been taken into account. In other words, the dialogue being called for may have already taken place in other quarters, and the lack of scholarly work by African-Americans in the field may indicate an informed judgment that biomedical ethical discourse is an esoteric and exclusive enterprise where African-American participation is not really welcome on any level.

I don't dispute that there is a distinctive African-American ethos that has a direct bearing upon how biomedical ethics is done. But the real question is not *whether* such a perspective exists but *why* it exists and whether its continued existence is predicated upon the persistence of racist oppression of African-American people. Given the reality of racism, we must not fall into a trap and let the discussion of uniqueness divert attention from the universals, where the African-American perspective is strictly valued on the ground of uniqueness and not fully appreciated for its universal significance as a critique of the destructive inhumanity of the dominant ethos. In my opinion, the authentic dialogue begins when we realize that both perspectives are operating within one moral universe and not two, and that each brings a valid critique to bear upon the other. Both must be subjected to scrutiny by similar standards — it is as erroneous to romanticize (uncritically) African-American culture as it is to overlook the racism that is endemic to European-American culture. The point is not that the African-American ethos is unique, but that it is *characteristically human* in ways that the European-American ethos is not. I will discuss the problems and limitations of principlism in bioethics from an African-American perspective — that is, taking into account the distinctive ethos, theology, and ethics of the African-American people, with a view toward understanding how honest dialogue among African-Americans and European-Americans can move us all toward a bioethics that is truly ethical.

The African-American Ethos

Based upon my own teaching and research in the area of African-American ethical discourse, I would like to offer a list of seven features that describe the African-American ethos or lifestyle and contrast them with opposite features that characterize the European-American ethos. I am indebted to one of my former doctoral students, Fr. George Ehusani, for helping me to understand and describe distinctive features of both African and African-American cultures. Although the following characterization of the African-American ethos is my own, these and other humanistic aspects of traditional African culture are discussed in detail in Ehusani's book, *An Afro-Christian Vision: "Ozovehe!" Toward a More Humanized World* (1991), with specific reference to his own ethnic group, the Ebira of Nigeria.

First, the African-American ethos is holistic, not dualistic, emphasizing that most matters are better understood in terms of "both-and" rather than "either-or." Second, it is inclusive, not exclusive, accepting of difference rather than seeing difference as grounds for discrimination or exploitation. Third, it is communalistic, not individualistic, especially valuing family and community over the individual in moral importance. Fourth, it is spiritual, not secular, rejecting any ultimate dichotomization of the sacred and the secular and acknowledging the pervasive presence and power of the unseen realm over what is seen. Fifth, it is theistic, not agnostic or atheistic, affirming not only the existence of God but also the relevance of belief to every aspect of life. Sixth, its basic approach or method is improvisational, not forced into fixed forms, with an openness to spontaneity, flexibility, and innovation, particularly in the realm of music and art. Seventh, it is humanistic, not materialistic, valuing human life and dignity over material wealth or possessions.

These features of the African-American ethos are largely derived from traditional African cultures, yet in America as well as in Africa, this life-affirming perspective is not always strictly adhered to or applied. However, the African-American ethos, notwithstanding the many exceptions and abuses that can readily be cited, is essentially holistic, inclusive, communalistic, spiritual, theistic, improvisational, and humanistic in ways that the European-American ethos is not, though exceptions would apply there as well. Moreover, even if it is an exaggeration to say that the European-American ethos is dualistic, exclusive, individualistic, secular, atheistic, inflexible, and materialistic, these characteristics are necessary and sufficient conditions for the propagation of racism, which can be regarded as the logical consequence of a worldview that readily expends both soul and spirit in the pursuit of wealth.

The roots of the African-American ethos predate by centuries the exploitative schemes Europe brought to Africa, Asia, and the New World in the form of slavery, imperialism, and colonialism. Still its best fruits are yet to emerge if and when African-Americans can resist cultural and ethical assimilation of European-American values that have spelled death to our ancestors and our children and can persuade ourselves and others to embrace African-American values that are more humane and life affirming.

The Problem of a Black Theology

Black theology is a term first popularized some twenty years ago by James Cone, an African-American theologian who authored *Black Theology and Black Power* in 1969, followed by numerous other books and articles on the subject. It is one of several specific cultural expressions of a broader genre known as liberation theology. Liberation theologies all begin with the analysis of oppression, affirm the personhood of oppressed people, and advocate social and political change to liberate the oppressed. Black theology, in particular, analyzes the oppression of black people, affirms the personhood of black people, and advocates their social and political liberation.

In his 1984 volume *For My People: Black Theology and the Black Church*, Cone critically assesses the development of black theology during the 1960s and 1970s, with a view to influencing its direction for the 1980s and beyond. His critique includes a series of generalizations concerning the dialogue between black theology and the liberation theologies of the world, each of which has direct relevance to the problem of principlism in relation to African-American thought. First, Cone asserts that "every theology is a product of its social environment and thus in part a reflection of it" (1984:172). Thus, European-American theology, as well as philosophy, brings a unique set of collective experiences and biases to scholarly discourse, despite any disclaimers to the contrary offered (or implied) in the interest of objectivity and universalism. The same is true for black theology and philosophy, except that African-Americans can more self-consciously accept the limitations of discourse that reflects social environment. Specifically, African-Americans are more aware of the limitations of their own voices and have a heightened sensitivity to the social context of others who seek to do theology and philosophy for the whole.

The second general statement Cone makes speaks even more specifically to the problem of principlism:

> Every theology ought to move beyond its particularity to the concrete experiences of others. No theology should remain enclosed in its own narrow culture and history. That has been the awful mistake of the dominant theologies of Europe and North America. They talk about God as if Europeans are the only ones who can think, and that is why they still have difficulty taking seriously liberation theologies in Asia, Africa, and Latin America, or that of minorities in the U.S.A. (1984:173)

Third, Cone concludes that:

> Every theology needs instruments of social analysis that will help theologians define the causes of injustice. How can we participate in the liberation of the poor from poverty if its causes are not clearly understood through social analysis? Social analysis is nothing but a way of uncovering the causes of evil and exploitation. It helps us to see more clearly and thus to know the nature of the evil we are fighting against. As long as theology remains ignorant of the causes of exploitation, it will not be able to effectively fight it. (1984:174)

Here he reveals participation in the liberation of the poor as the essential agenda of black and other liberation theologies. Of course, just as no theological or philosophical consensus exists as to what constitutes justice in the society, so also it may be difficult or impossible to agree upon how evil can be discerned. In any case, for Cone, evil is measured most precisely by the suffering of the oppressed. From the vantage point of bioethics, the social manifestations of that suffering include lack of access to health care resources and the inattentiveness of the dominant society to the special health needs of minority communities.

In view of our concern here for the cultural parochialism of principlism, it must be admitted that a strictly black or African-American theological perspective could have similar limitations. If there is only one God, in whose image all human beings are made, then reflection upon the nature of God is severely restricted in any theological discourse that only takes account of the experience of one race, culture, or gender. The African-American experience may provide an appropriate starting point for theology, because all theological reflection is grounded in the particularities of race, class, gender, and culture. Indeed, all theologies have a contextual point of departure and are rooted in the particularities of human experience, even if their conclusions point toward universal revelation and eschatological considerations. But the basic message and implications of black theology ought not be exclusive to the African-American community simply because historically the experience of suffering, rejection, and exploitation in relation to the dominant culture has been a major hermeneutical concern of African-American religion. In other words, African-American religion never intended to isolate itself morally from the dominant culture, but rather sought to stand as a witness against racism in the name of God. And to the extent that blacks and whites identify themselves as Christians, the relevant scriptural mandate to love one's neighbor as oneself has been habitually violated — whites have despised their black neighbors, and blacks, insofar as they have internalized this racial hatred and animosity, have not loved themselves. Cone addresses some of these issues in detail in his most recent book, *Martin & Malcolm & America: A Dream or a Nightmare* (1991), in the course of his theological analysis of the life and thought of Martin Luther King, Jr., and Malcolm X. Cone's closing exhortation draws on his evaluation of the joint contributions of these two great African-Americans to American religion and politics: "As Americans we (blacks, whites, Latinos, Asians, and Indians) should create a society which contributes to the well-being of all citizens, not just to the well-being of some" (1991:317–18). Indeed, this call to accountability ought to be extended to the whole community of bioethicists, African-American and European-American alike.

I accept as established historical fact that the black churches emerged in response to racism — not because African-Americans chose to exclude European-Americans from their worshiping communities, but because they were denied full participation in virtually every aspect of American life, including religion. Ironically, the black churches were forced into existence by white churches that excluded blacks from participation in worship on the basis of racism and related ideas concerning the inferiority of African-American religion and culture on the one hand, and the superiority of European-American religion and culture on the other. It is tragic that racism overruled love in the justification of racial separation in the religious realm. And since it remains true today — as Martin Luther King, Jr., claimed many years ago — that 11 o'clock on Sunday morning is the most segregated hour in America, then both black and white Christians must be held accountable for allowing racism, or the response to racism, to dictate their behavior and systems of values in relation to each other.

While it may be valid to uphold the particular cultural traditions associated with religious worship, any theology that exclusively addresses the perspectives of one group without giving attention to the interests and concerns of others is suspect. For example, it became characteristic of European-American religion to dichotomize and relativize any theological considerations that would question white hegemony. Rather than face the fact that slavery, terrorism, discrimination, and other manifestations of racism contradict the central teaching of the Christian faith — which is to love God and neighbor as oneself — in the interest of logical consistency, it became more convenient to invalidate any association between what one believes about God and what one does to others. While it is rare to find overt pronouncements of racist ideology in white religion, many seem to understand that songs, sermons, and liturgies about love of neighbor are not to be taken seriously with reference to blacks. Praxis and principle are necessarily divorced from each other. On the other hand, historically it has been in the best interest of African-Americans to lay full claim to the relevance of praxis to principle in a theological context where God exercises sovereignty over all peoples in all situations, and not only during worship or on Sundays. Also, it makes more sense to identify the separation of the sacred from the secular as an expression of the peculiarity or deviance of white religion than to single out the merger of the same as indicative of the distinctiveness of black religion.

If black theology and black churches have brought a distinctive perspective to American life, it grows out of their courage to address questions of theodicy brought to the fore by the experience of racism and their willingness to respond theologically to the reality of unmerited suffering by affirming the goodness of God, the evil capacities of humanity, and the promise of salvation offered through Jesus Christ to bring redemption, reconciliation, and wholeness to a broken world. Yet, the fact remains that any theology or any church whose existence is justified primarily on the basis of racism or its effects will bring serious deficiencies and liabilities to the ethical dialogue needed to formulate a bioethics that promotes justice, healing, and human dignity for all.

There are other black theologians whose work bears critically upon the prospects for increased dialogue between European-American and African-American bioethics. One is James Evans, president and professor of systematic theology at Colgate Rochester Divinity School and author of *We Have Been Believers: An African-American Systematic Theology*. In the book's introduction, Evans proposes a procedure for establishing an understanding of justice based on criteria developed by black theologians:

> One must have a set of criteria by which one can determine whether the present social order is just. These criteria must themselves be drawn from the content of African-American Christian faith, rather than from any extraneous philosophical norms of

good and evil, right and wrong. Therefore, one cannot introduce a notion of justice, for example, as central to ethical behavior if the notion itself is not central to the theological affirmations of African-American faith. (1992:8)

This method of resolving the question of whether or not there is justice in the social order speaks directly to the problem of principlism. Perhaps justice takes priority over every other ethical norm in this regard, where the European-American philosophical notion of justice is subject to correction or affirmation by the collective experience of African-American people, who know firsthand the consequences of justice ill-conceived, misapplied, and flatly denied.

A second significant work grounded in the norms of black theology is *Empower the People: Social Ethics for the African-American Church*, by Theodore Walker of the Perkins School of Theology at Southern Methodist University. This book presents an outline of a contemporary black social ethics, offering the symbol of "breaking bread" as a guide to interpreting and applying biblical and religious principles to the ethical dilemmas faced by the African-American community. Citing the title of a well-known Negro spiritual as a backdrop for the ritual mediation of meanings communicated by the symbol, Walker explains:

Our understanding of the witness of Scripture is that we ought to break bread together (bread being understood as a symbol for the various resources that nourish wholesome social existence), and moreover we understand from the biblical witness that this is the absolutely essential aspect of right relation to God — indeed, it is the ethic of breaking bread that in God's final judgment separates righteousness from unrighteousness. (1991:102)

His prescriptive analysis for the whole of African-American life draws on the African holistic emphasis in black theology and extends beyond the purview of blacks in the U.S. to embrace an ecological concern for the health and well-being of the entire world:

We know that the bread we ought to break internationally, nationally, and locally includes leadership, money, food, jobs, land, housing, righteous education, and socialization (including the use of such resources as religious ritual, music, and dance), vastly increased attention to male-female-family-church relations, health care, child care, home care, family care, elder care, power, and other opportunities and resources essential to the nurture, survival, fruitful increase, and empowerment of all the people...the ecological sensitivity that we can harvest from the cultural gardens of traditional African and native American peoples, and from the gardens of other traditional peoples, calls us to see that the well-being of people is fully related to the well-being of other life. In order to contribute to the well-being of all the people, including those who are not yet born, we must contribute to the nurture and fruition of the whole living planet. (1991:120)

Although Walker does not give a great deal of specific attention to bioethics, he clearly conceptualizes the global context in which bioethical dilemmas need to be analyzed and resolved, further affirming the need for African-American ethicists to work out both principle and praxis in creative dialogue with European-Americans and others who may not hold the same point of view with regard to what constitutes human well-being and who must take responsibility for it.

The Problem of a Black Ethic

The idea of a uniquely black ethic entails some of the same problems and limitations of black theology if it does not transcend its particularity at some points in order to bring critical commentary to bear upon the society at large. Although a number of ethicists and philosophers have sought to characterize the African-American ethic as it compares to and contrasts with its European-American counterpart, one of the most insightful analyses was published in 1971 by African-American ethicist Preston Williams. In "Ethics and Ethos in the Black Experience," Williams offers a three-part typology to describe the life experiences of blacks in a racist America: (1) victimization, based upon "the fact that every Black person in America is injured or cheated by the conscious and unconscious notions of white superiority in the American mind and social system"; (2) integration, achieved as an exception to the rule of racial exclusion by "the unusual Black who by the power of his intellect, drive or personality has forced his way into mainstream America in spite of the color of his skin"; and (3) black awareness, which goes "beyond integration to ask that all men recognize the existence of a spirit, a set of social structures and norms in Black life that are worthy of acquisition by Blacks and whites" (1971:104–5).

All three aspects of this typology — victimization, integration, and black awareness — should be taken into account when evaluating the relevance of African-American ethical discourse to biomedical concerns. Still, the fundamental assumption of the black awareness ideal, namely that black values and norms ought to be shared with and acquired by

others, especially commends itself as a worthwhile point of departure for
African-American participation in bioethics. Ultimately, the ethical question is not one of African-American perspective as much as it is a matter
of African-American participation and inclusion. Perspective suggests a
particular point of view, a unique angle or approach, while participation assumes an unqualified stake and role within the whole discourse.
It must not be forgotten that the hyphen in the term *African-American*
connects two irreducible dimensions of experience: first, the retention
of vestiges of African identity, and second, the struggle for acceptance
as Americans. Moreover, what is arguably the most distinctive ethical
claim that African-Americans have made against a racist America — that
is, the fundamental affirmation of human dignity regardless of social
condition — is clearly worthy of adoption by bioethicists who are con-
scientiously concerned with transcending the particularities of race and
culture in the pursuit of justice and human wholeness. Walker's ethic
of "breaking bread" suggests ways black theological ethicists can produce a prescription for human wholeness in dialogue with more secular
European-American thinkers.

> This black God-conscious social ethical prescription — that we
> break bread together — is understood to apply to every social cir-
> cumstance. It is at this point that black theological social ethics
> can offer a prescriptive word to the whole world...the ethic of
> breaking bread calls black theological social ethics to affirm the
> bread-breaking aspects of liberal and radical and other secular
> social ethical thought. (1991:102)

Can Bioethics Be Ethical?

An African-American perspective is ultimately a human perspective —
a concrete, particular witness to universal truth. The African-American
ethos should not merely be regarded as an interesting minority perspective or contribution, but rather as a perspective that informs the
shape and content of the whole discourse. In order to be truly ethical,
bioethics must be holistic, inclusive, communalistic, and humanistic, if
not also spiritual, theistic, and improvisational, which is to say that it
ought to reflect both the particularity and universality of the African-
American experience and not be grounded solely in the thought of
European-American philosophers.

To take a holistic approach in bioethics, emphasizing that most matters are better understood in terms of "both-and" rather than "either-

or," would enable the pursuit of a harmonizing relationship between Afrocentric and Eurocentric thought rather than rejecting one and replacing it with the other. Such an approach would seek to augment and humanize the deductive, rationalistic, individualistic ethics of European-American thinkers to take into account some of the religious, historical, and cultural factors that characterize African-American collective experience. Many African-Americans have no problem combining modern medicine with such remedies as prayer and folk cures in their own personal health care decision making; on the level of bioethical discourse, the same notion can be applied to include what appeals simultaneously to the rational faculties and to the religious sensibilities in pursuit of human wholeness. While the principlism of European-American bioethics seems not to allow for the peculiarities of African-American exceptions and examples in the decision-making process, a holistic bioethics that embraces both principle and praxis, African-American bioethicists can more easily envision harmonizing Eurocentric and Afrocentric thought since most African-Americans have by necessity acquired the habit of holding European-American perspectives in tension with our own experiences. An inclusive bioethics is ethical insofar as it sees difference as an opportunity to enhance the whole rather than as grounds for discrimination or exploitation. There is a critical distinction to be made here between the terms *inclusive* and *holistic*. A *holistic* bioethics seriously questions the characteristic dualisms of Western culture, whereas an *inclusive* bioethics promotes the self-conscious and intentional rejection of racist, sexist, or classist biases and practices. Therefore, to be inclusive is not the same thing as seeking diversity as an end in itself; rather, the desired outcome of inclusivity in bioethics is fruitful dialogue, genuine mutuality, and the sharing of power and resources.

It is no simple matter to move from exclusion to inclusion. In fact, inclusivity can emerge as a more sophisticated form of oppression when the morally problematic assumptions that produced the exclusive practices in the first place remain unexamined as "others" are invited to become assimilated into the dominant group.

One of the most important distinctions to be made between the European-American bioethics of principlism and the proposed African-American bioethics is that the former is highly individualistic, while the latter would be more communalistic. The failure to give attention to the moral importance of both the individual and the community in which that individual is situated is a serious shortcoming of much of modern bioethical discourse in the U.S. While some attention is normally given in such thought to the roles of family members in making treatment decisions and resolving ethical dilemmas, not much weight tends to be given to the influence of extended family, faith communities, neighbors, and peer groups, in such matters. For example, the subject in just two of thirty-five cases in the Beauchamp and Childress text is identified by race — a white male lawyer dying from emphysema who carried on his legal practice from his hospital bed (1983:301–4), and an unmarried white woman forced by court order to undergo a cesarean section (1983:312–13). It is unclear why race was a factor in either case. Although it could be that the editors made no decision to report or not report race consistently, given that the cases were drawn from a variety of sources, one wonders how race is to be understood as relevant to these cases. Is race mentioned in these cases to make a point about their social location or moral values? Or does the reference merely serve to reinforce racist assumptions that only white males work hard or only white infants are worth saving? Ethnicity is a key factor in defining and valuing community among African-Americans, so a communalistic bioethics would give attention to race in order to enhance understanding of the individual in relation to the group, and at the same time, would take care not to use racial referents to evoke unsubstantiated judgments against individuals.

A bioethics that acknowledges the pervasive presence and power of the unseen realm over what is seen and rejects any ultimate dichotomization of the sacred and the secular seems to me to have greater authenticity than the strictly secular European-American bioethics. Although African-Americans are not demonstrably more "religious" than other Americans as measured by church attendance, denominational affiliation, and the like, the health and justice issues of the African-American community cannot intelligently be discussed without specifically referring to the pervasive influence of religious institutions, leadership, and belief systems on people inside and outside the church. Typically, European-American bioethicists lift up religious affiliation as important only on the abstract level of individual belief rather than in the context of a community of persons giving support to each other in collective ethical practice. Furthermore, religion tends to be raised as a factor only when a serious conflict emerges between religious belief and medical advice. For example, in the thirty-five cases listed in the Beauchamp and Childress text, religion is only mentioned in relation to noncompliant, deviant, or criminal behavior, including two Jehovah's Witnesses who refused blood transfusions, an involuntary mental patient who mutilated himself upon direct orders from God, and the finding that among men committing impersonal sexual acts with one another in public restrooms, most of the married men were Catholic (1983:298–300;295–96;285–87).

Thus, one is drawn to the conclusion that religion is only noteworthy as a negative factor in bioethical discourse. It would be preferable for bioethicists to devote more careful and respectful attention to religion as context and as resource for persons engaged in health care decision making. Perhaps this can occur only if we return to a more theistic frame of reference for doing bioethics. Even if the agnostic or atheistic biases of individual European-American bioethicists must remain unchallenged, it seems necessary to cultivate an intellectual awareness of the ways African-Americans affirm the existence of God and the relevance of belief to every aspect of life. To reconsider the significance of the sacred in bioethics seems to be an essential step toward increased insight into a whole range of human attitudes and behavior with respect to health issues.

While it may seem far-fetched to expect European-American bioethicists to adopt improvisational approaches or methods in keeping with the African-American ethos, the question remains as to what extent justice can be served by rigid adherence to fixed forms and structures. Given the very difficult fiscal dilemmas now being encountered by public-policy makers on the federal, state, and local levels with regard to the allocation of health care resources, particularly for the uninsured poor, an openness to spontaneity, flexibility, and innovation is something to be desired and not to be feared or guarded against if bioethicists are to make any effective contribution to the creation of viable and just cost-cutting measures. Much of the improvisational ethic in African-American life derives precisely from the challenge of "making do" with limited resources to meet the needs of the individual or the community. It may be that the insights and proposals of those who have understood the conditions of poverty and oppression will provide a distinctive reality base for European-American bioethicists who are accustomed to doing scholarly analysis without taking assumptions other than those of the white middle class into account.

If the African-American ethos is truly humanistic, valuing human life and dignity over material wealth or possessions, then incorporation of this perspective into the bioethics of the dominant culture should result in the development of more humane and less materialistic approaches to health care dilemmas. This humanistic point of view seems to be missing from many systems now in place to administer health care in the U.S. How many medical schools prepare their graduates to understand ethics, culture, and religion in relation to the administration of medical care? To what extent are research and development priorities geared exclusively toward technological advances that will benefit a small segment of the society? If bioethics embraces the "bottom-line" logic of measuring human outcomes primarily in terms of social costs and benefits, how can a high regard for human dignity on its own terms be cultivated so as to humanize public policy? Commitment to the concept of human dignity on the part of bioethicists can help to counteract the American penchant toward applying inhumane measures to human problems, so that some members of the society are deemed more worthy than others to receive its benefits and blessings.

Conclusion

The African-American ethos can serve as a rich resource for ongoing research and dialogue with regard to pressing issues such as health care resource allocation, treatment-nontreatment decisions, patient-physician relationships, and management of reproductive technologies and interventions. Without a doubt, African-American ethicists have much to gain through continued conversations with European-Americans who remain firmly committed to principlism. It is hoped that this discussion will foster meaningful partnerships between bioethicists of European-American and African-American backgrounds as they undertake the common task of addressing the ethical dimensions of medical practice, resource allocation, and public policy. It remains my conviction that any bioethics that does not give priority to justice, equality, and human dignity in administering health care is unethical, regardless of how much care is taken by whom to be racially, culturally, or intellectually inclusive.

NOTE

1. I prefer to use the term *European-American* in place of *Anglo-American* because it compares more consistently with *African-American* with reference to continent of origin, and it avoids the typically American bias that regards *Anglo* as superior to and/or representative of the rest of Europe.

REFERENCES

Beauchamp, Tom L., and James F. Childress. 1983. *Principles of Biomedical Ethics.* 2d ed. New York: Oxford University Press.
Cone, James H. 1991. *Martin & Malcolm & America: A Dream or a Nightmare,* 317–18. Maryknoll, N.Y.: Orbis Books.

———. 1984. *For My People: Black Theology and the Black Church.* Maryknoll, N.Y.: Orbis Books.

———. 1969. *Black Theology and Black Power.* New York: Harper and Row.

Ehusani, George Omaku. 1991. *An Afro-Christian Vision: "Ozovehe!" Toward a More Humanized World.* Lanham, Md.: University Press of America.

Evans, James H., Jr. 1992. *We Have Been Believers: An African-American Systematic Theology.* Minneapolis: Fortress Press.

Flack, Harley, and Edmund D. Pellegrino. 1989. "New Data Suggests African-Americans Have Own Perspective on Biomedical Ethics." Kennedy Institute of Ethics *Newsletter* 3 (April): 2.

Walker, Theodore, Jr. 1991. *Empower the People: Social Ethics for the African-American Church.* Maryknoll, N.Y.: Orbis Books.

Williams, Preston N. 1971. "Ethics and Ethos in the Black Experience." *Christianity and Crisis* (31 May): 104–5.

~ 7 ~

A Feminist Critique of Biomedical Principlism

Christine E. Gudorf

Feminist approaches to biomedical ethics have developed primarily from women's lived experiences of alienation within the U.S. health care system over the last few decades, not from academic comparisons of the U.S. system with other systems or of the dominant ethical method — principlism — with other ethical methods. *Principlism* here denotes the most commonly taught approach to biomedical ethics within the training of medical professionals in the U.S., a largely deductive approach, sometimes augmented by case studies, which begins with a select set of principles that guide all decision making and activity.

Within the broad-based women's movement of the last thirty years, women have developed critiques of principlism's virtually total reliance on principles, of the specific principles used within biomedical principlism, and of the structure of the health care system that gave rise to principlism. All three of these critiques are based on the often negative consequences of the health care system for women and other groups historically estranged from the corridors of power in the health care system. I concentrate here on presenting a general feminist critique of the method of principlism and of the adequacy of its principles. This involves sketching feminist reforms to principlism and to the present health care system.

By the 1970s, feminists had recognized a number of problems women faced in the contemporary health care system. These included (1) the medicalization of childbirth, with its attendant alienation and disempowerment for women, illustrated in the mid-twentieth century both by increased rates of cesarean sections and induced labor and by arbitrary hospital rules regulating visitation and excluding spouses from birthing; (2) the acute disproportion in the rates of women's diagnosed depression, mental illness, and institutionalization compared to those of men; and (3) the standardization of radical mastectomies and radical hysterectomies for a wide range of breast and uterine abnormalities (Sherwin 1992:143, 151–52).[1] As late as 1990 women still received different and inferior medical care compared to that received by men: they are 30 percent less likely to receive kidney transplants, 50 percent less likely to be referred for diagnostic testing for lung cancer, and 90 percent less likely to be referred for cardiac catheterization *for the same symptoms and conditions.* Moreover, medical researchers have largely ignored the study of diseases and medications in women (McMurray 1990). At the same time, women are often overtreated with tests, surgery, and drug prescriptions (Weaver and Garrett 1983). Women divided — and still divide — on how to approach these and similar issues of discrimination; that division became clearer during the 1980s. Susan Sherwin describes that division when she differentiates between a "feminine" analysis, which seeks to restore an excluded feminine dimension, and a "feminist" analysis, which sees the basic problem as one not of exclusion but of distortion — the distortion of power, of relationship, of maleness and femaleness, which constitutes patriarchy (Sherwin 1992: chap. 2).[2] While acknowledging that the two analyses are closely connected, Sherwin posits that they locate the origin of the problem differently. The feminine analysis sees the problem in biomedical principlism as a historical focus on the masculine as generic, a focus that ignores the feminine, with the consequent exclusion of feminine approaches from social institutions and systems. The feminist analysis, on the other hand, maintains that principlism, because of its reliance on principles and a specific set of principles, functions to create and sustain a unique social system.

Feminine Analysis: Restoring the Excluded "Feminine"

Moral psychologist Carol Gilligan has illustrated this feminine approach in her work comparing the moral development of males and females (Gilligan 1984). Gilligan argues that the dominant model of moral development (Lawrence Kohlberg's) was developed from research on an all-male population under the mistaken assumption that there was one human pattern for moral development (Kohlberg 1969, 1973). Her own research demonstrated that instead of relying (as Kohlberg had shown morally mature males do) on abstract moral principles as the guides for discrete, autonomous individuals, females attempt to make pragmatic choices that safeguard the persons and relationships about which they care. Gilligan argued that this alternative, feminine model of moral decision making based on care should be accorded equal status and regard with the masculine model based on principle.[3]

Similarly, philosopher Sara Ruddick has suggested that the maternal approaches of women to persons and situations be appreciated as a good and perhaps more adequate model for moral choice than prevailing masculine ones in many of the problematic areas of modern life which require peacemaking and conflict resolution (Ruddick 1984). In her controversial book *Caring,* moral theorist Nel Noddings makes a claim that caring is characteristic of women and is superior to men's reliance on abstract principles of justice as a moral model (Noddings 1984). Virginia Held shares the view of Gilligan, Noddings, and Ruddick. She writes that dominant understandings of the self are alien to women because they are based in autonomy rather than relationality, and, like Ruddick, urges that we model all moral decisions on the relationships between mothers and children "instead of importing into the household principles derived from the marketplace" (Held 1987:41–56). All these perspectives lift up relational approaches of women to moral choice as equal or superior alternatives to male reliance on abstract principles. They see male reliance on principles as proceeding from a model of the self that is autonomous, a model in which relationship is external to and not constitutive of the self.

Feminist Analysis: Reversing Patriarchal Construction of Reality

Jean Baker Miller and many other commentators point out that this difference between autonomous and relational persons is based primarily in power, and not gender, differences (Miller 1986: chap. 1). Only dominant persons can afford to be autonomous and guided solely by abstract principles; subordinates need to be relational at many levels to survive. Furthermore, autonomous selves who rely on principles for grounding moral choice delegate nurturance and other communitarian functions to others who are subordinate to them. Subordinates need to understand dominant persons on whose goodwill they depend; at the same time, their greater vulnerability requires stronger interpersonal networks of support. Our society values the bodily service and nurturance functions delegated to subordinates (women and other racial or ethnic and class subordinates) less than those functions delegated to the dominant group.

The fact that subordinates serve these lesser functions is then used to justify domination over them: these subordinates, it is said, are so embedded in relationality, in the particular context, that they are unable to "transcend" the concrete and allow themselves to be guided by abstract principle (Pateman 1980:20–31).

It is not surprising, then, that bioethics developed out of the ethical questions posed by the most dominant group in health care (physicians) and into a field of study utilizing a deductive approach based on principles. Nor is it an accident that the central principles in bioethical principlism, to cite Beauchamp and Childress's *Principles of Biomedical Ethics,* begin with autonomy and include nonmaleficence, beneficence, justice, veracity, and confidentiality (Beauchamp and Childress 1979). More *social* principles — mutuality, community, solidarity, empathy, nurturance, wholeness or integrity, and relationality itself — are not lifted up, despite our knowledge of their importance for individual as well as community growth, health, and healing.

The principles chosen in bioethical principlism reflect the primary experience and social status of their framers. The experience and social status of women and other less powerful groups would suggest other values and principles — values and principles more likely to call into question the structure and function of the health care system. At the very least, a feminist bioethics both modifies the principle of autonomy — ethicist Sarah Hoagland proposes "autokoenony" to assert the integrity of the person *in community* (Hoagland 1988) — and complements the principle of justice with community and mutuality.

Feminist analysis, as distinct from feminine analysis, does not insist on the recognition, appreciation, and inclusion of the traditionally feminine in existing systems and institutions so much as it understands both the "feminine" and the "masculine" as produced by patriarchy and therefore alienating in some ways for women. Many feminists have pointed out that not all women or even all groups of women identify with what has traditionally been understood as feminine; black women in the U.S., for example, have for the most part experienced neither the cult of "true womanhood," with its emphasis on sexual purity, nor the nonparticipation in the paid workforce that are often taken for granted by white women in describing the feminine.[4]

Feminist analysis asks systemic questions about which specific groups suffer and which benefit, and how the system maintains such suffering and benefit patterns, to ascertain what restructuring needs to be done. Such questions turn up major differences between women, as well as major differences between men and women. For example, ethicist Susan Sherwin points out that black women in the U.S. are four times more likely than white women to die in childbirth and three times more likely to have their newborns die (Sherwin 1992:226). Black women are twice as likely to die of hypertensive cardiovascular disease, are twelve times more likely to contract AIDS, and four times more likely to die as a result of homicide. Even though they have lower rates of breast cancer incidence than white women, black women in the U.S. are more likely to die of it (Sherwin 1992:226).

Feminist analysis agrees with feminine analysis at two points: both reject the assumption in principlism that the application of any body of abstract principles to experience adequately discloses the good, and both recognize the inadequacy of the body of dominant bioethical principles for expressing and revealing the normative experience of women. But feminist bioethics then goes beyond these two criticisms and insists that both the principlist method of ethics and its specific principles emanate from a social system characterized by a pattern of layered domination and subordination. The *basic* problem with the principlist model is not that it relies on abstract principles, nor that its particular principles emanate from male experience of the normative, but that both the reliance on principle and these specific moral principles function to regulate and maintain an unjust social system oppressive to women and other marginalized groups.

Increasingly, feminists reject the Noddings-Gilligan dichotomy that opposes care and principles. Feminists understand the principle of justice, for example, as intrinsic and necessary to women's welfare.[5] Moreover, real nurturance includes rational calculation. The rational and the affective do not conflict but complement each other in humans; their separation distorts human nature. The need is to connect the use of principles with an examination of the concrete situation of those most at risk. The linkage of these two processes gradually results in modification of both the body of relevant principles and their interpretation.

It was not merely blindness to the existence of feminine perspectives that allowed the medicalization of childbirth over the last hundred years. Rather, the greater social power and status of men allowed an ambitious new profession of male physicians to protect their own interests through redefining childbirth as illness requiring rational scientific intervention not obtainable from midwives they depicted as mired in superstition (Hunter College Women's Studies Collective 1983:455; Betts 1974:50–53; Ehrenreich and English 1973; Anderson 1977:240–44). This medicalization of childbirth gave them greater power and control within medicine and society, increased their income, and, through their control of both surgery and drugs, allowed them in the mid-twentieth century dramatically to reduce the inconvenience of obstetric work through inducing births and doing cesarean sections, despite the risk to mothers and infants.

Similarly, the hospital rules that long restricted visitation, even by spouses, to new mothers and infants, and excluded spouses from delivery existed clearly for the convenience of the hospital staff (Hunter College Women's Studies Collective 1983:293–95). As soon as a few voices of protesting women in the sixties began to coincide with a dropping birthrate, causing hospitals to compete for maternity patients, all these rules — and the trend from noninduced vaginal childbirth to induced and surgical births — began to reverse (Boston Women's Health Collective 1984:380–81, 385–86; Gordon 1990:440). It never occurred to most health care workers until the late sixties and early seventies that justice, beneficence, or nonmaleficence could have any connection with the issue of who could or could not be with a maternity patient during her delivery and hospital stay, much less that there might be grounds for challenging her doctor's choice of delivery method.

The visitation policy was not simply a matter of sexual discrimination, for the chief beneficiary of the rules was the nursing staff, which was also female. Visitation policy, like the process for deciding manner of delivery, was primarily an issue of power within the structure — who has it, and who doesn't. Changes in visitation policy occurred at a time when the power of nurses within hospitals was declining, squeezed between, on the one hand, increasing specialization of doctors (which located more resident doctors in hospitals), and on the other hand, the development and expansion of the role of professional hospital administrators. The most dominated group was pregnant mothers and their families, who had no voice within the health care system itself and who were rendered even more silent and powerless by their understanding of doctors and nurses as experts.

Apparently, until women began drawing attention to the fact, the psychiatric profession never recognized that the overwhelming disproportion of women in the patient population could result from sexist discrimination. Feminists began insisting that an important link existed: on the one hand, more women than men were diagnosed as depressive, were maintained on mood-changing drugs, and were institutionalized (and for less serious causes) (Chesler 1972; Brandon 1972:17–18; Fabricant 1974; Foucault 1980). On the other hand, characteristics and behaviors deemed appropriate for males in our society were those associated with mental health and normal adult adjustment, while those understood as appropriate for women were understood as immature, unhealthy, and defective (Chesler 1972).[6] Because the focus for applying the principles of bioethics was that of the doctor in relation to an individual patient, there was little examination of the diagnostic criteria or comparison of the treatment of men and women, and therefore no grounds for deciding that justice was being denied women.

The biomedical ethics texts of the sixties and seventies emphasized the principles that should govern the doctor-patient relationship (Curran 1978:64–68). Virtually the only social issue regularly considered was the issue of allocating scarce resources, and even on this issue, the focus remained until the late seventies and early eighties on the allocation of kidneys and dialysis machines to this patient rather than that patient. Bioethicists rarely focused on the *structure* of the health care system as a whole until the 1980s.

Of course, the principles approach to bioethics has developed a great deal over the last few decades. For example, doctor-patient issues have had to share the bioethical focus with systemic issues in health care as the principle of justice has been applied beyond the situation of the in-dividual medical practitioner. Today, for example, probably the most serious health care problem in this nation is the size, and continuing growth, of the medically uninsured sector of the population. Their plight is now widely recognized, but it is very important to understand *how* their plight came to be recognized, because this process points the way to possible solutions.

Millions of Americans have always been uninsured; this is the major reason that medical care for the urban poor has for decades con-sisted primarily of care given in hospital emergency rooms and has not included prenatal or other preventive care. But in recent years, the num-ber of uninsured grew to about 40 million persons, or 18 percent of the population, for a number of reasons. First, states cut back Medi-caid eligibility, so that today Medicaid covers only 40 percent of those with incomes under the federal poverty line, while it covered 63 per-cent of that group in 1975 (Callahan 1990:73–74). Second, well-paid blue-collar jobs with medical benefits disappeared in great numbers as production began to migrate overseas, leaving many unemployed and without coverage. Third, many employers began laying off full-time workers with benefits to hire part-time workers who were ineligible for benefits such as health insurance. Furthermore, many employers simply stopped providing health insurance as a benefit, or paid only a small part of the premium, so that some employees' families could not afford the remainder of the premium and thus were not covered. Finally, in the last decade, insurance companies have begun to cut back on cover-age of the chronically ill by refusing to include them, or even persons in high-risk categories, in the pool of the insured. Persons with heart con-ditions, high blood pressure, kidney failure, asthma, and emphysema, not to mention those who have AIDS or are HIV-positive, are being disqualified for coverage by a variety of company regulations and are fast becoming uninsurable. The size of the uninsured group became so large that public funds to reimburse hospitals and doctors for emergency care for the uninsured needy were overwhelmed. *Health care providers raised their prices again and again* to cover the cost of caring for the uninsured. Those who had health insurance were unwittingly paying for those who didn't.

At this point, the issue of the uninsured became a concern for hospitals, city governments, employers, and insurance companies, who have in many ways come to replace physicians as the dominant force in health care. When health care costs increase so much that insurance companies can no longer pass them on because the number of companies willing to offer insurance to their employees shrinks, then insurance companies have a big problem. Thus the uninsured became a "public" issue worthy of political attention when they became a concern to powerful social institutions — *not* when citizens experienced medical and economic need.

Recognizing the genesis of the problem, then, we must note what is really at stake in the public debate over a national health care plan for the U.S. Will our plan be aimed primarily at the welfare of the neediest (the chronically ill, persons with AIDS and other terminal illnesses, the unemployed, underemployed, and other poor)? Or will it simply work to preserve the comparative wealth and power of insurance companies, employers, and the ranks of the health care system, without either decreasing the level of care afforded to the privileged or significantly increasing the budgetary deficit?

Proposed reform plans claim to be motivated by a desire to obtain coverage for the uninsured. But many plans fall short of this goal. Former president Bush's January 1992 proposal, which created tax credits that could be transferred into insurance coverage for the uninsured, would do nothing to help the two neediest groups of uninsured: the unemployed, who do not pay taxes and therefore cannot use tax credits, and the chronically or terminally ill, who cannot get insurance companies to issue them policies regardless of the cost of premiums. A feminist analysis can be helpful here.

From the perspective of feminist ethics, the only adequate bioethics is one that includes this simple principle: promotion of the common good includes the good of *all* persons in the community. This principle would shape a feminist approach to health care reform. Christian ethicist Margaret Farley proposes the feminist hermeneutic principle: "whatever diminishes or denies the full humanity of women must be presumed not to reflect the divine or authentic relation to the divine, or to reflect the authentic nature of things, or to be the message or work of an authentic redeemer or a community of redemption" (Farley 1985:296). With this statement, Farley is rejecting centuries of thought in which the good of women was not directly pursued but was assumed procured through such things as just wages paid to fathers and husbands, through social reverence for motherhood, and through the development of bioethical reflection around beneficent male experts who control the bodies and health of women. The common good must directly include the concrete and complete welfare of all persons as persons and not as assigned social roles. What is good for children, for the institution of the family, for husbands, or for the economy is not necessarily good for women or for other groups historically at the margins of power structures.

Feminist liberationist theologians and ethicists sometimes make this point with slightly different language, insisting on a *preferential option for the poor and marginalized* rooted in Judeo-Christian faith (Fiorenza 1983: chap. 1, esp. 32). The language of preferential option originated not in the women's movement but in the Latin American liberation theology movement, which shares with feminism this starting point for reflection: the concrete condition of those groups at the bottom of the society (Gutiérrez 1979:169–221, esp. 200–206). For feminism and all liberation theologies, the test of any society's justice is the welfare of those at the bottom of the sociopolitical and economic ladder.

The welfare of women has continually been neglected and attacked without the principle of justice coming into play. The double standard in sex — for example, women's double burden of employment and domestic work, the enrichment of men and impoverishment of women by divorce, as well as the sexist treatment of women in the health care system — have all continued without challenge from standard understandings of justice (Andolsen 1985:3–18; Sidell 1986:13, 104–7). Many violations of justice remain, for the most part, politically invisible because they are part of the structure of society and therefore taken for granted. This suggests that we must augment principles of justice with a hermeneutic of suspicion when approaching social reality: specifically, to make violations of justice visible, we must approach any social system with a suspicion that the powerless and marginalized of society are discriminated against, and we must use social analysis to test for such discrimination. For example, analysis of the health care system is especially critical for feminist reflection on new reproductive technologies. Many feminists reject any evaluation of these new technologies apart from the prevalent power structures in our health care system. They suspect that although the new technologies may not in themselves threaten women or other oppressed groups, their implementation may, simply because the present controlling elites control the technologies.

The feminist addition of the hermeneutic of suspicion to the principles approach integrates the strengths of traditionally feminine processes of moral discernment (concern for concrete persons and relationships) with the strengths of the traditionally masculine processes of moral discernment (the rational application of universal principles). A second procedural change important to feminism is the insistence that principles (and the values upon which they stand) should not be ranked in hierarchical order (for example, autonomy over beneficence). A ranking that is appropriate in one situation is not appropriate in all others, for the values are differently embedded — and under different degrees of threat — in different situations. To insist on a hierarchical ranking of values or principles is to insist on the priority of one social group's perspective over all others. The refusal to rank values and principles makes feminist bioethics more open to the particularities of the situation than many other types of principlism.

Feminist liberation theology also challenges the implicit assumptions about God in theological forms of bioethical principlism. One assumption, for example, lies in the tendency to regard principles as revealing truth. Feminist liberation theologians view this tendency as evidencing an image of deity as giver of rules and principles, which in turn reveals his (masculine) nature as ruler and judge. They further see this as a legalistic misunderstanding of the nature of Jewish and Christian revelation and point out that rules and principles are not an exclusively privileged medium for revelation in this tradition. Divinity, divine activity, and divine intentions have even more frequently been communicated through stories of divine activity, stories of human lives and communities, and stories of the interaction between divinity and humans.

The insistence on principles as revelatory is theologically linked for Christians with a focus on Jesus as the Word rather than on Jesus as the embodied divine figure whose historical life is presented in the Gospels. The focus in liberation theology on the historical Jesus, with all the attendant difficulties in recovering that historical figure, has arisen from an understanding that Christian principles and rules must be derived from lived experience. Lived experience should not be captive to principles or rules divorced from the life experience from which they sprang. Is this not what Jesus meant in Mark 2:27, when he insisted that the Sabbath (law) was made for people, and not people for the Sabbath? The centrality of the Mosaic law in Judaism — itself begun in the First Commandment's reference to the Exodus story — was overthrown within early Christian history when the Council of Jerusalem in the Book of Acts agreed with Peter and Paul that the law did not bind Gentile Christians. Before rules delineated membership and before principles stated the core beliefs of Christians, a young Jew walked around Galilee with his followers, telling parables and working miracles to exorcise demons and to heal, feed, and raise people from the dead. Why should those parables and accounts of Jesus' activities apply to contemporary bioethics only through principles and not as stories?

Feminist liberation theologians tend to understand divinity as relational, even as the ground of relationship, rather than as something properly approached only through law or principles. Because divinity — and therefore reality — is basically relational, principles become most useful when joined to recognition and appreciation of the unique person with whom one is in relationship. For example, in health care, the principle of informed consent is an important way of recognizing patient capacity and responsibility for decision making. But any attempt to make informed consent real for any specific patient will entail dealing with the particularities of that patient, her physical situation, her fears and anxieties, the limits of her intellectual understanding, her lifestyle, and her relationships.

Embodiment

The central principle that feminism has contributed to an understanding of health care is embodiment. Western Christian culture has understood women primarily as body and men as rational soul. This culture has understood body not only as inferior to the spiritual mind-soul but as subject to that rational, spiritual mind. While salvation required both men and women to resist the temptations of the carnal body, this task was viewed as much more difficult for women, because they were proportionately much more carnal than men. Thus Augustine understood men to be made in the image and likeness of God by themselves, but women to be made in the image and likeness of God only when joined to a man.[7] Virginity, according to St. Jerome, was a tremendous aid to salvation for women, because it allowed them to escape from the "feminine" condition of subjection to the flesh and become "virile."[8] Even more necessary than virginity, however, was subordination to male authority. Although everyone had to submit to (male) religious authorities, women, in addition, were required to submit to husbands "as to the Lord" (Ephesians 5:22).

Women's experience in Western history has led twentieth-century feminists to reject both sexual dualism (male over female) and spiritual dualism (mind over body) and to insist instead on the integrity of the body and the mind-soul. Christian feminists insist that Jesus Christ both modeled the complete integration of the body with the mind-soul and demanded that Christians follow his example (Nelson 1983: 24–32). Today, feminists are the major group calling for the recognition of human embodiment — the understanding of the human person as co-extensive with, and inevitably influenced by, the particularities of one's human body.[9] Because all human knowledge and experience are mediated through the body, our bodies are not merely something that we possess and can control. Our bodies *are* us. One of the ironies of human history is that Western Christianity seems to have waited, in a state of body-denial, for two millennia for feminist theology to give meaning to the Incarnation by proposing embodiment and rejecting the body-soul dualism that made Incarnation impossible.

The principle of embodiment carries a number of implications. First, respect for each person requires respect for each *embodied* self. This not only makes activities like physical torture immoral but further insists that both social standards of bodily beauty and medical interventions designed to change the appearance of those bodies must answer to this principle. Such respect is especially important for women, who are generally more oppressed by narrow cultural standards that define the beautiful body. Eating disorders such as bulimia and anorexia nervosa can be viewed, then, not only as diseases that can kill but as deadly *symptoms* of a wider problem of socialization around values in our society. In addition, much of contemporary orthodontics, as well as various kinds of cosmetic surgery, becomes morally questionable.

Much more significant, however, is the change that the principle of embodiment makes in how one understands one's *responsibility* toward one's body. If my body is a possession, like a car, then when I suspect that something is wrong, I take it to the expert who specializes in bodies, and turn it over to the expert's care. But if my body is myself, I cannot delegate responsibility for care to someone else. I must be responsible for myself and care for myself, because in so doing, I create myself. Such an understanding raises questions about the word *patient* as used in bioethics, especially the understanding of the patient as passive, dependent, and trusting of professional medical expertise. Barring personal incapacity, it simply is not moral to consign responsibility for one's self to another person. Sickness requires consulting experts, receiving advice, collaborating — not surrendering control over oneself. Surrendering the self cannot be a model for achieving self-health, for self-health must include personal integrity. When "informed consent" is used as evidence of the patient's surrender of his or her embodied self to the control of physicians and hospitals, the dignity of the embodied person has been violated.

Allied to the acceptance of one's body as a constitutive part of the human self that demands respect is the rejection of understandings of normal bodily events and functions as diseases or illnesses requiring medical intervention. This means not only that aging and death are to be regarded as normal and not in themselves demands for medical intervention but also that processes in female body life (menstruation [including premenstrual syndrome], childbirth, and menopause) are not to be medicalized as dysfunctions requiring intervention (Sherwin 1992: chap. 8). Of course, excessive bleeding, anemia, or pain associated with menstruation, premature childbirth, toxemia, and other abnormalities can require medical intervention. The point is that the female functions of menstruation, childbirth, and menopause are not *in themselves* disorders. And because they are simply natural female processes, women need to take primary responsibility for them. They should have access to complete information about them and about their most common dysfunctions so that, if a problem does occur, women can *consult with* physicians instead of abdicating responsibility for their bodies to physicians.

Emphasis on embodiment pushes toward wellness-oriented health care and away from the crisis-centered health care that has characterized our society. Wellness-oriented health care must approach the human person as an integrated person — not as a machine with a malfunctioning part. Such health care would include, much more than at present, an emphasis on educating the general public in nutrition, exercise, environmental health hazards, stress management, overall mental health, and other general aspects of lifestyle that affect health.

Finally, the principle of embodiment implies a need for greater sensitivity to the connections between humans and the rest of nature. Feminists generally agree on this point, and from this general agreement, *ecofeminism* has developed as a school of thought.[10] Yet feminists divide over the relationship of *women* to nature. Is the perception of women's greater closeness to nature accurate, or is that closeness historically learned? Writers such as Carolyn Merchant and Susan Griffin have chronicled early understandings of earth as female. They show, too, how modern society has viewed scientific progress: as advances the rational human mind has made in probing, discovering, and controlling nature understood as female — as fertile, creative, nurturant, chaotic, and disordered (emotional) (Merchant 1980; Griffin 1978). The issue is, as earlier between feminine and feminist analysis, whether women (usually by virtue of their fertility and their menstrual cycle) are materially closer to nature, or whether closeness to nature was part of the role that patriarchy forced on women (Washbourne 1977; Downing 1989:119ff).

Sherry Ortner explains that two of the principal duties historically assigned to women mediate the gap between nature and culture: women have taken raw foodstuff and raw (newborn) human life and transformed (civilized) them for the world of culture, so that food becomes meals, and children enter into the customs and patterns of the society (Ortner 1974: 67–87). Women constantly move back and forth between nature and culture, with one foot in each. But, Ortner argues, this pattern is assigned, and it should be changed. Men and women are equally linked to both nature and culture.

A third feminist position rejects the very dichotomy between nature and culture. It identifies this division as the basis of our ecological disaster and insists that men and women depend equally upon nature, since all culture is transformed nature (Roach 1991: 47–59).

Conclusion

Feminism, then, employs a qualified type of bioethical principlism. One of its basic principles is that the moral status of any health care system must be tested not only against abstract principles such as justice, individual integrity, community, mutuality, and embodiment but also against the concrete and comprehensive well-being of the least powerful, most marginalized members of society. In addition, feminism rejects the nonrelational implications of principlism's autonomy, substitutes individual integrity for autonomy, and insists on adding principles that are both more social and more relational, such as mutuality and community. Finally, the feminist principle of embodiment seeks to emphasize the particularity and materiality of human existence, and the consequent need to take context seriously in ethical reflection. For feminists, ethics, whether in the biomedical field or any other, is inseparably connected to spirituality. Ethics is not limited to a search for justice, much less for stable social order. Rather, ethics is oriented toward the achievement of full humanity for all, toward what Western religion has called the Reign of God and what many secular ecofeminists describe as *human communities* — communities that are just, peaceful, cooperative, and sustainable within themselves, between themselves, and in relation to the rest of creation.

NOTES

1. I am indebted to Susan Sherwin's book for many of the following analyses. Other sources on the standardization of radical mastectomy and hysterectomy are Boston Women's Health Book Collective 1984:478–83, 488–96, 513–16 and Hunter College Women's Studies Collective 1983:448, 454. For lack of space I cannot further develop this issue here.

2. While the logic behind the "feminine" label is clear (this position does advocate valorizing traditionally feminine traits and behaviors) the "feminist" label is more polemical, since it seems to define feminism in ways which exclude those advocating "feminine" analysis. Such exclusion is questionable, since this group both self-identifies as feminist and has made major contributions to feminist thought. Here I use the distinction only with reference to the analysis, and not to exclude from the feminist ranks those using "feminine" analysis.

3. Gilligan was not particularly clear about distinguishing the "is" from the "ought to be" in describing men's and women's moral processes. She not only wrote about the need to valorize women's present model of moral choice (the feminine one) but also explained the evolution of both the feminine and the masculine model with reference to Nancy Chodorow's thesis on the effects of female caretaking of young children during the period of gender identification (Chodorow 1979). This latter is significant because Chodorow clearly advocates the inclusion of male caretakers along with female caretakers during this period so as to *integrate* the present male and female experiences and *eliminate* the present dichotomy between masculine and feminine patterns of moral decision making. Thus Gilligan seems both to valorize the feminine model and to argue that it needs to be eliminated.

4. For this and other issues at stake between white feminists and black womanists, see Thistlethwaite 1991.

5. See, for example, the primacy of justice in the work of Beverly Harrison which points to the role of anger as a response to the violation of justice; Harrison 1985:3–21.

6. This is also true of physicians who are not psychiatrists; see Corea 1977.

7. See Augustine, *De Trinitate* 7.7, 10, quoted in Ruether 1974:176.

8. See Jerome, Epistles 130, 10, in Ruether 1974.

9. Probably the best example is the Boston Women's Health Book Collective's *The New Our Bodies, Ourselves* 1984. For a theological treatment see Nelson 1979. Nelson's approach to embodiment is feminist.

10. See, for example, Caldecott and Leland 1983; Daly 1978; Diamond and Orenstein 1990; Plant 1989; Grey 1981; Salleh 1984:339–45; Kheel 1991:145–64.

REFERENCES

Anderson, Sandra F. 1977. "Childbirth as a Pathological Process: An American Perspective." *MCN: The American Journal of Maternal Child Nursing* 2:240–44.

Andolsen, Barbara Hilkert. 1985. "A Woman's Work Is Never Done: Unpaid Household Labor As a Social Justice Issue." In *Women's Consciousness, Women's Conscience: A Reader in Feminist Ethics,* ed. Barbara Hilkert Andolsen, Christine E. Gudorf and Mary D. Pellauer, 3–18. Minneapolis: Winston Press.

Beauchamp, Tom L., and James F. Childress. 1979. *Principles of Biomedical Ethics.* New York: Oxford University Press.

Betts, Doris. 1974. "Still Life with Fruit." *Ms.* 2:50–53.

The Boston Women's Health Book Collective. 1984. *The New Our Bodies, Ourselves.* New York: Simon and Schuster.

Brandon, Sydney. 1972. "Psychiatric Illness in Women." *Nursing Mirror* 34:17–18.

Caldecott, Leonie, and Stephanie Leland, eds. 1983. *Reclaim the Earth: Women Speak Out for Life on Earth.* London: Women's Press.

Callahan, Daniel. 1990. *What Kind of Life: The Limits of Medical Progress.* New York: Simon and Schuster.

Chesler, Phyllis. 1972. *Women and Madness.* New York: Avon.

Chodorow, Nancy. 1979. *The Reproduction of Mothering.* University of California Press.

Corea, Gena. 1977. *The Hidden Malpractice.* New York: Morrow.

Curran, Charles. 1978. "Medical Ethics: History and Overview." In *Issues in Sexual and Medical Ethics,* ed. Charles Curran, 64–68. Notre Dame, Ind.: University of Notre Dame Press.

Daly, Mary. 1978. *Gyn/Ecology: The Meta-ethics of Radical Feminism.* Boston: Beacon.

Diamond, Irene, and Gloria Orenstein, eds. 1990. *Reweaving the World: The Emergence of Ecofeminism.* San Francisco: Sierra Club.

Downing, Christine. 1989. "Artemis: The Goddess Who Comes from Afar." In *Weaving the Visions: New Patterns in Feminist Spirituality,* ed. Judith Plaskow and Carol Christ, 119ff. San Francisco: HarperCollins.

Ehrenreich, Barbara, and Deirdre English. 1973. *Witches, Midwives and Nurses: A History of Women Healers.* New York: Feminist Press.

Fabricant, Benjamin. 1974. "The Psychotherapist and the Female Patient." In *Perception and Change,* ed. Violet Franks and Vasanti Burtle. New York: Bruner-Mazel.

Farley, Margaret. 1985. "Feminist Theology and Bioethics." In *Women's Consciousness, Women's Conscience: A Reader in Feminist Ethics,* ed. Barbara H. Andolsen et al., 296. Minneapolis: Winston Press.

Fiorenza, Elisabeth Schüssler. 1983. *In Memory of Her: A Feminist Theological Reconstruction of Christian Origins.* New York: Crossroad.

Foucault, Michel. 1988. *The History of Sexuality,* vol. 1, Introduction, trans. Robert Hurley. New York: Vintage.

Gilligan, Carol. 1984. *In a Different Voice: Psychological Theory and Women's Development.* Cambridge: Harvard University Press.

Gordon, Linda. 1990. Rev. ed. *Woman's Body, Woman's Right: Birth Control in America.* New York: Penguin.

Grey, Elizabeth Dodson. 1981. *Green Paradise Lost.* Wellesley, Mass.: Round-table Press.

Griffin, Susan. 1978. *Women and Nature: The Roaring Inside Her.* New York: Harper Colophon.

Gutiérrez, Gustavo. 1979. "Theology from the Underside of History." In *The Power of the Poor in History,* 169–221. Maryknoll, N.Y.: Orbis Books.

Harrison, Beverly. 1985. "The Power of Anger in the Work of Love: An Ethic for Women and Other Strangers." In *Making the Connections: Essays in Feminist Social Ethics,* ed. Carol Robb, 3–21. Boston: Beacon.

Held, Virginia. 1987. "Non-Contractual Society: A Feminist View." In *Science, Morality, and Feminist Theory,* ed. Marsha Hanen and Kai Nelson. *Canadian Journal of Philosophy* 13 (supplementary volume): 41–56.

Hoagland, Sarah Lucia. 1988. *Lesbian Ethics: Toward New Value.* Palo Alto, Calif.: Institute of Lesbian Studies.

Hunter College Women's Studies Collective. 1983. *Women's Realities, Women's Choices.* New York: Oxford.

Kheel, Marti. 1991. "Ecofeminism and Deep Ecology: Reflections on Identity and Difference." In *Covenant for a New Creation: Ethics, Religion, and Public Policy,* ed. Carol S. Robb and Carl J. Casebolt, 145–64. Maryknoll, N.Y.: Orbis Books.

Kohlberg, Lawrence. 1969. "Stage and Sequence: The Cognitive-Development Approach to Socialization." In *Handbook of Socialization Theory and Research,* ed. D. A. Goslin. Chicago: Rand McNally.

———. 1973. "Continuities and Discontinuities in Childhood and Adult Moral Development Revisited." In *Collected Papers on Moral Development and Moral Education.* Moral Education Research Foundation, Harvard University.

McMurray, Richard J. 1990. "Gender Disparities in Clinical Decision-Making." *Report to the American Medical Association Council on Ethical and Judicial Affairs.*

Merchant, Carolyn. 1980. *The Death of Nature: Women, Ecology, and the Scientific Revolution.* San Francisco: Harper and Row.

Miller, Jean Baker. 1986. *Toward a New Psychology for Women.* 2d ed. Boston: Beacon.

Nelson, James B. 1983. *Between Two Gardens: Reflections on Sexuality and Religious Experience.* New York: Pilgrim.

———. 1979. *Embodiment: An Approach to Sexuality and Christian Theology.* Minneapolis: Augsburg.

Noddings, Nel. 1984. *Caring: A Feminist Approach to Ethics and Moral Education.* Berkeley: University of California Press.

Ortner, Sherry B. 1974. "Is Female to Male as Nature Is to Culture?" In *Woman, Culture and Society,* ed. Michelle Zimbalist Rosaldo and Louise Lamphere, 67–87. Stanford, Calif.: Stanford University Press.

Pateman, Carole. 1980. " 'The Disorder of Women': Women, Love and the Sense of Justice." *Ethics* 91 (October): 20–31.

Plant, Judith, ed. 1989. *Healing the Wounds: The Promise of Ecofeminism.* Philadelphia: New Society.

Roach, Catherine. 1991. "Loving Your Mother: On the Woman-Nature Relation." *Hypatia* 6, no. 1 (Spring): 47–59.

Ruddick, Sara. 1984. "Maternal Thinking." In *Mothering: Essays in Feminist Theory,* ed. Joyce Trebilcot. Totowa, N.J.: Rowman and Allanheld.

Ruether, Rosemary R. 1974. "Virginal Feminism in the Fathers of the Church." In *Religion and Sexism: Images of Women in the Jewish and Christian Traditions,* ed. R. R. Ruether, 176. New York: Simon and Schuster.

Salleh, Ariel Kay. 1984. "Deeper than Deep Ecology: The Ecofeminist Connection." *Environmental Ethics* 6:339–45.

Sherwin, Susan. 1992. *No Longer Patient: Feminist Ethics and Health Care.* Philadelphia: Temple University Press.

Sidell, Ruth. 1986. *Women and Children Last.* New York: Penguin.

Thistlethwaite, Susan. 1991. *Sex, Race and God: Christian Feminism in Black and White.* New York: Crossroad.

Washbourne, Penelope. 1977. *Becoming Woman.* San Francisco: Harper and Row.

Weaver, Jerry L., and Sharon D. Garrett. 1983. "Sexism and Racism in the American Health Care Industry: A Comparative Analysis." In *Women and Health: The Politics of Sex in Medicine,* ed. Elizabeth Fee. Farmingdale, N.Y.: Baywood.

~ 8 ~

PRINCIPLISM AND RELIGION
THE LAW AND THE PROPHETS

Courtney S. Campbell

The controversy over the status of principlism in biomedical ethics contains more than a hint of familiarity in the moral memory of theological ethics. In the mid-1960s, approximately at the dawn of contemporary bioethics, a vigorous debate transpired in academic forums, religious communities, and even among the general public over the acceptability of "contextualist" morality or "situation ethics" (Cox 1968). Joseph Fletcher, among others, charged that traditional religious morality, as expressed in commands, principles, and rules, fostered a "legalistic" attitude toward moral choices in medicine, particularly regarding reproductive issues, abortion, and euthanasia. Fletcher's own *Situation Ethics* set up a dichotomy between principles and persons, which he resolved on the side of the sovereignty of rational moral agents. The norm of love or *agape* was to direct moral choices contextually, thus liberating persons from a legalistic reliance on principles. Paul Ramsey, on the other hand, while likewise affirming the centrality of *agape,* maintained that love was typically embedded in several moral principles, or "in-principled," which prevented a slide into moral relativism.

Fletcher and Ramsey, of course, were not only significant theological ethicists, but also prominent figures in the emergence of biomedical ethics, and echoes from that not-too-distant debate surely resonate in the present dispute over principlism. Bioethical critiques that portray a principlist methodology as a form of "ethical engineering" (Caplan 1982:155–68) reflect concerns about a mechanistic and legalistic morality similar to the patterns that emerged in the theological discussion. The controversy over the ascendancy of personal choice has come full circle, in part because respect for personal autonomy is now incorporated within the ethics of the medical profession, and in part because the coupling of choice and love affirmed by Fletcher has gradually dissolved, such that on many accounts, self-determination seems either the *only* or the *supreme* principle of biomedical ethics.

Moreover, just as the theological debate defied simple polarization (Gustafson 1971:104), so also the dispute over principlism in biomedical ethics involves quite diverse groups of ethical methods, often united more by what they deny than what they affirm. I will use the term *principlism* to refer to an account of moral reasoning and justification in which moral principles and rules, derived from or validated by a more general ethical theory, are applied to concrete situations ("cases") of conflicting moral demands to provide a guide for particular actions and a basis for judgment about those actions. On this specification, it becomes clear that diverse critiques of principlism have directed their objections at several quite different targets. Some, emphasizing justification of decisions within the framework of ethical theory, charge that principlism lacks the integration provided by a unitary moral theory. Others, less concerned with the foundations of morality, have argued that the principles themselves are too general to illuminate the moral realities of clinical practice. Still others contend that principlism slights the necessity for a thick description of persons and moral agency. Finally, some have claimed that the sociological and political presuppositions of principlism limit its gender and cultural applicability.

A dispute over the normative status of principles, then, invokes the moral memory of a theological controversy. It is important, however, not to overdo the parallel. The theological debate was possible because of a common discourse and shared moral orientation (for example, about the theme of love) within the religious traditions. The principlist debate in biomedical ethics, meanwhile, is concerned in part about moral discourse *across* communities and whether the principles themselves validly express some trans-communal moral values. This quest for a common ground of moral discourse has culminated in another contemporary trend in biomedical ethics: the marginalization of religious perspectives. This feature is displayed in nearly all the prominent bioethics teaching anthologies, in which readings and themes oriented by religious considerations are virtually absent; in the claims of prominent philosophers that a successful bioethics "does not need theology" (Engelhardt 1985:88); and even in the metaphors of "mantra" and "ritual incantation" critics use to characterize principlism, which displays a striking form of insensitivity or ignorance toward certain patterns of religiosity.

The contemporary debate over principlism thus provides an occasion to draw on this theological memory for critical insight and to address a perennial question about the relevance of religious perspectives for biomedical ethics. I will begin by proposing an analogy between bio-ethical principlism and moral law, though distancing this interpretation from the theological criticism of "legalism." The theological limitations of principlism will then be explored through three moral meanings of prophecy. The witness of the biblical prophet may take the forms of *exposing hypocrisy, preserving memory and re-membering,* and *embodying promise.* The first two modes of witness invoke values already present within a moral community's discourse; here, the question focuses on the distinctiveness of the witness. The form of promise, in contrast, may invoke different values based on a distinctive vision of the human good, and raises the question of the relevance of these values for an audience who does not share the vision. Prophetic promise does offer a rich context of meaning and ultimacy that is especially necessary to the realm of medicine, in which issues of the nature and identity of the self, the experience of dependency, pain, and suffering, and the reality of death and human destiny are standard fare. The marginalization of religion therefore may indicate a bioethics that is increasingly meaningless.

Principlism as Moral Law: A Theological Critique

Critics so characteristically bury principlism without praise that its considerable appeals as a moral methodology for biomedical ethics need display. Its objectives are comparable in some formal respects with those of natural law morality, among which is the construction of common ground for public moral discourse. The formulation of general principles and norms aims to offer a morality that is public in the sense of being "available to all intelligent, reasonable, and responsible members of [a] culture despite their otherwise crucial differences in belief and practices" (Tracy 1986:115). This availability is constituted in part by a reliance on publicly accessible reasons as the basis for judgments, a role filled by the specific principles themselves. Thus, a diverse audience of reasonable and responsible persons can invoke normative principles such as non-maleficence, beneficence, justice, and respect for personal autonomy to establish moral obligations and to serve as standards for moral justification and criticism. We can then see in principlism both a substantive and procedural framework for moral discourse in the world of medicine.

This would be no small achievement in any context, but perhaps especially so in a fragmented moral culture such as our own. Little binds particular moral communities together except perhaps the tenuous bond of citizenship, and we have no shared, substantive vision of the personal or collective good of human life, but rather find ourselves in dialogue with moral strangers with particular and contrasting visions. In such a setting, the challenge of sustaining moral discourse, whether the participants make their moral home in a religious community, a professional tradition, or a secular philosophical perspective, can be substantial.

The principlist response to pluralism characteristically has been to stress the moral significance of shared *procedures* at the risk of adopting a stance of metaphysical neutrality or agnosticism about the nature of the good life. We can, on the principlist account, be "friendly strangers" (Childress 1989a:43), because of a shared commitment to procedural values of moral reasoning and accountability, as well as to institutional procedures that express convictions about the equality of persons, and the presence of a general trust that others will respect the common principles and rules of the moral life. The public affirmation of a substantive position rooted in a particular vision of human nature or destiny may, by contrast, risk divisiveness and disruption, a moral babel that threatens to subvert the moral reliance on publicly accessible reasons espoused by principlism.

To be sure, the question of what we consider a publicly accessible reason, or how we come to determine common principles that ought or do govern our lives and choices in the moral world of medicine, is not, as we shall see, a theologically neutral matter. We need first, however, to develop the proposed analogy of principlism with moral law somewhat further to cast both its potential and perils in sharper theological relief.

While principlism takes seriously our intuitive sense of personal responsibility and public accountability for actions, the metaphors of principlism reveal that a legal model of reasoning informs the content of responsibility. In the principlist method, moral agents "weigh and balance" principles that carry "presumptive" status to resolve "cases" of moral conflict. They "appeal" to principles to "defeat charges of moral liability" and to "defend" their choices and actions. The moral agent in medicine is also on trial before the community of public moral discourse.

The analogy with law also seems appropriate to the specific substantive principles, insofar as the obligations they prescribe amount to expectations of minimal decency. To borrow language from Judith Thomson, principlism offers an ethic for "minimally decent samaritans" rather than for saints, heroes, or "good samaritans" (Thomson 1971:47–66). This is perhaps the loftiest level principlism can achieve in the company of friendly moral strangers; even so, a minimalist morality that stresses, for example, respect for patient autonomy is an advance over the paternalistic pretensions of professional medicine. We might well wonder whether a culture that did not contain provisions for not harming others (for example, nonmaleficence), minimally promoting their welfare (for example, beneficence), giving persons their due (for example, justice), and acknowledging their interests in bodily integrity and life (for example, respect for persons) could sustain fully a common moral life. Even so, we should also recognize that a rich moral community, constituted by intimates rather than friendly strangers, and a common quest or vision rather than moral agnosticism, will seek to exceed moral minimalism through the expression of ideals, virtues, and aspirations, both personal and collective. A moral community needs principles and laws that serve as boundaries by which to *live* and a shared sense of ends and virtues by which to live *well*.

If principlism is agnostic about the good, it nonetheless appears to assume a realism about "the bad," namely, the fallibility and self-interested bias of human nature. Procedures of public accountability and justification are necessary because we have historically revealed ourselves as poor judges when our private interests are at stake, with a propensity for arbitrariness, rationalizations, and preferences that are only self-validated. In theological language, principlism assumes a fallenness to human nature, and if that moral anthropology is valid, then risking what Stephen Toulmin calls a "tyranny of principles" may be preferable to the anarchy of autonomy (Toulmin 1981:31–9).

The anthropological realism that principlism presupposes is perhaps best captured by H. Richard Niebuhr's image of "man-the-citizen, living under law." The moral self in this image is involved with legislating, obeying, and administering: "We come into being under the rules of family, neighborhood, and nation, subject to the regulation of our action by others. Against these rules we can and do rebel, yet find it necessary — morally necessary, that is — to consent to some laws and to give ourselves rules, or to administer our lives in accordance with some discipline" (Niebuhr 1963:53). This moral necessity to an ethic of principles, rules, laws, etc., reflects an acknowledgment of our common finitude and fallibility that must be constrained if we are to fashion a viable moral culture.

Yet, this focus on the minimalism and constraints of principlism may be overly narrow theologically. An influential tradition of religious discourse holds, for example, that moral law has not only a preventive and regulating function, but also a pedagogical function, and this could imply an instructive or teaching role for principlism in medicine analogous to the role of law for "sanctification" in the religious life (Calvin 1960:360–62). This theological correction would not challenge the fundamental realism about human finitude and fallibility, but rather concerns openness to human possibilities for growth and transformation of moral character. It indicates, then, a complementary rather than contradictory relationship between principles and virtues.

We are not, in any case, merely submissive (or rebellious) citizens in the ethics of principlism, but also judges who participate in a common calling of evaluating our own actions and choices as well as those of others. That judicial status is embedded in the principlist stress on "justification," which is likewise open to differing theological understandings. The model and even language of justification may for some traditions be theologically suspect because it suggests that we have arrogated to ourselves what belongs to God, namely, the role of judge over our fellows. We may, and bioethical principlism typically does, focus on acts, or external morality, rather than on the motive or internal character of the agent. A theological critique might affirm God alone as the source of justification of human beings and portray assumption of this role as a reflection of a "works-righteousness" consciousness and a "playing God" mentality, that is, the wrong of pride. It seems possible to contend, however, that the necessary task of distinguishing between justified and unjustified choices in the moral world of medicine does not infringe on the sovereignty of God over justifying persons in the religious world of salvation.

Alternatively, the judicial emphasis in principlism might be seen as an occasion for the exercise of *interpretation*. The necessity of interpretation in biomedical ethics is displayed when we focus on the content of the normative principles. We should, I think, be able to find a consensus about the existence of a general obligation not to harm others, as expressed in the principle of nonmaleficence. However, once we move from recognizing this obligation to considering its practical relevancy, that is, once we experience a moral context that requires us to ask questions about "what counts as harm?" or "which others did you mean?" our initial common consensus will evolve into a moral argument characterized by a process of interpretation, for neither the stringency nor the scope of nonmaleficence is immediately self-evident. We should then see the community of friendly strangers that principlism presupposes not simply as an audience of justification but also as participants in substantive interpretation.

This process, Michael Walzer has suggested, is somewhat analogous to the task of the judiciary, in that it "closely resembl[es] the work of a lawyer or judge who struggles to find meaning in a morass of conflicting laws and precedents" (Walzer 1987:19–20). The search for moral content will always depend in part on a common set of principles, perhaps codified in a sacred text in a religious community or a constitution in a political society, but the interpretive process will also always seek to bring those principles and the precedents built upon them into a meaningful practical equilibrium with ordinary, everyday moral experience. A dialectical and mutually corrective relationship emerges between principlism and our experience, with the principles serving to guide or refine our conventional *modus operandi,* but yet always open to substantive discovery and re-interpretation in light of our ongoing experience of the moral life.

Such an approach, relying on both the settled and the situational, the embedded and the experienced morality, can confirm or challenge conventional positions. We may, to draw on the moral world of medicine, have reached a tradition of consensus that, based on principles of nonmaleficence and beneficence, patients should not be required to undergo "extraordinary" or disproportionate medical interventions. The meaning of these criteria for any particular circumstance will, however, require interpretation, as for example, when we encounter a patient whose life is sustained only by nutrition and hydration provided by medical means. This particular method of sustaining life was introduced in the late 19th century, and only recently routinized within medical practice. Prompted by some very vexing medical situations (for example, persistent vegetative state) and wrenching court cases, we have in the last decade witnessed and participated in an interpretative inquiry that has sought to discover whether such a method is to be understood as a medical treatment and thus could be removed according to the non-medical criteria of the extraordinary treatment standard, or is instead a form of basic care that responds to essential human needs.

The analogy I have proposed of principlism as a form of moral law should be distinguished from the earlier theological critique of principlism as "legalistic," that is, an inflexible, mechanical, and contextually insensitive morality that reached prospective closure on moral choices. I have wanted to suggest a contextual sensitivity at the core of bioethical principlism, namely, the difficult endeavor to find common ground for moral discussion in a pluralistic society. Moreover, the necessity of interpretation forecloses the prospects of formulating advance answers according to some moral logarithm; on the contrary, in some versions of principlism, reaching closure can be annoyingly difficult. Nor does the proposed analogy suggest a uniqueness to principlism: The recent revival of a casuistical method clearly builds on a model of reasoning in the common law as appropriate to the moral life more generally.

Nevertheless, the analogy does highlight several features of principlism that are of theological significance. First, the principles of biomedical ethics are (or, are at least defended as) "prescriptive" rather than "illuminative" principles for moral choices in medicine. That is, they hold a binding or obligatory status that carries more moral weight than a maxim or summary statement of the moral wisdom of past generations. At the same time, the generality and the plurality of the principles require interpretation in light of our experience of the moral life, and thus do not permit giving these prescriptive principles the status of moral absolutes.

Second, the common but minimalistic character of the morality that principlism seeks to explicate means, on one hand, that it expresses values shared with traditions of religious ethics and, on the other, that it does not encompass the moral entirety of such traditions. Principlism includes religious morality to some extent: The religious themes of love of neighbor, stewardship and justice, and the image of God (*imago Dei*) certainly overlap with the central principles of biomedical ethics. However, the correlation is not complete: First, love requires more than a minimal concern for the welfare of others; it does not exist only when there is no or minimal sacrifice to self-interest. Second, we have not fully done justice in a theological account if we limit our moral horizons to a voluntarily assumed contractualism; we must instead expand those horizons by encompassing gift-oriented, covenantal relations or a preferentialism for the voiceless and vulnerable in a society; and finally, autonomy may limit a person's moral interest to making discrete decisions rather than to engaging with the full character and integrity of the person. This overlap and yet tension between principlism and religious morality requires fuller explication.

Part of this tension is revealed by both the principlist commitment to agnosticism about the common human good and its anthropological assumption of human finitude and fallibility. The first feature seeks to preserve consensus about morality, but as a consequence fails to place moral choices in medicine, and in the moral life as a whole, in a broader context of ultimacy that gives such choices purpose and meaning. We mislead ourselves to think we can resolve the question of the ethics of physician-assisted suicide and active euthanasia, for example, by the principles of beneficence and respect for autonomy without recourse to some account of suffering, dignity, and the nature of the self. The second feature conveys a realism about human nature that could easily find a home in much traditional theological anthropology, but it may yet fail to give us a full portrait of the moral self. These tensions will shape the lines of inquiry in the subsequent sections.

Principlism and Prophetic Criticism

To that community of friendly strangers (agents, citizens, judges) found in principlism, the moral discourse of a religious tradition is expressed in the form of a *prophetic witness*. I wish to emphasize two dimensions of this prophetic witness. The first is that it implies a complete and total relativizing of traditional structures and practices, including those of medicine. The witness seeks to describe things as they *really* are and this revealed reality means we cannot ascribe ultimacy to the way things are in the present. This first dimension assures a critical nature to the prophetic witness: it articulates a profound disparity and incongruence between the moral world we live in and that world as it could or should be. It delivers (to draw again on legal imagery) an "indictment" of the status quo (Gustafson 1990:130). One theological criterion of adequacy for a principlist morality, then, is the extent to which it can sustain this critical dimension of a prophetic witness.

A second aspect of moral prophecy is an offer of promise and hope, or what is often referred to as a sense of destiny or eschatology. The witness reveals not only the relativity of our present situation, but the fullness of things as they should (and really will) be. This reality is promised, and it thereby offers hope and direction for the future, not in the sense of a detailed blueprint of programmatic steps, but rather in the articulation of a broad vision of human destiny and ultimacy. The working out of the promise over time is our responsibility as persons and communities. A second criterion of theological adequacy with respect to principlism, then, is the extent to which it can sustain a sense of ends and destiny that gives meaning and purpose to our moral lives.

Let me first develop the critical dimension of a prophetic witness by examining two models used by proponents of principlism to establish the common principles of the moral life. One influential approach might invoke the philosophical method of detachment and disinterested reflection. We divest ourselves from particular interests and parochial convictions, especially our own, in order that we may see more clearly into the nature of the moral life. On this very prominent model, we should be able to discern the binding principles of morality from "no particular point of view" (Nagel 1980:83).

A principal feature of this view of the moral world is that it gains for us precisely that sense of critical distance otherwise unavailable when we are immersed in everyday life. We need to "step back" or "out" of the stream of our lives, deliberate and reflect in a disinterested manner, and then carry this critical consciousness back with us into moral experience as we engage in justification and criticism of actual practices. We can perhaps concede that the model of detached reflection provides this distance, but it does not come without loss.

We first can't achieve such a vision without some kind of division of the moral self, exemplified best by appropriations in biomedical ethics of the Rawlsian notion of the "veil of ignorance," particularly in the area of resource allocation.[1] Our morality toward others turns out to be a morality toward a projected image of one's rational and self-interested self. We gain critical clarity at the expense of personal particularity, and so formulate a morality that turns out to be alien and foreign to the persons we know ourselves to be. We construct a self-interested morality from the mind that has no grounding in our selves as *embodied and relational* persons.

More problematic theologically, the moral view generated by detached reflection marginalizes the religious or spiritual self. As Kent Greenawalt observes in summarizing the suppositions of a Rawlsian method: "...citizens in a liberal democracy should resolve both value and factual questions that are relevant to justice without relying on particular religious convictions" (Greenawalt 1988:53). Religious convictions and worldviews are particular, and are expressed from "somewhere," namely an ongoing moral tradition embodied by a particular community. The veiled, compartmentalized self required by the model of detached reflection, thus, can't accommodate them.

Proponents of this model aren't, to be sure, entirely comfortable with the conclusion that the morality constructed through detached reflection would be foreign and alien to who we are. Thus, they attempt to show in manifold ways how this morality is also coherent with our considered judgments learned through everyday moral experience. We might, of course, then wonder why it was necessary to split the self to construct a morality that may turn out to merely reflect what we already knew and (perhaps) already do. The possibility of criticism within such an account rests finally on this discrepancy between knowledge and action.

This criticism suggests, in any event, a second approach, not so much a disinterested "step back" from life to reflect as a "step forward...into the thicket of moral experience" (Walzer 1987:24). This plunge into particularity may enable us to see the principles of biomedical ethics less as abstract statements of transcendent universals and more as constituting an "*embedded* common morality" (Childress 1989b:88). In this version, principlism expresses obligations that persons from *any* particular point of view could recognize and adopt, be it comprised of a religious, professional, secular, or civic tradition of morality. An embedded principlism enables us to retain a unified self and construct a rooted, lived-in morality that should reflect our embodied and relational experience of the moral world. Moreover, as this common morality is in part embedded in formative religious practices and traditions, this approach does not seem to require marginalizing the religious to the outer boundaries of civic discourse. Instead, religious norms or values, among which are the dignity and equality of persons, can be institutionalized over time in various social practices, including those of medicine.

The embeddedness of such a morality may make it seem incapable of sustaining a sense of critical distance and even a critical self. Nevertheless, as Walter Harrelson suggests, a critical prophetic witness involves judgments on actions and practices that violate the inherited, generally accepted norms of a moral community. The biblical prophets deliver a critique not from "up there" or "nowhere" but by citing the historical standards of the faith community (Harrelson 1986:508–12). The prophetic witness seems like a discovery when in reality it is a *recovery* of the moral tradition. Similarly, an embedded principlism can rely on the accepted norms of common moral life (the principles) as a standard for moral assessment and criticism. We can be critical, for example, of businesses that market health care products without full disclosure to consumers of the possible risks of the product, or physicians who do not inform their patients of alternative treatments, because such firms and professionals, in company with the moral community of friendly strangers, assume and rely on a principle of informed consent as part of a shared morality. To violate such a principle betrays our sense of trust; to be secretive about the violation is to betray the commitment to public accountability.

The capacity to *expose moral hypocrisy*, which is a core ethical feature of a prophetic witness, therefore presumes some common ground for judgment. The prophetic indictment would not be acknowledged in the absence of shared standards or publicly accessible reasons regarding determinations of guilt and innocence. Both the critical capacity and the shared standard are challenged by a question about the validity of the embedded morality itself. Why, for example, we might ask, should informed consent be part of this morality anyway? This is hardly an idle inquiry, since though informed consent is now taken to be a cornerstone of moral medical practice, the history of medicine reveals it was not always such.

The moral critique of professional paternalism has often been articulated through a grand theoretical construct of informed consent, sometimes invoking philosophical notions of "social contract," and occasionally religious themes of "covenant." However, an equally persuasive case can be made for a principle of informed consent within medicine by *remembering* and interpreting the traditions of personal rights and the radical equality of persons embedded in the moral culture of which medicine is a part. A common civic tradition affirmed by friendly moral strangers can provide sources of justification and criticism of practices within specialized professional communities. This critical recollecting and interpreting of shared values in light of ongoing experience points to a second characteristic of a prophetic witness, its role as *memory of the moral community*.

The prophetic memory is particularly significant when moral light needs to be cast upon what has heretofore been darkness, which is frequently the situation in a medical culture driven by an ideology of unrestrained technological progress. Informed consent itself takes on entirely new significance when the practice of medicine can actually benefit people, which was not the case until quite recently, but doing so requires the invasive procedures of innovative medical technology (resuscitation, in vitro fertilization, transplantation, among others). The ever-present challenge of the new and innovative in medicine can threaten to erode our sense of ethical direction, as expressed by the commanding presence of the "technological imperative." The moral logic of that imperative is that we now have entered a transmoral realm, an era in which technology creates its own values. Yet, we find this moral rupture inadequate and instead seek continuities over time in our experience of moral problems. The presence of medical technology does not mean the end of morality as much as the need for interpretation; it signals that the values underlying our embedded morality have come into conflict. The responsibility of bringing these underlying values to the surface of moral discourse so that they can bear directly on innovations in medicine is the prophetic calling of recollection and memory.

I have wanted to contend that a prophetic witness in biomedical ethics need not assume the philosophical model of disinterested, detached reflection. Nor is the prophetic witness necessarily an alien voice; we are just as likely to find a prophetic witness of moral hypocrisy or moral memory drawing upon the embedded, shared values of a culture. In this respect, a prophetic figure or community is less a detached outsider and much more a "connected critic" (Walzer 1987:37–40). I shall address subsequently whether these forms of a prophetic witness are necessarily religious. It is sufficient for now to indicate that these forms illuminate how religious perspectives *are* relevant in biomedical ethics, for we need not look very hard before finding recent examples of both in public moral discourse.

The Roman Catholic critique of proposals to legalize physician-assisted suicide and voluntary, active euthanasia has often appealed to a "consistent ethic of life." As formulated by Joseph Cardinal Bernardin, the basic values of this ethic, such as the sanctity and dignity of human life, are already present in society's moral, legal, and professional ethos. Their origins may lie in the formative religious traditions of Western culture, but they have over time come to form an embedded and shared morality. Moral hypocrisy is displayed when we seek to validate a practice of euthanasia while affirming these common values.

Yet, the *public* (and not merely religious) significance of this ethic lies in its claim that moral consistency is required across a whole range of "life" issues, including abortion, euthanasia, capital punishment, and war. Even advocates of abortion rights, for example, have conceded they would find the moral claims of their opponents more compelling were the commitment to human life advanced comprehensively rather than compartmentalized; otherwise, the appeal to "pro-life" values on abortion really does seem to reduce to an "anti-choice" position. A pro-life perspective that restricts its moral horizons to a single issue may be open to the charge of hypocrisy, then, with respect to other social practices where the value of human life is no less equally threatened.

The consistent ethic of life, of course, is concerned not merely with moral criticism but also with re-collecting and illuminating the embedded morality of society. A further example of prophetic memory is illustrated in an *amicus* brief filed in 1990 by the United Methodist Church in the *Cruzan* case before the U.S. Supreme Court.[2] The brief asked the Court to find in favor of Nancy Cruzan's parents' request to withdraw her feeding tube, a conclusion it held would represent "a broad and deeply held traditional moral consensus," including such core values as "liberty of conscience." As with the consistent ethic of life, it is the "connectedness" of the critique, its reliance on common values, that gives it moral authority in public discourse, though perhaps not ultimately persuasive efficacy.

This latter proviso is necessary because in a community of friendly moral strangers, we may well dispute whether these (and similar examples of prophetic witness) properly interpret the embedded morality or have remembered well enough. Yet, such disputes, whether they occur within a religious community, as in Catholic critiques of the consistent ethic of life, or between religious traditions, as in denominational diversity over proposals for active euthanasia, or between religious and secular traditions, are carried on as interpretive arguments. That is, the possibility of an argument presumes the reality of some shared public standards; otherwise we would not know whether or about what we were arguing. The argument itself contests the content of those standards.

Prophecy and Priestly Routinization

This account of a prophetic witness may appear so broad as to lose any distinctively "religious" features; after all, if the common normative principles of a community constitute the substantive standard of moral criticism, theoretically any reasonable and responsible person who affirms such principles could engage in such a critique, and practically, each of us does. The preceding analysis may then appear to expand the prophetic while eclipsing the religious.

I am not entirely persuaded that this is a valid conclusion. I want to suggest first that the religious traditions of prophecy illuminate the *form* of moral criticism. The prophet speaks to or bears witness against the community in the name of the community's own values. The community's discovery is the prophet's recovery. The model provides an important contrast to alternative approaches that have recently been influential in biomedical ethics. Such approaches hold either that no common values exist and so moral discourse is really a chimera, or that the embeddedness of the values in our discourse calls primarily for clarification rather than for critique. I have wanted to contend instead for the integral relation of common values and moral criticism: the possibility of the latter presumes the presence of the former. The religious traditions of prophecy can then provide a valuable reminder regarding the conditions of moral critique in biomedical ethics.

At the same time, the critical edge of an embedded morality can be diminished. As suggested by Max Weber's account of routinization or rationalization in the development of religious traditions (Weber 1964), for example, certain institutionalized settings of biomedical ethics, such as hospital ethics committees, research review boards, or policy commissions, can risk softening the sharpness of an embedded principlism. A concern with outcomes and conclusions, particularly consensus on policy, can impede processes of substantive moral argument and assessment of various proposals for the question under consideration. Clearly some consensus is necessary to a moral medicine. Principlism can nonetheless run a risk of moral routinization because of its focus on procedures to secure agreement among friendly strangers who disagree about, and thus may not discuss, their ideas of the good. Thus, the emphasis on consensus, on not only shared values but common conclusions, may foster a subtle shift in the moral focus of principlism from critique to legitimation, from restraint to regulation, from indictment to implementation.

Following Weber's language, moral discourse oriented by a practical demand for consensus may come to reflect less of a prophetic and more of a *priestly* ethic. The prophetic witness serves as the basis for priestly activity, in that the priestly form systematizes the content of prophecy and adapts it to practical needs, but the realm of ethical concern is different. The prophetic indicts sins, the priestly constructs a ritual for their confession and forgiveness. The prophetic witnesses to what is not (but should be), the priestly seeks legitimation for what is. The prophetic provides a vision of medicine's ends, the priestly administers and sanctions its means. The priestly is no less necessary, but it is less critical.

Sustaining a balance between a critical and a routinized morality, however, requires a historical embodied community that lives out the tensions between standards and conduct and preserves moral memory through its practices and traditions. Such a community can offer (in Weber's term) *exemplary* prophecy (Weber 1964:55). The moral constituency presumed by philosophical principlism, however, characteristically requires the legal fiction of an audience of "reasonable persons." It is at best a shadow of the kinds of historically viable religious communities present in our culture. These traditions serve as living exemplars of ethical interpretation and exposition, and an embodied moral wisdom or memory.

The religious character of a prophetic witness may then be defended by these three claims regarding the form of moral criticism in biomedical ethics, the routinization of a critical morality, and the exemplary prophecy of an embodied morality. Their relevance can be assessed by considering the evolution of the principle of respect for autonomy in biomedical ethics discourse. It is an overstatement to contend that the very appeal to autonomy should be considered theologically suspect and a symbolic infringement on theonomy. Respect for personal autonomy implies (or should imply) a defining premise of a liberal democratic society, namely, its commitment to religious liberty (Greenawalt 1988:14–29). It is a principle that provides social space for freedom of religious expression. Moreover, such an appeal correlates with the anthropology of the *imago Dei* regarding the moral agency of the self.[3] Nonetheless, the many languages of individualism in biomedical ethics, expressed in diversity over whether the moral principle and obligation we are concerned with is that of "autonomy," "respect for autonomy," or "respect for persons," indicate that the correlation is not one of moral equivalence.

In an earlier medical context dominated by traditions of paternalistic beneficence, an appeal to a principle of autonomy provided a necessary moral critique. Autonomy has subsequently become so routinized, so embedded in the discourse of biomedical ethics, that its moral role has shifted from criticism of professional action to legitimation of patient choice. Indeed, as displayed in the expanding support for physician-assisted suicide and active euthanasia, respecting a person's self-determined choice has come to suggest an *immunity* from public moral scrutiny. The claim that such a decision is a "private" choice seeks to remove it from the realm of public accountability, and indeed, from the realm of publicly accessible reasons. The appeal to privacy, as an expression of personal autonomy, makes it increasingly difficult to determine what moral grounds there would be for not acquiescing in autonomous choices, so long as such choices allow equal autonomy for others.

The routinization of autonomy has not come without moral loss in other ways as well. The autonomous self of biomedical ethics is constituted primarily by the mind, or the legislative will: As H. Tristram Engelhardt, Jr., describes the sociology of our moral relationships, "It is...mind meeting mind in order to create a fabric of obligations" (Engelhardt 1986:129). Moreover, the moral questions about limiting autonomy almost always revolve around "losing one's mind" in some sense. That is, we are concerned about conditions or criteria of competence, of comprehension of information, of contexts of coercion.

What we have neglected to notice is that in the process of constructing a bioethics of mind, what we've really lost are our bodies, emotions, and senses. The self has been split after all into one part self-interested chooser and one part "property," to be used and disposed of at "will." The self we are so concerned with respecting turns out to be disembodied, that is, unlike any self we know and experience. This creates a striking paradox, for if we are not to find a principle of self-determination morally alien, we need to formulate some substantive account of the "self" the principle presupposes. In its stead, however, autonomy offers a truncated self that chooses without any clear sense that we have moral criteria to assess the choice.

A prophetic witness, expressed in the moral memory of a historical and embodied religious tradition, here seems vital to a critical biomedical ethics. That witness calls the moral community to *remember* its collective consciousness of the transcendent dignity of the human person, and in so doing, to *re-member* the moral self. The anthropology of the *imago Dei* offers a moral depth to the self that can facilitate this collective remembering and re-membering. The *imago Dei* does express distinctive capacities for reasoning and rationality, to be sure, but also invokes characteristics of human creativity, the capacity for relationship and community, and responsible, compassionate stewardship for others, *all* of which are experienced through an embodied self. This is not to downplay the diversity of religious interpretations of the self, but it is to contend that this basic anthropological claim precludes a reduction of the self to a rationally self-interested chooser, the ascendent model of the self in biomedical ethics.

Moreover, the presence and practices of a living community witness to the radical *dependency* of human beings. We are born vulnerable and completely reliant on others for our being and quality of being, for care, nourishment, and sustenance. We acquire a sense of self-identity and integrity in our relationality with others and through the dialogue of I-Thou relationships. We learn through our experience of illness, aging, and mortality that powers beyond our control govern our lives, and thus, qualify our aspirations to independence. Our experience of vulnerability and dependency sustains our capacity for compassion. The commonality of dependency itself gives rise to a community of moral equality.

Prophetic Promise

I have wanted, then, to suggest the possibility of a distinctive religious presence in biomedical ethics because the prophetic tasks of exposing moral hypocrisy and expressing moral memory require a lived and embodied ethical tradition and a community with a history that makes it capable of remembering. Yet a third (and perhaps more prominent) image of a prophetic witness is iconoclastic: The moral tradition of a community is not so much recovered and remembered as shattered and replaced by a morality rooted in a new vision of communal life and social order. This vision of prophetic promise invokes understandings of ultimate human destiny and meaning, both personal and collective. It offers hope for transformation from present societal conventions and practice toward a just and peaceable community. It provides a moral critique of the present state of affairs, to be sure, but the source of that critique is less embedded ethical standards than the affirmation of promise and transformation; indeed, the critique is unintelligible without the promise. In this respect, little accommodation seems possible with a morality that assumes agnosticism about the human good; the prophetic promise seeks to make such questions unavoidable in moral discourse.

A prophetic promise thus presupposes a very particularized vision of the good. While it involves a sense of transformation that is transcendent — that is, of going beyond the present to the more fundamental reality of the promise — unlike the philosophical method of detached reflection, it is a substantive vision pronounced from "somewhere" rather than a morally agnostic view pronounced from nowhere. Yet, this very particularity of the promise looks at first to be a vice more than a virtue when we consider its relevance for the moral concerns of the community of friendly strangers. Indeed, in Weberian language, such an account may be perceived as "irrational" when measured against the general norms for publicly accessible reasons for decisions (Weber 1958:296); in more contemporary language, this vision of the moral world invites moral incommensurability.

The prophetic promise of transformation seems to assume, then, the character less of the connected critic and more of the marginalized voice in the wilderness. Since the promise and the moral critique are integrally related, one who disagrees with the sense of ultimate ends envisioned by the promise may disavow the critique as well. The strong inclination, then, will be to dismiss the prospects for public relevance of this form of prophetic witness.

We cannot ignore, of course, the regularity with which radical breaks from a religious, political, or cultural tradition occur, that issue in new forms of community with distinctive practices and ways of life. The appeal of a prophetic promise is recurrent rather than aberrational, as persons may seek to embody the reality of the promise in the reality of the present. Such a community does offer exemplary prophecy in that its practical expression of a prophetic promise, its moral practices and patterns of life, can witness to alternative ideals and meanings in human relationships. A tradition that takes seriously its formative narratives regarding, for example, hospitality to the stranger and embodies those as part of its common life can, through its practices of personal and collective care, both indict the social scandal of treating the medically indigent as abandoned outcast and display constructive social alternatives. Perhaps the reasons for such practices are not publicly accessible, but the patterns of care and of life can be.

Moreover, even in a pluralistic society committed to common ground for moral discourse, the practice of medicine unavoidably raises what Kent Greenawalt refers to as issues of "borderlines of status," which in turn expand the standards of public accessibility. When does life begin and when does it end? Are persons in persistent vegetative state dying or already dead? What characteristics are necessary for an entity to be considered part of the moral community? When we confront such borderlines, Greenawalt contends, "everyone must reach beyond commonly accessible reasons to decide many [such] social issues and...religious bases for such decisions should not be disfavored in comparison with other possible bases" (Greenawalt 1988:113, 144–72). In resolving such issues, appeals turn on metaphysical (if not explicitly religious) or at least particularistic convictions that are not publicly shared.

The above discussion suggests we need to distinguish between a publicly shared position and the public relevance of a position that is not commonly shared. David Tracy, for example, has argued that we misplace the question of the relevance of religious discourse in the public realm if we focus only on questions of "origins," that is, on the particularistic and unshared source of an account of morality. Because of claims to divine authority or revelations, the traditions of religious ethics fall precisely into this category of origins, which for some biomedical ethicists becomes a license for dismissal. The obsession with origins is misdirected in two important respects, however. First, because our very notions of "public" and of "rationality" turn out to be historical and communal (particularistic) constructs, we risk rendering public moral discourse vacuous and incoherent, and seeing "reasonable argument...exit from the public realm" (Tracy 1986:119). If such a moral discourse were valid (and our experience of the moral life as well as philosophical principlism presume that morality is in fact worth arguing about), no legitimate reason would exist for giving preferential status to a philosophical or a professional morality while marginalizing a religious ethical tradition, since the origin of each is particular.

Furthermore, the obsession with origins makes us lose sight of "effects," or the ways in which a particular tradition informs and shapes public discourse. On Tracy's account, for example, "every classic work of art or religion is highly particular in both origin and expression yet deeply public in result" (Tracy 1986:119). That is, such works disclose perspectives and interpretations of reality and the moral world that are capable of being shared and communicated in the company of friendly strangers. This disclosure may occur in part through narrative discourse and story telling; a story about a traveler who is assaulted and robbed, ignored by passers-by, and finally cared for by a stranger and adversary can assist the broader community in its interpretive quest to understand obligations of assistance and rescue, and the relations between morality and law. A philosopher like Judith Thomson achieves a very public effect by recourse to a very particular story like the biblical parable of the Good Samaritan (Thomson 1971:62–4). The stories themselves do not of course resolve the issue, but they can dissolve preconceived assumptions and answers by helping us see a moral problem or situation in a new way or perspective. In so doing, we are relying on the interpretive skills of analogy and imagination to bring the story from its original context (for example, as a response to a question about the meaning of love) to public relevance.

A witness of prophetic promise, which would certainly qualify as "highly particular" in source or origins owing to its rootedness in a specific, substantive account of the good, may nevertheless contain public relevance through "effects." Yet, why should we expect a particular vision of human destiny, perhaps embedded in a narrative or embodied in a community, to have any public results? The answer, I wish to contend, is that the promise of transformation, no less than the other forms of prophetic witness, must reach and engage common human realities. It does so less by the ultimate destiny and values it posits as by the *questions* presupposed by those values. That is, the promise is one particular response to questions of common concern for all persons.

Our moral selves are constituted not only by reason, will, embodiment, creativity, and sociality, but also by a distinct capacity for self-transcendence. We do "stand back" from the ebb-and-flow of daily life and reflect, not in the disinterested way of the philosophical method of detached reflection but in a profoundly personal and interested manner on the nature and purpose of our lives. We engage the kinds of questions thrust upon us in ultimate situations: our experience of origins and our perplexities about identity; the lived realities of unfairness, dependency, frustration, and evil; the presence of pain and suffering; and our anticipation of death and destiny. These ultimate situations, and the questions of *meaning* they elicit, are inescapably common human concerns, and it is precisely these questions that a prophetic promise must engage in the evolution from particular origins to public effects. Though the ultimate values and vision may not be shared, the ultimacy of the questions such values presuppose is.

It is, moreover, such questions that are unavoidably embedded in the practice of medicine. We cannot escape coming up against our finitude and dependency, against the reality and limits of our embodied selves, against the meaning of our mortality, as we experience cycles of illness and recovery, or protracted periods of pain and suffering, or the process of aging that culminates ultimately in our deaths. This has several important implications for a prophetic presence in biomedical ethics. First, philosophical principlism and philosophical approaches to biomedical ethics more generally have not, by their own admission (Engelhardt 1985:79–91), devoted sufficient attention to such matters; it should not be surprising, then, if we find such approaches to be humanly lacking or incomplete.

By contrast, a quest for meaning has historically been at the core of religious communities and their ethical traditions. The relevance of the prophetic promise for biomedical ethics thus lies in according greater prominence to this quest and in offering particular but substantive understandings of its nature. For example, we know (though we frequently engage in denial) that we will die; we assert in response our desire/right to a "death with dignity." We will, however, likely find ourselves perplexed as persons and caregivers as to how to achieve such a death, unless we have resources that enable us to understand what it is to *live* with dignity, and how dignity is related to our aspirations of control over both our living and dying, and to our common experience of dependency.

As the prophetic promise is rooted in a vision of ultimacy and destiny, it can offer a context of meaning for the central experiences and questions of our lives. Without that context, it's unclear why a question about the manner of dying would even arise personally, let alone be a matter addressed in public policy forums, or encouraged through advance directive legislation. I want to consider these themes through two primary illustrations.

The Quest for Meaning and Biomedical Ethics

In a society of friendly moral strangers, our procedural commitments often entail that questions in biomedical ethics are reduced to an issue of the boundaries of public intervention in private choice or, in the language of principlism, a conflict between beneficent paternalism and respect for personal autonomy. So long as the individual is competent, informed about the nature of his or her actions and its potential risks for self-imposed harm, and deliberating voluntarily, a heavy burden of moral proof is imposed on others, whether it be family, professional caregivers, or even the state, to justify restrictions on personal choices.

The contemporary controversy over legalized euthanasia is a prime illustration of this boundary issue, and yet the principlist framework for resolving the conflict seems inadequate because embedded in the central moral arguments are convictions and questions about human nature and destiny. Thus, the permissibility of euthanasia often first rests on an appeal to the basic dignity of patients, which can be met only by the exercise of control and empowerment over dying. This coupling of human dignity with an ideology of control may be problematic, especially as so much of our lived experience is beyond personal control and choice. Are we only fully human when we achieve mastery of the contingencies of life? It is also a striking paradox that one asserts control only to subsequently relinquish it to the other person, who has consented to take life. We affirm liberty of the self to be subject to the power (medical and moral) of another.

It is also argued that euthanasia is a morally compassionate and humane response to the problem of patient pain and suffering. This appeal coheres nicely with a medical ethos that has taken as a primary objective the eradication of pain and suffering. Thus, in a culture conditioned to expect magic bullets to provide instantaneous technological relief and remedy, the protracted pain and suffering present in dying can be experienced as an unbearable personal burden and an assault on this dominant medical ideology.

We need to ask, however, whether such a moral claim seeks to ensure us an immunity from our humanity. Not all pain is pointless; not all suffering is purposeless. While we naturally experience a reflexive, inward response to our own (experience of) pain and suffering, it can also turn us outward, enabling our capacity to respond with a compassionate presence to the bodily and psychic afflictions of others. This appeal for legalized euthanasia seems thus to reflect a flight from compassion rather than an expression of compassion (McCormick 1991:1132–34).

While much pain is susceptible to medication and relief (indeed, physicians who perform euthanasia in the Netherlands contend *all* pain is medically manageable), and the need for more research into pain control is undisputed, in an important sense the suffering experienced in terminal illness is technologically incorrigible. The common failure in the ethics literature on euthanasia to differentiate between "pain" and "suffering," and instead to portray suffering as but an extreme on a pain continuum, reflects an attempt to *medicalize* suffering. Yet, suffering defies such medicalization because people experience it as a crisis or threat to the identity and integrity of the self, one that understandably becomes particularly poignant and acute with the onset of terminal illness. The self we once knew and experienced seems to fade both in memory and bodily capability; even if we retain some sense of who we were, we become less sure of who we are or will be.

The moral problem is thus the pretensions of defining suffering as a medical problem. As William F. May suggests, some "problems" in biomedical ethics can be solved, but others have to be faced and lived through (May 1991:3), and suffering is clearly among the latter. It seems tragically misguided to believe we can achieve the medical end of eliminating suffering by eliminating the sufferer. We need simultaneously to discuss whether eliminating suffering should be an end of medicine. This is not to dispute the truth of the observation of Dr. Rieux in *The Plague* that it is preferable to relieve suffering than portray its excellence; it is, however, to suggest that the medicalization of suffering contains its own moral logic that bears examination.

My point here is not to resolve the controversy over legalized euthanasia, but rather to indicate that it invokes deep substantive questions of meaning that the moral horizons of a principlist framework obscure. The "problem" does not merely concern the legitimacy of restrictions on private choices, but the nature of the self — its dignity, identity, and integrity; the paradox of self — and medical mastery over the human condition; the place of suffering and death within medicine; the ideal of a good death within human life as a whole. Such questions of meaning give us some context within which to locate the ethical issue. They enable problem "seeing," which is a necessary complement to the principlist preoccupation with problem "solving." Unfortunately, where we most need a collective conversation, we find a moral void, and the agnosticism of principlism renders it existentially empty or alien when we confront the ultimate situations of our lives.

Another illustration of how the boundary limits of principlism unavoidably open up to a deeper, meaning-full level of discourse is provided by debates over public policies to address the scarcity of transplantable organs. One alternative that has gained increasing support is an organ market, which (subject to procedural safeguards) would allow for commerce in bodily parts between vendors and buyers. For some proponents, such an approach seems consistent with respecting autonomy, and current legal restrictions and moral objections express a well-intentioned but finally misguided paternalism. Opponents, meanwhile, raise the specter of exploitation and inequity, and the moral loss that would attend transforming a "gift" and community-affirming model into one governed by principles of consumerism and *caveat emptor.*

An organ market may or may not "solve" the problem of organ scarcity, but when the question is reduced to a conflict between principles of autonomy and altruistic beneficence, we risk a severe case of moral myopia. One context of meaning for the organ scarcity problem concerns the social embeddedness of autonomous choices, as dramatically illuminated by a recent situation in which a Turkish father sold his kidney to pay for his daughter's operation. This prompted assessments of organ sales as "utterly repugnant" and the proposal of legislation to prohibit such sales (Kinsley 1989:88). What is really repugnant, however, is the kind of social inequality that allows a person's alternatives to be limited to "your kidney or your daughter's life." The denunciation of the sale misses the point about the need to rectify the deeper social injustice. The provision of goods to meet basic human needs, including needs for both health care and education, is required before we can say a choice is made autonomously rather than under duress.

A second context of meaning has instead to do with a very basic concern about the relation of self-identity and embodiment. That is, if personal identity is distinct from one's body, we are much more likely to see the body as comprised of "parts" (a mechanistic metaphor) available for exchange in a commercial market, or as "property" (an economic-legal metaphor) that can be alienated, transferred, and used according to rights of self-ownership. Alternatively, if embodiment is intrinsic to self-identity, we may see the selling of an organ as a symbolic selling of the self.

The property metaphor reflects not only a capacity for alienation (transfer) *of* the body, but also a condition of alienation (estrangement) *from* the body. This latter condition is present, I have already suggested, in our efforts in biomedical ethics to construct a morality for disembodied persons. The consequence of this disembodiment is not merely a different picture of the self, but rather a self that shuns deeper questions of meaning precisely because it lacks depth. Indeed, as Morris Berman suggests in his provocative *Coming to Our Senses,* the profound sense of hollowness we experience in our lives, the void of meaning in contemporary culture, is attributable to our lack of being "rooted" or "grounded" in bodily experience (Berman 1990:19–62).

It's not the case then that the quest for meaning is an intellectual journey that engages and stimulates the mind. Rather, the quest is unintelligible when we alienate the body from the self. To the extent that it reflects this condition of estrangement, it should be little wonder that contemporary biomedical ethics, including principlism, has minimal room for questions of purpose and ultimacy, nor again, that we find these models of moral experience humanly incomplete or unsatisfying.

The quest for meaning within biomedical ethics, and thus the relevance of biomedical ethics to human experience, therefore requires a shift in our appraisal of the body. Seeing the body as merely a machine or tool for medical manipulation, or as private property for personal disposal, does not do justice to the sentiment of respect and dignity appropriate to an embodied self. The prophetic promise of the body as "temple" or "sanctuary" calls us instead to re-member the self through remembering the body. The tasks of remembering, in both senses, are very much embedded in the current gift model of organ procurement and transplantation; indeed, it might be seen as a paradigm practice of remembering. It quite literally involves a process of dismemberment to obtain an organ and a re-membering of the body of another (and thus of the person's self) through the transplant operation. Moreover, relatives who give permission for the donation of organs often speak of their deceased loved one as "living on" in the recipient; that is, they are engaged in a process of memory and remembering. A context that holds such profound human meaning and moral depth is unlikely to be sustained if we transform organ transplantation into a practice of commerce governed by the rules of selling assets and property.

Reclaiming the Prophetic Voice

This exploration of three moral meanings of prophecy in biomedical ethics has suggested ways in which moral themes in religious traditions would not so much supplant as supplement principlism. It also clearly implies the prospects of connections between these themes and other emerging critiques of principlism. The characteristics of voice (witness), memory, and body, for example, are likewise prominent features of feminist perspectives in medical ethics. The central role attributed to interpretation in a prophetic account is of course at the core of hermeneutical approaches. The reliance on exemplary character and story as a prophetic witness evolves from particularistic origins to public effects also suggests common ground with approaches that emphasize the role of virtues or narratives. A dialogue between these various paradigms is not only possible but promises mutual influence. Furthermore, while religious traditions do not have a moral monopoly over the three forms of prophetic witness, they are nevertheless best socially situated to express a credible witness in biomedical ethics because they are visible, embodied communities of moral discourse and meaning.

In a very fundamental sense, the presence of theological voices in biomedical ethics offers a window through which we can view the larger question of the place of religious convictions in a liberal, pluralistic society. The moral and political premises of such a society can of course be contested, and influential theologians have explored this alternative. I have instead tried to illustrate how, even if one accepts the principlist premise of common ground for moral discourse, embedded in the practice of medicine are "borderline" questions in which recourse to religious convictions may be necessary and appropriate. When these borderlines must be resolved for purposes of public policy, religious perspectives need not be compartmentalized from the ethical, but rather translated into concepts that reflect the embedded morality and ethos of the society. The public resonance to the "consistent ethic of life" morality displays this approach most prominently and persuasively. At the same time, it is important to resist efforts to make biomedical ethics co-extensive with the realm of public policy.

The presence of a prophetic witness, embedded in particular communities, is in any event important to the vitality of contemporary biomedical ethics, lest its discourse become increasingly distanced from human experience and increasingly meaningless. The moral agnosticism of principlism and a bioethics of the mind do not do justice to our embodied, relational self that quests for meaning and purpose. The practice of medicine makes an encounter with both body and quest unavoidable;

we thus neglect the witness of religious traditions and communities at the peril of who we are and can be.

NOTES

Acknowledgments — The author wishes to acknowledge the constructive criticism made on this paper by participants at a conference at the Park Ridge Center in October 1991, as well as that offered by Dr. B. Andrew Lustig of the Center for Ethics, Medicine, and Public Issues, Baylor University.

1. In *A Theory of Justice*, John Rawls is concerned to identify the principles a rationally self-interested person would choose in a hypothetical original position to govern basic social and political institutions. The fairness and impartiality of this process, notwithstanding self-interest, is ensured by a veil of ignorance, in which participants are ignorant of their personal characteristics and social endowments, their social position, and their historical period; see Rawls 1971:136–42.

2. Brief of the General Board of Church and Society of the United Methodist Church as amicus curiae in Support of Petitioners, *Cruzan v. Director of Missouri Department of Health*, 1989:1–5.

3. The biblical creation narratives relate that human beings are created in the image of God, and subsequent narratives ground the prohibition of taking human life in this same theological anthropology. Subsequent theological discussion has sought to identify those features by which we image God, thereby asserting a conception not only of person but also of God and their relatedness. Some theologians have concentrated on reason and free will and the effects of human fallenness and sin on our rationality and freedom. Still others have focused on the wholeness of an embodied self. The image of God provides a theological ground for values of freedom, equality, the sanctity of human life, and stewardship. An insightful discussion of the relevance of the image of God for bioethics is found in Bouma et al. 1989:27–66.

REFERENCES

Berman, Morris. 1990. *Coming to Our Senses.* New York: Bantam Books.

Bouma, Hessel III, Douglas Diekema, Edward Langerak, Theodore Rottman, and Allen Verhey. 1989. *Christian Faith, Health, and Medical Practice.* Grand Rapids, Mich.: Eerdmans.

Brief of the General Board of Church and Society of the United Methodist Church. 1989:1–5.

Calvin, John. 1960. *Institutes of the Christian Religion,* II.vii., ed. John T. McNeill. Philadelphia: Westminster Press.

Caplan, Arthur L. 1982. "Applying Morality to Advances in Biomedicine: Can and Should This Be Done?" In *New Knowledge in the Biomedical Sciences,* ed. William B. Bondeson, H. Tristram Engelhardt, Jr., Stuart F. Spicker, and Joseph M. White, 155–68. Dordrecht: D. Reidel.

Childress, James F. 1989a. "The Normative Principles of Medical Ethics." In *Medical Ethics*, ed. Robert M. Veatch, 27–48. Boston: Jones and Bartlett.

———. 1989b. "Ethical Criteria for Procuring and Distributing Organs for Transplantation." In *Journal of Health Politics, Policy and Law* 14:87–113.

Cox, Harvey, ed. 1968. *The Situation Ethics Debate*. Philadelphia: Westminster Press.

Engelhardt, H. Tristram, Jr. 1986. *The Foundations of Bioethics*. New York: Oxford University Press.

———. 1985. "Looking for God and Finding the Abyss: Bioethics and Natural Theology." In *Theology and Bioethics: Exploring the Foundations and Frontiers*, ed. Earl E. Shelp, 79–91. Dordrecht: D. Reidel.

Greenawalt, Kent. 1988. *Religious Convictions and Political Choice*. New York: Oxford University Press.

Gustafson, James M. 1990. "Moral Discourse about Medicine: A Variety of Forms." *The Journal of Medicine and Philosophy* 15:125–42

———. 1971. *Christian Ethics and the Community*. Philadelphia: Pilgrim Press.

Harrelson, Walter. 1986. "Prophetic Ethics." In *The Westminster Dictionary of Christian Ethics*, ed. James F. Childress and John Macquarrie, 508–12. Philadelphia: Westminster Press.

Kinsley, Michael. 1989. "Take My Kidney, Please." *Time* (13 March): 88.

May, William F. 1991. *The Patient's Ordeal*. Bloomington: Indiana University Press.

McCormick, Richard A. 1991. "Physician-Assisted Suicide: Flight from Compassion." *The Christian Century* 108 (4 December): 1132–34.

Nagel, Thomas. 1980. "The Limits of Objectivity." In *The Tanner Lectures on Human Values*, vol. 1. Salt Lake City: University of Utah Press.

Niebuhr, H. Richard. 1963. *The Responsible Self*. San Francisco: Harper and Row.

Rawls, John. 1971. *A Theory of Justice*. Cambridge: Harvard University Press.

Thomson, Judith Jarvis. 1971. "A Defense of Abortion." *Philosophy and Public Affairs* 1:47–66.

Toulmin, Stephen. 1981. "The Tyranny of Principles." *Hastings Center Report* 11 (December): 31–9.

Tracy, David. 1986. "Particular Classics, Public Religion, and the American Tradition." In *Religion and American Public Life: Interpretations and Explorations*, ed. Robin W. Lovin, 115–31. New York: Paulist Press.

Walzer, Michael. 1987. *Interpretation and Social Criticism*. Cambridge: Harvard University Press.

Weber, Max. 1964. *The Sociology of Religion*, trans. Ephraim Fischoff. Boston: Beacon Press.

———. 1958. "The Social Psychology of the World Religions." In *From Max Weber: Essays in Sociology*, ed. H. H. Gerth and C. Wright Mills. New York: Oxford University Press.

~ *Part Three* ~

Currents in U.S.
Biomedical Ethics

~ 9 ~

EXPERIENCE AND MORAL LIFE
A PHENOMENOLOGICAL APPROACH TO BIOETHICS

Richard M. Zaner

This essay veers away from the prevailing view in biomedical ethics: the applied, or principlist, view. Working within clinical settings for the past decade has convinced me that it is erroneous to begin with presumptions, even the presumptions that physicians are supposed to be governed by beneficence and patients by autonomy. These are important notions, to be sure, and cannot be ignored in an essay grappling with the many complex issues intrinsic to clinical encounters. It is nonetheless perhaps more productive to probe these encounters in more depth than has been usual, before making up one's mind about such austere matters as ethical principles.

As it seems untoward to introduce a Grand Duchess to assembled personages too early in the evening, so does it seem premature to address such grand issues as "principles" at a time when ethical deliberations within clinical life have only just begun. Too much remains obscure and likely to be overlooked following that course. A genuine phenomenology of clinical life and work must first be attempted, the multiple themes and characteristics of illness and medicine unraveled — a project of major proportions — before we can probe the highest, or most foundational, notions in moral life and ethical theory, much less determine their bearing on practical life.

So far as I can tell, only a handful of serious efforts have been made to understand the complicated discipline of medicine. Among the finest came almost at the beginning of Western medicine: Galen's attempt at a synthesis of Plato, Aristotle, and ancient medicine. The only similar attempt at a theory of medicine in our times — Scott

Buchanan's lucid *Doctrine of Signatures* — fell on deaf ears when published in 1938 and has been mostly ignored since. A thoughtful probing of Galen's vision, Buchanan's Aristotelian interpretation certainly deserves study by any who would pretend to understand medicine and its moral issues. Its reprinting (Buchanan 1991) is a seminal event that can occasion the reflection so much needed within present-day biomedical ethics.

Another caveat is appropriate. As I have suggested elsewhere (Zaner 1981a), matters pertaining to the spirit are vital to any venture into issues of health and illness, grief and loss, life and death. For my present purposes, such questions had to be put aside, but a full discussion of ethics and medicine must at some point come to grips with those weighty questions. A true phenomenological approach, of course, can never decide issues in advance, but must take them up when, and if, the proper wits and grace are granted. Now to the matter at hand.

Consider any one of the quite typical "case presentations" reported in current medical journals. For instance:

> A 22-year-old healthy nonsmoking man presented after coughing up a cup of bright-red blood. The initial history and physical examination were unremarkable. A chest roentgenogram, arterial blood gas levels, the complete blood count, indexes of coagulation, the platelet count, and the blood urea nitrogen concentration were all normal. (Conetta, Tamarin, et al. 1987)

Other diagnostic tests and results are reported, as is the bare fact that the patient was "additionally questioned," though nothing of what was then elicited is reported.

We might well wonder just who this man is, whether he has any family or friends, what he does for a living, where he was and what he was doing before going or being taken to the hospital, and how he got there — or any number of questions prompted simply by the fact that this "case report" is not about rocks or twigs but about a sick person. How is it that sick people are "presented" in this manner? What is meant when it is said that his history is "unremarkable"? Indeed, what is presented: the person or merely "the disease"?

To ask such questions is to invite an exploration into the heart of modern medicine (Baron 1981). It is, indeed, to invite thinking about "cases" in a somewhat different manner. For instance, consider another type of case report.

A Clinical Encounter

Some time ago, our maternal-fetal unit asked me to consult on an "abortion problem." A twenty-two-year-old married woman had been referred for evaluation and management of her first pregnancy. An ultrasound (US) by her private obstetrician had showed something unusual, though he wasn't sure what it was. He determined that her pregnancy was in its twenty-second week (plus or minus two weeks), and this was confirmed by a second US, which also noted a myelomeningocele along with possible ventricular dilatation (spina bifida with patent spinal lesion and protrusion). Informed of these results, the woman was also told that the radiologists couldn't be completely certain of their diagnosis; for greater accuracy, serial US would be needed, to see whether the hydrocephalus was developing. The possibility of an abortion was mentioned: the woman was told that abortion was at that time a therapeutic option but that Tennessee law prohibits abortions after twenty-four weeks' gestation (without documented threat to her life). Because she was rapidly approaching the cutoff date, waiting for even a week might prohibit abortion. On the other hand, an alpha-feto protein (AFP) test could provide further information, with results available in a day or so. The test was done, and the woman was informed that her alpha-feto protein levels were elevated, strongly suggesting the presence of spina bifida. She was also told that, as with the US, the diagnosis was still not 100 percent certain, because AFP tests show a "statistically significant" number of false positives (as well as false negatives). With these two indications in hand, nevertheless, a therapeutic abortion was offered.

At one point, one physician told me that "she seems angry, and feels that we're being deliberately unclear" about the tests. He thought her "agitation" and "anger" were directed at him for offering a "therapeutic abortion," and because of the "ethical controversy" about this, he thought I might help. She seemed to me indeed agitated, anxious, and angry, but it was not clear that these emotions were directed at the physician.

On meeting the couple, I first told them that my role was to help them to think carefully about their situation in light of their own beliefs. It was clear that they understood matters quite well: there was a "good chance" that their baby had multiple congenital anomalies; abortion was one option for them, but if they did not opt for abortion now, they would shortly not have that option. If the pregnancy continued, there was a "good chance" that labor might have to be induced before full term, possibly by cesarean section (because of fetal head size), with neonatal care thereafter: shunting the hydrocephalus, surgery to close the spinal lesion, ventilator assistance, and so on.

As it turned out, their feelings were quite directed, but not at the physician for being unclear or suggesting abortion, not at themselves (even though it was unplanned, they had welcomed the pregnancy), and not even more globally at God or "things." Something else disturbed them: "How in the world can we decide what to do? The doctor just doesn't understand what it's like for us. It's not that we are opposed to abortion, but what if the tests are wrong, and there is nothing wrong with our baby? But if the tests are right, and we don't abort, that's not right, either; it's just not right to bring a baby into the world with so much going against it! Put yourself in our shoes: is it right to force a baby to be a hero just to stay alive...and for how long? What will its quality of life be, with all the pain and suffering it will have? We know we've got to decide, but it's just not fair!"

Clearly, the "problem" was not abortion, neither for them nor the physician. The issue seemed to them a harsh dilemma. Any decision they made at that time, verging on twenty-four weeks, would be irreversible yet could be based only on uncertain information. My suggestion that the hard issue for them concerned that "basis" hit home immediately: "How," the husband blurted out, "can anybody be asked to make such a decision when the tests could be wrong?" His wife continued, "But how can we decide to continue with the pregnancy if the tests are right?" "I know they're only trying to do their best," she continued plaintively, "but the way they talk, we don't know what to think. Once we've decided, we can't 'undecide,' and the basis for it is just not certain enough for that kind of decision. For that, you ought to be able to be more certain!"

My observation, given as gently and sincerely as I could, that "moral life is unhappily like that: sometimes very critical matters have to be decided on the basis of uncertain evidence," was received with understanding, but with anguish as well. We probed the options if pregnancy were continued and the baby did have patent spina bifida, as well as the other possibilities if it did not. Most important, I thought, was for them to be very clear that they had thought about each of the possibilities as thoroughly as they could, so that in the aftermath of their decision, they would be less likely to berate themselves with thoughts of "if only we had..."

They should not, I suggested, demand more of themselves than was reasonable at the time, and they had to make their decision within these circumstances. I also reminded them that not deciding would still be a crucial decision. "You mean," the woman responded, "that all we can do is just decide, even if it turns out we are wrong?" "No," I said, "but you have to try to figure out just what they're telling you about the US and the AFP test: they said there is a 'statistically significant chance' that the AFP was a 'false positive' and that the radiologists were '75 percent confident' of their interpretation." "But what does all that mean?" the husband asked. "Precisely," I responded. "If 'statistically significant' is translated, it means something like 3–5 percent." "What?" the woman broke in. "Then there's a 95–97 percent chance the test is right?" "Not only that," I responded. "The radiologists think their reading is very likely correct — 3 out of 4 chances. Put that together with the AFP test: both are more likely correct than not."

They understood that "uncertainty" was not a single thing but rather presented them with the need to consider chances and risks, to weigh and consider information in the light of "likelihoods" — not too differently from how many of us think about weather reports. To some, a "30 percent chance of rain tomorrow" means it will rain on them; to others, that it won't; while still others. . . .

Moral life invariably involves deliberating about chances, risks, and likelihoods within a specific situation and its particular circumstances, and on that basis having to choose. Because choices involve accepting responsibility, moreover, it is best that we weigh and consider as thoroughly as possible what makes our lives worthwhile. "If the unfortunate turns out," I concluded, "then however much sadness and anguish you feel, at least you'll have the strong, clear sense that you did the best you could have done, in the light of your best understanding of the situation you actually face."

I have obviously shortened the actual conversation with the couple, and an equally key part of this "consult" involved the physicians and nurses. It was important, after all, to clear up the misunderstanding, to stress how the couple had interpreted the statistical formulation of uncertainty, and to be very clear about the basic moral issue they faced.

Disclosing the Moral

This "case" involves a number of experiences and interpretations. The couple, the physician, and I experienced the couple's difficulties, and each of the parties involved experienced relationships with the others. Moreover, everyone involved interpreted the experience as having a "moral" dimension.

From the outset, the encounter was a temporally unfolding context consisting of a complex set of interrelationships among persons

variously experiencing and interpreting one another.[1] Of particular significance were the perils to the fetus and the pregnancy, and these evoked
moral as well as medical concern. The doctor's initial construal of the
situation as *moral* arose from a rather typified understanding of "bioethics problems" — abortion being a main item on the canonical list. In
fact, however, the couple's concern did not stem from moral anger over
 abortion but from their having to make an irreversible decision on the
basis of uncertain diagnostic information.

They understood that dilemma to be the centering moral issue, and
five subthemes shaped their situation: (1) the couple's concern to do
right, to be good, and to act justly; (2) the prospective baby's future
implied by any decision reached; (3) the doctor's concern to do right, to
be good, and to act fairly in relation to both the developing fetus and its
parents (with a concern also to act consistently with professional codes
and established practices); (4) the couple's distress over the confusing
uncertainties; and (5) the doctor's dismay over the anger he thought was
directed at him.

In general, then, they understood *moral* implicitly and at times even
explicitly as connected with doing right, being good, and acting fairly as
they made the decisions and considered the consequences (so far as these
could be known) implied by each alternative. Both the couple and the
physician were primarily focused on the developing fetus and, although
in different ways, on the couple themselves (their well-being now and
in the aftermath).[2] On the other hand, neither of them was focally concerned about the doctor, although trust and physician competence were
doubtless background issues.

Within this encounter, then, *moral* has initially two main senses: a
concern for the *present* welfare (right, good, justice) or detriment (wrong,
bad, injustice) of others; and a concern evoked by alternative decisions
about the welfare or detriment of people in relation to the *future*, that is,
the aftermaths of present decisions for each of the parties individually,
for the relationship between husband and wife, and for the baby.

Disclosing Experience

Although their experiences were textured by different feelings and
thoughts, each of the individuals felt caught up in a perilous adventure.
Their involvements had the sense of uncertain and forbidding paths and
eventualities, of a troubling trial or test.[3] To listen to the wife's words,
for instance, was to be immediately alerted to hazards faced by her baby
and by her and her husband (indeed, dangers to their marriage), and

to their sense of alarming inability to know what to do. Implicit in the passionate words of the doctor about "anger" were an alert — "watch out when you're dealing with this couple, for they are difficult, given to anger" — and a clear warning that, because abortion was the presumed "problem," one needed to be on guard for the well-known controversies abortion always provokes.

Thus, harbingers of possible pitfalls and precarious risks marked the doctor's and the couple's conversations and physiognomic expressions at the outset. The couple's poignant plea for help in understanding things and reaching a decision, for instance, harbored a prominent sense of vulnerability. Though *they* had to make the decision, they had to trust *others* — the doctor and the radiologists — for the information without which no right, good, or just decision could be made. The doctor, on the other hand, already conversant with ultrasound diagnosis and AFP tests and their interpretation, seemed both cautious and impatient. Although aware of potential risks, and apparently ready for the matter to be decided, he nevertheless seemed to them reluctant to proceed with any alternative. Yet he seemed confident that the diagnosis was correct. He did confide in me that he knew very well what the future looked like for such a fetus and that he was inclined toward abortion. He seemed somewhat disturbed that things were not immediately obvious to the couple. He doubtless communicated that peculiar mixture of caution and impatience to the couple. His mixed message may well have prompted their strong reactions, which the doctor saw as "anger" toward him, and even their sense that "the doctor just doesn't understand what it's like for us."

The Doctor-Patient Relationship

What interests me about such cases are the *relationships* between the people involved. That is not, of course, a focal concern for either patients and families or physicians. Although the relationship may come up at some point for either party (as when someone asks either of them how they got along), neither has that as a central topic of concern. The doctor is concerned with and is accountable for the welfare of his patients; the patients want their distress and difficulties resolved.

This relationship (indeed, every helping relationship) is special in several ways. First, although the wife and the doctors were complete strangers, the initial history, physical examination, and ultrasound procedure involved highly intimate contacts. Not only her body but also her very self and family life were, in Pellegrino and Thomasma's words, "probed and violated in closer proximity and more intimately than is usually permitted even to those the patient loves" (1981:185). Thus, even though they are utter strangers, Eric Cassell points out, "the usual boundaries of a person, both physical and emotional, are crossed with impunity by physicians" (Cassell 1985a, 1:119). The social and historical context — institutional setting, licensure requirements, professionalization of health care, and so on — that yield typical expectations for such a relationship may often, though not always, ameliorate these physical and personal probings.

Second, the relationship is asymmetrical, with power (the ability to "do something") on the side of the doctor: knowledge (about fetal development), technical skills (doing c-sections), access to resources (ultrasound equipment and radiologists), social and legal legitimation (license to practice obstetrics) belong to the physician (Lenrow 1982). None of these were part of the couple's stock of knowledge. Indeed, like most patients, they did not even know how to assess whether those who professed this range of power were in fact capable. So far as they were strangers, moreover, neither doctor nor patient had (or could have) any prior understanding of the other's beliefs and values — beyond the sort of *typified* knowledge we all share as members of the same culture — much less whether they *shared* any values (about abortion or mental retardation, for instance).

Third, if the physician is thus asymmetrically advantaged, the patient is correlatively disadvantaged — that is, uniquely vulnerable. In this case the disadvantage had multiple forms: not only was the wife compromised by the difficult pregnancy; she and her husband were also in a state of distress and confusion. Centered on the fetus and the pregnancy, they were also "in the hands" of the doctors, forced to place trust in instruments, medications, procedures, and most of all, people — within circumstances in which, on the other hand, trust was problematic. Contrary to embedded social understanding and medicine's long history of solitary decision making by doctors, the couple themselves faced the awesome prospect of making irreversible decisions on an uncertain basis for their still only potential infant. They had to decide now, and they knew full well that whatever they chose, they alone were responsible for the aftermath. Other features of the relationship are thus understandable: the need for accurate, understandable communication of pertinent information and the delineation of available alternatives (along with respective likely aftermaths); their need for help to identify and articulate not only the real issues to be faced but also their own moral beliefs, aims, and values; and the doctor's misunderstanding and poor communication.

Forms of Feeling and Moral Experience

Like many clinical encounters, this situation was remarkable for the range of passionate feelings expressed by the main characters. These feelings harbor remarkable significance. In the first place, the feelings manifested in our case were *evoked* strictly by the fetus's condition (to a lesser degree, the parents'), were *directed* to the fetus as "now presented," and were *aimed* at the range of possible future prospects (as efforts to "do something" for the fetus and parents). In this complex sense, the feelings were *oriented expressions of moral concern,* efforts to do the right thing, to be good people, and to act fairly toward everyone concerned. They were efforts to be responsive to the present and responsible for the future.

Second, the wife at one point blurted out: "The doctor just doesn't understand what it's like for us." Then, almost in the same breath, she seemed to plead with me: "Put yourself in our shoes: is it right to *force* a baby to be a hero just to stay alive?" As I understood it, she really meant the latter for the doctor as well, if not primarily: to understand "what it's like for us," he and I needed to put ourselves in their shoes.

I agree (Zaner 1988:297–307) with Herbert Spiegelberg (1986:99–104) that this common expression intimates an act having profound moral cognizance. What this moral cognizance is and how best to characterize it, however, are singularly difficult issues. In what follows, I can only scratch a few of its fascinating surfaces. Clearly the wife was appealing both to me and to the doctor to do something she regarded as quite vital to her and her husband. On the negative side, she was not asking the doctor to think about their situation *as if it were in fact his own.* The question was *not* "what would you do if you were I?" She was not asking for an act of imaginative identification (for the doctor to become the person facing the situation and try to feel their pain). Nor was she asking him to consider what he would do if he and his wife faced such a situation. To "put yourself in our shoes," I understood them to mean, would entail seeing things as they saw them and yet remaining oneself.

Not to belabor the obvious, she was urgently asking the doctor to *understand* their situation *from their point of view;* more accurately, they wanted him to *be understanding.* To do this, Arthur Kleinman insists, the doctor has "to place himself in the lived experience of the patient's illness," to understand the situation "as the patient understands, perceives, and feels it" (Kleinman 1988:232–33). This act seems to involve supposing something contrary to fact, not only a kind of "fiction deliberately flying in the face of the facts," but even "contrary to all normal possibilities" (Spiegelberg 1986:100). At the same time, they were not asking the doctor to pronounce moral judgments about them should they choose abortion, for instance.

On the face of it, to "put yourself in my shoes" seems absurd: how could one person — with his unique bodily wherewithal, experiences, history, frame of mind — assume the place of another person — with a different personal, bodily, social, and historical situation? In a sense, of course, each of us does this all the time. Thanks to socially derived and typified everyday knowledge, each of us knows in general ways what it's like, for instance, to be a letter carrier or lawyer even though we are neither, to drive a semi or a tractor even though we do not drive, to use a wrench or operate a crane even though we have done neither, to suffer acute pain or be faced with an urgent dilemma even though we are currently experiencing neither. As Alfred Schutz has pointed out, moreover, our everyday knowledge of the life-world is incredibly rich and detailed even while it is also unevenly distributed (Schutz and Luckmann 1973). Despite the inadequacies, inconsistencies, and inconstancies of commonsense knowledge and understanding,[4] then, they are for the most part quite sufficient in the context of daily concerns — we get along for "all practical purposes," as we say. But when someone asks us to "put yourself in my shoes," to understand something from their perspective, we generally do not go beyond such taken-for-granted forms of understanding.

Sometimes, though, something more is demanded, and ours is a good case in point. The couple urgently asked the doctor to understand their predicament as they actually faced and experienced it: to 'feel with' them, as it were, from their own perspective and from within their own moral framework.

To put yourself in someone else's shoes involves several critical steps: helping the person articulate and understand what his or her own moral framework includes and how he or she orders it; identifying the most pressing issues, given the basic ordering of values and commitments; and weighing the alternatives with a view toward their aftermaths and their consonance with the person's beliefs. Providing that kind of help requires disciplined self-knowledge (including frequently practiced, disciplined reflection to delineate one's own feelings, moral beliefs, and social framework), followed by a rigorously disciplined suspension of it — a kind of practical distantiation that undergirds the act of compassion or affiliative feeling.[5]

Strategies for Decisions

The couple's anxiety and confusion clearly needed attention. Certainly, they would be better equipped to make decisions if they could be helped to translate into their own framework such terms as "statistically significant chance" or "75 percent confidence level" (and, of course, to get the doctor to understand how differently things appeared from their perspective). It was equally important, though, for them to understand the situation from the doctor's perspective: how did he understand those terms and phrases — the uncertainty — and what were the implications for a course of action?

As the doctor pointed out to them, he was not "100 percent certain" of the accuracy of ultrasound and AFP tests. At the same time, he understood his responsibilities to the couple: he felt quite strongly that he was there to help. He wanted to do the right thing for them, and he hoped that what he thought was "good" would also be good for them. Here, it seemed to me, the key to the physician's approach was the peculiar blend of caution and impatience.

His sense of uncertainty deeply textured his efforts to do the right thing. In different terms, the physician's responsibility to seek the patient's good — beneficence, as it is often termed — is contextually determined and shaped by the balance of certainty and uncertainty (both diagnostic and prognostic). Statements in clinical medicine have to do only with probabilities; they apply only to a population of patients sharing certain characteristics with the individual patient. Accordingly, one can never know in advance where on the frequency-distribution curve any individual patient will be. Yet, to be technically correct, one must be able to predict as closely as possible where each patient is located on that curve. That prediction is never, or rarely, certain; uncertainty in various forms is always present. Accordingly, "optimization of decision and action in the face of uncertainty is the central characteristic of clinical decisions" (Pellegrino 1983:164). Celsus's definition of medicine as the "art of conjecture" is right.

In our case, the doctor had to proceed with caution, both because the prognostic and the diagnostic pictures were uncertain and because he did not at the time fully appreciate what the couple wanted. Uncertainty on both counts is textured with caution and leads to a decisional strategy: decisions must be the *least irreversible possible*, given the particular circumstances.

Following this strategy, the doctor weighed a number of factors: the possible diagnoses, the probabilities that each diagnosis is correct, the possible prognosis for each diagnosis, and the possibilities for action in the event of error (in diagnosis, side-effects, and so on). In doing so, the physician attempted to balance the contextual determination of beneficence with the least irreversible decisional strategy and identify a total therapeutic strategy. At the same time, even having on hand the impressive body of medical knowledge about such matters — including knowledge about the diagnostic determinations and therapeutic alternatives (what is wrong and what can be done about it), the doctor was also obliged to assess alternatives in light of the couple's beliefs, values, and wishes.

For example, knowing a good deal about the probable outcomes for nonaborted infants with multiple congenital anomalies, the doctor believed that he and the couple might well find themselves facing even greater problems if they let the twenty-four-week cutoff point pass. If the pregnancy continued (for whatever reason) and the diagnosis was confirmed, the fetus's head size might soon dictate the need to terminate the pregnancy. If the woman refused to have a cesarean section (not unusual), the termination would have to come sooner — and this would place all the severe difficulties of prematurity on top of the neurological ones already diagnosed. But if fetal head size were too great for vaginal delivery and the woman continued to refuse a cesarean section, only one of two options would be available: to seek a court-ordered cesarean (which he earnestly did not want and probably would not pursue) or to perform cephalocentesis (puncture the fetal brain to drain enough cerebral-spinal fluid to permit vaginal delivery). The latter would doubtless mean fetal death — but even if it didn't, severe, life-threatening impairment (and even neonatal death) would be very likely.

Hence the doctor's feelings of caution and impatience arose as much, if not more, from his medical understanding as from his sense of what the couple felt. Because he felt that he had to communicate everything to the couple, he had tried to convey something of that likely progression of events. At the mention of, and possibly even emphasis on, abortion, he thought he detected anger. Although he had continued with the rest of the potential outcomes, it seemed to him that they were stuck on abortion. What the couple had fastened onto, however, was instead the need to decide quickly, and at the same time the uncertainty — hence, the pressing need to get clear, to attain a deeper understanding of alternatives and outcomes. Caution and impatience are inevitable if also uncomfortable mates.

Although the couple seemed clearheaded to me — as did the physician when I talked with him — my "go-between" role was not sufficient. It was thus imperative (and surprisingly easy) to arrange for several conferences between the couple and the attending physician (several nurses and consultants also attended), so that their different perspectives and concerns could be aired. The second meeting was memorable for its quiet candor and the couple's eventual acceptance of the diagnostic evidence: although it was not certain, they recognized that it weighed heavily on the side of severe fetal damage. Abortion, for all its difficulties now and for the future, was the only reasonable option for them.

An Experiential Approach to Illness

A great deal more could be unraveled from this encounter itself. A number of themes, however, are already evident.[6]

As Robert C. Hardy (1978) indicates, several themes run through patient and family experiences of illness.[7] First, sick and distressed people *want to know what's wrong with them* (or their family members). Second, they also want to know *that the people taking care of them really care.* Others have noted this *"need to know and understand and the need to feel known and understood"* (Engel 1988:124).

Of course, many people have difficulty finding out what's wrong. Some fear being regarded as pushy; some are not in a good position to question those who take care of them; others simply don't know how to talk with doctors, nurses, and others. Candid communication is difficult in hospitals in any case. Illness, pain, suffering, fear, timidity, and ignorance can compromise it further. Still, those preoccupations come through with striking clarity, along with a surprising readiness by many patients to understand the many dilemmas, failures, and mistakes that can occur.

From the patient-family's perspective, illness forces a break with the usual flow of daily life and the typical ways in which the body is experienced. To come under the care of a physician, especially within a hospital or clinic, is to be transformed from "person" to "patient." Correlatively, one's illness narrative becomes a "case," and the patient is placed within numerous and unavoidable trust relationships. As noted earlier, being in a place of health care obliges the patient to rely on other people who, in their efforts to take care of the patient, inevitably work within parameters of relative uncertainty, ambiguity, and fallibility. Patients and providers are, moreover, most often strangers to one another, yet they are in circumstances that invariably involve intimate actions regarding the patient's body, self, personal life, family relations, and social life.

Relationships with helpers are essentially *asymmetrical,* with power on the side of the helpers. Yet not only does illness single out (and at times threaten) the individual as "this" unique person; it harbors the promise of recovery (ultimately, self-recovery) and is marked by various forms of gratitude. Each of these themes is briefly detailed in the following section, to suggest the main results of a phenomenology of the illness experience (Zaner 1988:53–91, 224–42, 283).

Dimensions of the Illness Experience

1. *Interruptions in daily life.* Included among the numerous recipes of commonsense life (Schutz 1967:3–47) are many by which we learn to identify, monitor, label, and communicate bodily functions and dysfunctions. Daily routines (edging grass, talking with friends, getting a drink of water) can become destabilized, suddenly or gradually, through illness. Whether these interruptions appear as ordinary (straining to read a street sign), puzzling (experiencing weight loss even when one is eating properly), or dramatic (being awakened by acute abdominal pain), the familiar can seem quite strange, and the apparently innocuous (for example, a lump) may become the occasion for panic.

Illness thus has a unique way of cutting into the fabric of daily routines. The person's life may become altered: temporarily, as with a broken leg, or for longer times, as with diabetes; trivially, as when one has flu, or grievously, as with cancer. Whichever it may be, the person's affected part, up to then silently in the background, may come to dominate awareness or hover over one's experience. The person can no longer take for granted something that has hitherto been taken for granted.

Even the usual flow of time and shape of space are affected. Ordinary actions — reaching out, going toward, embracing, listening, looking — are altered; and the usual ways of expecting, hoping, greeting become confounded. "The future, either short-term or long-range, takes on a brittle quality. One finds one's plans disrupted and possibilities withheld" or perhaps put on hold (Rawlinson 1982:75). Illness is unsought; it singles us out as vulnerable and affects our vital sense of ourselves.

2. *Unavoidable trust.* Impaired in some way in the ability to do for oneself, the sick person enters a complex network of unavoidable trust relationships — involving other people but also medications, procedures, equipment, regimens, and the like. A woman who had a botched surgery was dismayed: "You have to trust these people...like you do God. You're all in their hands....I trusted him not to let an inexperienced person mess up my life" (Hardy 1978:40). Having no choice but to trust in all these ways, communication takes on acute significance. A man with lung cancer emphasized: "When the doctor told me I had

this tumor, frankly, it alarmed me, but he did it in such a way that it left me with a feeling of confidence" (Hardy 1978:9). A diabetic underscored the point: "If you can't communicate and you can't understand your disease, then you don't have confidence in the medical help you are getting" (Hardy 1978:236).

3. *Caring for suffering.* Clinical encounters evoke the need for responsive care from those in whom trust is invested. Eric Cassell (1991:30–47) addressed this directly, reporting a case in which it was clear that a woman with disfiguring cancer not only was in acute pain but was suffering acutely over her sense of disfigurement, her inability to understand why she hurt so much, and her anxieties about her future and ultimately her death.

A narrow focus on disease and pain, Cassell points out, may obscure the crucial dimensions of suffering. "People in pain frequently report suffering from pain when they feel out of control, when the pain is overwhelming, when the source of the pain is unknown, when the meaning of the pain is dire, or when the pain is apparently without end." Moreover, suffering is intensely personal: it is perceived "as a threat to [persons'] continued existence — not merely to their lives but their integrity as persons" (1991:36). Even in the absence of pain, people may suffer from a sense of having lost themselves in relation to the surrounding world — objects, events, other people. Detecting the sources of suffering requires candid discussion of a person's sense of her body and self, circle of intimates, social life, and goals. Without candid dialogue, the person's own moral sense cannot be understood.

The unavoidable necessity of placing trust in others evokes a correlative need to be genuinely cared for. Sick people and their families generally understand quite well the need to establish good relations with nurses and doctors. Often this need translates into a desire for accurate, adequate, and understandable information conveyed promptly, sensitively, and continuously. The failure to establish such relations with clinicians correlates with patients' feeling of compromise and abandonment. The correlate of patients' trust is responsive care.

4. *Soundings of uncertainty.* Illness provokes a need to know and to understand: What's gone wrong? Is it serious? What does it mean for me and my family? Now and in the future? Is it curable? Treatable? And, if so, by what means, at what risk, and at what cost? What should be done?

Each of the three main aspects of clinical judgment (Pellegrino 1979) — determining what is wrong, what can be done about it, and what ought to be done about it — involves uncertainty and ambiguity and thus fallibility (Gorovitz and MacIntyre 1976). Contrasted with this is the sick person's quite understandable desire to know with as much certainty as possible what should be done. Although specific and effective treatments exist for some diseases (for example, penicillin for pneumococcal pneumonia), clinical judgments are often not so clear and are even less clear when the clinician takes the person's experience and interpretation of illness into account.

For patients seeking to know what is wrong, and what can and should be done about it, it is rarely appropriate merely to cite statistical probability patterns for classes of diseases or persons, for uncertainty and ambiguity more often give people the sense of being "at a loss," adrift, unable to "take one's bearings" or to know "what to hold onto." The experience is thus notable for its prominent sense of peril, its existential urgency, and for candid conversations concerning decisions, at times critical and irreversible, that must be made, often on the basis of relatively incomplete, uncertain, or ambiguous data.

5. *Intimacies among strangers.* To enter the world of medicine is often to enter forbidding and alien environs. Invariably, the patient is surrounded by strangers (other patients and hospital personnel) and by strange equipment, schedules, and procedures. Sociologically and architecturally, hospitals and clinics seem to enhance more than to ameliorate this strangeness. Stripped of familiar clothes, possessions, and surroundings, and told they must wait while clothed in anonymous gowns, patients are then asked to discuss the most intimate details of personal and bodily life to whoever is assigned to their "case." They are then poked and probed, swabbed and stuck, palpated and felt, in intimate and even humiliating ways — all in the service of being "cared for."

Illness is itself alienating. It disrupts the usual routines of daily life, including the ways in which one's own body is experienced. It may evoke other forms of strangeness — for example, new and peculiar feelings in one's body — that are difficult to convey even if one is sensitively encouraged to talk about them.

When communication is between or among strangers, the experience can be even more confounding. In a society in which relationships among strangers predominate, communication tends to be designed more for temporary ease of social passage and commerce than for intimate disclosures. For the hospitalized patient, talking and listening are often only exercises in remoteness, more sham than real. Yet it is precisely the sick person and family who need to know what's wrong and need to know that the caregivers genuinely care — a major index of which is candid, sensitive discourse (Zaner 1990). Without that, there is little basis for confidence in other people and no basis for trust, and lack of trust can only mean that an essential part of the therapeutic relationship is missing or threatened. To be a patient is thus often to find oneself in a deeply ironic predicament: intimate actions of touching, feeling, talking, and probing, which typically attest to personal intimacies, now go on between strangers, and thus they have a very different significance in the relationship between helper and patient.

6. *Power and vulnerability*. The fundamental asymmetry of power that characterizes the relationship between healers and patients presents compelling difficulties within the complex, bureaucratic institutions of health care. Though understandable and unavoidable, the asymmetry itself disadvantages patients. The mother of a partially sighted girl, for instance, noted how "overpowering" physicians can be: "They've got the edge on you" (Hardy 1978:92). "You're all in their hands, and if they don't care for you, who's going to?" a surgical patient plaintively asked (Hardy 1978:40). Here, Pellegrino seems right on target: patients seem "condemned to a relationship of inequality with the professed healer, for the healer professes to possess precisely what the patient lacks — the knowledge and power to heal" (1982:161).

Yet this inequality or asymmetry is constitutive of the helping relationship. Doctors have special knowledge and skills (through education and training) in the ways of the body. They have access to resources (people, technologies, medications, institutions, funding) and are socially and legally legitimated and protected (through licensing and statutes) to act on behalf of sick people.

Strongly enhanced by formal institutionalization, social legitimation, and legal authorization, this inequality of power is intensified by the sick person's illness; it places the patient in a position of supplicant. The patient is a petitioner whose appeal is precisely an endorsement of the very phenomenon that constitutes the inequality. The ability to treat, heal, or restore is the more difficult when the participants are strangers to one another, and thus cannot in any way assume that they share values, attitudes, desires, or aims.

7. *Illness as individuating*. The illness experience is centering: unlike most things in a person's life, illness uniquely singles him or her out as "this" individual — at times quite disturbingly. Bodily pain, the exacting scheduling of medications and diets, the unavoidable dependence on people and things (sometimes for one's very life), the anxiety over future prospects, the forced reordering of personal and family life, the way the disease preoccupies, the riveting focus of pain and strange new feelings only barely known, if at all — all these sharply and poignantly bring the person face to face with himself, his own human frailty and fragile hold on things, his very life and therefore death.

Especially in grievous illness, the person is marked out as *able to die*. In the midst of robust life, death is made *present* by illness, suffering, loss, and grief. In the familiarity of daily life, the awesome and radically strange suddenly appears: illness is experienced as a rudimentary threat.

With these telling glimpses of loss and death, illness confronts the person with what and who she is, was, and hopes to be, with finality. Wanting to know and wanting to be cared for are thus special appeals through which the person seeks recognition, affirmation, and appreciation of this singular person she is or hopes to be. To want to be cared for, in this deeply personal sense, is to want fundamentally to be this self in the presence of those who take care of her precisely in her vulnerability and suffering. As theologian Stanley Hauerwas carefully emphasizes, "it is our capacity to feel grief and to identify with the misfortune of others which is the basis for our ability to recognize our fellow humanity" (Hauerwas 1986:25). Trust on the part of the ill includes wanting to know and to be with those who help, as the persons *they* are, in their very caring for the vulnerable, trusting person.

8. *Illness: helping and promise.* The dyad of trust and care harbors promise, and not only that the sick person may recover or be comforted. It promises, too, the recovery of ourselves as the persons we are, patients and helpers alike. Even dying can provide the occasion for this recovery of selves. Illness may be the mask that loss and death at times wear, giving brief but arresting glimpses of chilling nothingness; it may be experienced as deeply dreaded but feared or perhaps embraced with grace. Here, the physician and nurse have their most significant task, as Cassell observes: to give patients "in this final stage of life the same kind of control that can be taught in earlier stages of living" (1985b:302).

The helping relationship is thus more akin to an educational process than is usually thought. Illness bodes loss of control — of self, bodily functioning, and social action — and of connection with valued persons. Caring for the distressed harbors the promise of self-recovery of both patient and helper, for both become learners in the process, even if, as strangers asymmetrically related, conditions cannot allow for more than situations of temporary trust. The physician in, and because of, the relationship is able to take advantage of the disadvantaged patient, as the Hippocratic Oath evidently recognized (Edelstein 1967:4–63). Indeed, it may well be precisely this sense of power to take advantage that constitutes the moral core of medicine: that one *can,* but *ought not,* take advantage (Zaner 1988: 202–223).

9. *"Telling" illness: gratitude and luck.* A forty-two-year-old coronary bypass patient interviewed by Robert Hardy stated:

I wouldn't take anything for this total experience, wouldn't trade it with anyone. This will sound stupid, I'm sure, but it was one of the best things that happened to me in my whole life.... It brought back what I would consider for myself, not necessarily for others, a new system of values.... Life itself has more meaning for me, each day, each breath. (Hardy 1978:229)

The experience was profoundly religious: "You're sort of released, you let go and let your Maker have His way." This patient also spoke of "relief upon arriving [at the hospital] before I was completely gone and was finally in the hands of others."

The ways in which illness is individuating are underscored here in another way. First, while grievous illness makes one unusually reliant on others, patients also exhibit a kind of gratitude. This textures the experience quite as much as the diminishment and even humiliation that illness often includes. "I am deeply grateful," a patient with end-stage renal disease reported, "that I am offered two possible methods of survival" — transplantation and dialysis (Coene 1978:7).

Second, a sense of their good fortune marks these patients' lives, especially when they are lucky enough to have supportive and responsive families, friends, employers, doctors, and nurses. This sense of good fortune has other dimensions. One of the bypass patients, for instance, emphasized: "I've been lucky in a lot of ways" (Hardy 1978:212), noting his "luck" in being able to take the surgery and the "luck" in living in a town offering the medical facilities and talent needed for his problem. Here, we see a kind of knowledge, an intimate realization of what the bypass patient calls "the total experience": fear, pain, uncertainty, confusion, as well as the multiple forms of relief and comfort. It is this "total experience" that he and others seem compelled to share, to talk about as a perilous adventure and as a kind of "good fortune." This sense of "good fortune" may well harbor a subtle yet keen sense of obligation — to those who gave care but also to others who are similarly afflicted. As Albert Schweitzer expressed his "other thought" in ethics: "I must not accept this good fortune as a matter of course but had to give something in return" (cited in Spiegelberg 1986:220), an idea that Spiegelberg interprets as an appeal for awakening "a moral sense that is usually dormant but that on special occasions can be brought to the surface" (Spiegelberg 1986:226).

Even though eager to talk about their experiences, such patients still may seem acutely aware of possible embarrassment: "This will sound stupid, I know," says one, and another knows he runs the "risk of sounding a little starry-eyed." That is, "telling" truly about one's illness experience seems always awkward, difficult, embarrassing: so intimate and profound are the experiences, and on the other hand, the language available for "telling" so inadequate. Here is a painful, poignant expression of the radical gap between the individuating characteristic of illness, and the forms of expression readily available to anybody; the gap between unique experience and typifying language, between the individual and the common — all deeply characteristic of the illness experience.

The Clinical Encounter

Experience is the point of departure and return for theory: its ground and ultimate "test," what it must at once illuminate and elucidate. Experience, however, is not univocal: the patient experiences, as do all those involved in the case. Consider merely some aspects of our patient's experiences: she experienced her body, her past, her hopes, plans, and fears; her developing fetus; what her husband did and said, as well as what her physicians (and all the others involved, including me when I entered the scene) did and said. Everyone's experiences are similarly complex.

Nor is this all. Every situational participant not only experiences but *interprets* the encounter within his or her own biography (Schutz and Luckmann 1973). These encounters are also socially framed by prevailing values, written and unwritten professional codes, governmental regulations, hospital policies, unit or departmental protocols, and so on — any or all variously contributing to "what's going on" in any specific case (Zaner 1988:29–52).

To simplify matters, consider only the patient and her physician. Each is a *self* and thus is *reflexively interrelated* with the other. Each experiences and interprets the other and at the same time experiences and interprets the relationship itself (Zaner 1981a:217–39). For example, this woman experienced her pregnancy and her developing fetus, and this experience was complicated by the ways she experienced and interpreted what her physicians (and others) told her. Similarly, her physicians experienced and interpreted her "anger" to be directed at them and concerned with abortion. Both experienced and interpreted the *relationship* itself. Regarding diagnostic data, for instance, she said "I know they're only trying to do their best" (interpreting the relation as "trying to help"); her physician said, "She seems to think we're being deliberately unclear" (the relationship was "not going well").

To probe clinical situations phenomenologically is to work somewhat like a detective: deliberately alert to the multiple ways in which participants interrelate and variously experience and interpret one another and, within that relationship, the relationship itself. Even a brief moment reveals a number of interrelated voices, each with its own emotional, volitional, valuational, and cognitive tonality, and each demanding to be heard and understood so that decisions can be made and aftermaths borne. The ethicist's involvement is thus a *work of circumstantial understanding;* reflection on this and other cases is a matter of *phenomenological explication.*

When one enters such a scene with the idea of trying to help, one is faced with the prominent need to sort things out, to ask "What's going on?" One cannot do this beforehand: one never knows in advance which issues must be dealt with, or just how the discovered issues are to be managed. The problems are strictly those of the people in the situation — that couple and their physicians. Similarly, alternatives, decisions, and outcomes are strictly theirs. Any encounter presents its own set of issues, moral and other — they are *context-specific* in the sense that working with and on behalf of such persons, helping them and advising them, requires a strict focus on the *situational definitions* (Zaner 1988:251–82). To understand these, one can only do one's best, so far as possible without interpretive predispositions, to understand the concrete ways in which the participants themselves experience and understand their situation and endow its various components with *meaning.* One goal was obvious: to identify precisely what was at issue for each of those involved, working toward a common understanding of problems, needed decisions, and acceptable solutions.

Phenomenological method suggests that in such clinical situations, *moral issues are presented for deliberation, decision, and resolution solely within the contexts of their actual occurrence* (Zaner 1988:242–48). Determining what's troubling the people requires cautious, attentive probing of their discourse and conduct, the setting, and other matters presented in the specific context. Nothing can be taken for granted. The couple's puzzlement, for example, about the "statistically significant" was central to their "anger," indicating (at least in part) what needed to be addressed; it could not have been gleaned in abstraction from the actual circumstances.

Thus *every situational constituent, including any moral issue, is presented solely within an ongoing relationship between patient and physician* (Zaner 1988:29–91) — at least, in its minimal form. That relationship is not itself, however, the focus for either patient or physician. The physician is concerned to help the patient (or at least to do no harm). The patient's concern is to have distress relieved, injuries healed, disease resolved, or at least to be comforted and cared for. Clinical ethics addresses that *relationship itself.*

These points can be expressed in formal phenomenological terms: (1) The "method" involves *epoché* and *reduction*. Gaining genuine knowledge or science requires that one "put out of action all the convictions we have been accepting up to now, including all our sciences," so as to "immerse oneself in the scientific striving and doing" specific to the pursuit of science (Husserl 1960:7). This idea, at first perhaps only a "vague generality," can be taken as a clue (*Leitfaden*) for reflective consideration. It is a sort of "precursory presumption" guiding reflection: what is it that one *claims* or *aims at* when one strives to be "scientific"?

Crucial to the undertaking is a rigorous reflective "attitude" or "orientation" (*Einstellung*) that enables one "to immerse oneself in" (*sich einleben in*), thereby becoming reflectively cognizant of the practice[8] specific to science, with its inherent claims and end. This methodical shifting to a reflective orientation is the *epoché*; rigorously maintaining it throughout the course of inquiry is the *reduction* (Husserl [1913] 1982).

(2) Every endeavor includes the possibility of this reflective-attentive shift — whether or not it is actually undertaken. Precisely because the practitioner experiences the field of medicine, he can recognize what MacIntyre (1981:175) terms the "goods" internal to it (its "standards of excellence" or "virtues") and may even periodically reflect on it. On the basis of such experiences and reflections, one can (and sometimes must) stop and think about the field and one's involvement.

Reflection in a strict sense requires a specific shift of focal attention (*epoché*) — away from active involvement in clinical cases for their own sake to considering them as examples of the practice — a shift that needs to be *sustained* throughout the reflective project. To stop and think about the efforts and actions specific to any field is, on the basis of one's own pertinent experiences, to become reflectively attentive to its inherent "intention" (Husserl [1913] 1982:125–41). This complex reflective act might be termed a sort of *practical distantiation,* circumstantial understanding, or more simply, phenomenological reflection.

There is nothing mysterious here; it is something each of us does many times in our daily preoccupations with more or less skill and attention. The method, Husserl once observed, is the very same as that which "a cautiously shrewd person follows in practical life wherever it is seriously important for him to 'find out how matters actually are'" ([1929] 1969:278–79). Just such seriousness was evident in our case; it was *vital* that the couple understand what they faced so that they could decide and act. They engaged in at least a form, perhaps only the first stages, of reflection — "stages," for they did not proceed any further with it. Their reflections were (Husserl might have noted) only the "beginning" of wisdom, but it is "a wisdom we can never do without, no matter how deep we go with our theorizings" ([1929] 1969:279).

(3) The "seriously shrewd" person must judge on the basis of sound *evidence*. She must judge "on the basis of a giving of something itself, while continually asking what can be actually 'seen' and given faithful expression" (Husserl [1929] 1969:278–79). Whether one has practical concerns (trying to have a baby) or theoretical ones (interpreting diagnostic tests), to seek sound judgment requires a concerted effort to know just how matters actually stand. Both the woman and her physician had a vital interest in knowing so that they could then decide which action was best for them and the baby.

Whatever may be at issue, to come to know something is to take it to be "thus and so," to take up some position toward it — for instance, to know it "fairly well," "sort of," "surely," "not at all well." To take a position is to appeal to some evidence that is supposed to ground or account for the position taken — the more vital the issue, the more crucial the need for solid evidence as grounding.

Evidence is not a sort of rare and special "datum," a magical wand or a conferral from on high having special privilege or guarantee (Husserl [1929] 1969:161, 177, 180, 289). To the contrary, evidence is a matter of *relevant experience* and is essentially contextual. Evidence about fetal hydrocephaly cannot be the same as evidence for alleging that the couple was "angry."

Even if there seems to be good evidence for believing that something is this or that, the possibility of error or deception is not precluded. The *possibility of deception* is inherent in the evidence of experience (in Husserl's broad sense) and "does not annul either its fundamental character or its effect." Not even genuine evidence provides "an absolute security against deceptions" ([1929] 1969:156, 157, 284–89). In ethics, especially clinical ethics, there is a clear demand for addressing uncertainty, error, deception, and ambiguity.

As experience in the generic sense (*Erfahrung*), evidence refers to the particular ways in which some affair (anger or hydrocephaly) is experienced or through which one is able to become aware of or to encounter that affair — and on that basis, come to know it, and make claims about it. *Evidenz* is strictly correlated to the modes of givenness (*Gegenbenheitsweise*), the ways in and by means of which the things allegedly known are encountered as "they themselves," as Husserl says, "in person" (*leiblich*).[9]

In our case, this need for good evidence was prominent. The family obstetrician first referred the couple on the basis of the ultrasound and clinical examination. The center's obstetricians saw the first ultrasound and obtained another, as well as the AFP test and, together with radiologists and others qualified to read such images and laboratory findings, came to the judgment that the fetus had severe problems. The couple, on the other hand, barred by their lack of knowledge of such things, could base their beliefs and concerns only on what they were told by the physicians ("hearsay" evidence, even if from "experts"). But the physicians' notion that the couple "seemed angry at us for mentioning 'abortion'" was not well grounded; the belief was quite wrong even while the claim that they were "angry" was correct. Clinically assessing this situation led immediately to the various claims and the evidence provided for the respective beliefs and claims, and then to the location of other, more appropriate beliefs and claims and their respective reasons or evidences.

(4) To consult as an ethicist on such a case is to be focused on the situation (people, setting, circumstances, issues) itself, *for its own sake.* The ethicist's concerns are strictly therapeutic: to help the couple understand what they face and what they have been told, and especially to help them become more aware of their own moral views so that they will be more likely to reach decisions commensurate with those views. On the other hand, this and other encounters may also be submitted to philosophical reflection, such as what has concerned me here. For that, the clinical encounter must be considered strictly *as an example* that, taken along with other examples, helps make certain themes prominent. These themes can in turn be systematically considered in further reflective work, leading ultimately to a more embracing philosophical understanding.

I have mentioned only several phenomenological notions — epoché and reduction and evidence. Much has been left out: the intentionality of experience, the differences among the relatively inexplicit awarenesses and active ones, the meaning of "feeling," encounters with others, and inner-time consciousness, to mention but a few (Zaner 1970; 1981a). A full phenomenology of clinical life has thus been only suggested. Nevertheless, this approach is remarkably fruitful, eminently practical, and above all faithful to the subtlety and complexity of these encounters.

In the Aftermath

Although some aspects of the experience of doctoring have been delineated in the literature,[10] more emphasis and detail have been given to the patient and family's side of the therapeutic dyad. That is a serious shortcoming because the central phenomenon, after all, is the relationship between doctor and patient. I have tried to provide here some insight into at least one constituent of that relationship — the patient-family's experience of distress — realizing that no firm conclusions can yet be drawn about the full phenomenon. Without anticipating what might come out of that more complete study, then, the following summary of my approach thus far can be given.

An accidental disruption in the routine flow of life, illness renders the person uniquely vulnerable, placed within a complex network of unavoidable trust relationships. It disrupts the person's usual ways of relating with other people, making the ill person unusually reliant on others who, in the nature of the case, work within situations that are relatively uncertain and ambiguous, and with people who are fallible. These others, usually strangers working within settings mostly unfamiliar to the sick person, possess or profess the power to know "what's wrong," "how to deal with it," and "what to expect." At the same time, to become ill is to recognize that we do not (or perhaps cannot) know "what's happening," "what's wrong," and "what should be done about it." Furthermore, we desperately need assurance that these strangers really do know what they profess to know, really can do what they profess to be able to do, and really care for us while taking care of us.

The experience of illness is thus shot through with complex moral dimensions. On the one side of the relationship is the vulnerability and *appeal* of the ill person; on the other, the *response* from the professed healer or helper.[11] Their asymmetrical relationship itself places the helper in a position in which he or she is able to take advantage of the multiply disadvantaged sick person, but precisely that is what ought not be done — an "ought" understood in the very beginnings of medicine's history, seen as needing an oath and covenant, and secured in most "codes" since that time.[12]

While clearly "disabling," illness or distress is at the same time among the most powerful and morally "enabling" (Zaner 1981a:181–237) of our experiences — enabling of keen and rigorous sensitivity that is a critical requirement of a fully humane and scientific medicine. As the couple in our case manifestly demonstrated during our several conversations, even significant loss is not always and only negative. For although they did eventually opt for abortion and thus lost the child they hoped to have, and even though they continued to suffer from the uncertainties of their experience, they nonetheless demonstrated gratitude, a sense of recovery, and an orientation toward the future marked by a sense of promise. More subtly, they seemed grateful, in a way, even for having been through the experiences of pregnancy, diagnosis, and discussion. Indeed, although they did not believe that abortion was a desirable outcome, they were grateful even for that, as seemed evident in their words after the abortion was over and they learned that their infant not only had a large myelomeningocele and hydrocephalus but also an omphalocele (open abdomen with organs lying outside) — and, in all likelihood, still other anomalies that would have made it all but impossible for the infant to live very long after delivery. Behind their words was a keen sense that it would not be right to "make such a child live" with no hope of correction.

Even while undergoing the grief of loss, the couple was already receptive to the doctor's advice to begin thinking about another pregnancy, though, wisely, they felt they should wait some time before actively considering that. Much of this "enabling" side of distress, understandably, did not fully emerge until several months later, when the couple visited us again and acknowledged their gratefulness for the detailed conversations with everyone, and for having been kept completely informed. Like others, they felt good for having been helped to understand things, and while the prospect of getting pregnant again was naturally colored by their previous experience and the uncertainties, their parting words were impressive: "There's much we don't understand, but we still feel we know a whole lot more than we did before all that; it helps to understand, and it makes life all the more precious when you realize all the risks there are just in getting into this world."

NOTES

1. In this respect, the clinical encounter is a special form of *contexture:* a "whole" that is neither a "sum," a "more than," nor reducible to parts, but rather a system formed of mutually interdependent and interdetermined constituents (see Zaner 1981a:67–91; Gurwitsch 1964:145–49, 317–35).

2. In a way, one could say that both abortion and continuing the pregnancy until delivery forced the couple to think of themselves in light of the prospect of becoming parents, of what William May calls "parenting" (May 1984).

3. These terms are not in the least forced as the etymology of *experience* suggests. Experience as such I take to be *intentive* in Husserl's comprehensive and original sense (Husserl [1913] 1982: secs. 33–46, 87–96 *passim;* and Husserl [1929] 1969: secs. 59–64, 70, 84–89, *passim*).

4. At the same time, insofar as we aim to be rigorous in our descriptive explications of experiences such as these, or any others, it is imperative that wherever we use the common tongue as a means of expression, "we require...a new legitimation of significations by orienting them according to accrued insights, and a fixing of words as expressing the significations thus legitimated. That too we account as part of our normative principle of evidence..." (Husserl [1950] 1960:14).

5. In this respect, understanding another is, as Spiegelberg remarks, a "type of phenomenological reduction" (1986:102; Husserl [1950] 1960: secs. 27–32).

6. That is, the phenomenological method of free-fantasy variation must now be expressly pursued (Zaner 1973a; Husserl [1913] 1982: secs. 69–71).

7. Hardy interviewed sixty different people, in each case a different illness; most involved patients, but some involved families of patients (Hardy 1978).

8. MacIntyre's definition of "practice" is apropos: "By a 'practice' I...mean any coherent and complex form of socially established cooperative human activity through which goods internal to that form of activity are realized in the course of trying to achieve those standards of excellence which are appropriate to, and partially definitive of, that form of activity, with the result that human powers to achieve excellence, and human conceptions of the ends and goods involved, are systematically extended." Science, among other activities, is specifically included (MacIntyre 1981:175).

9. Thus Husserl can say that evidence *"consists in the giving of something itself,"* along with the discipline of giving it faithful linguistic expression, which he includes in his "normative principle" of evidence (Husserl [1950] 1960:14).

10. Arthur Kleinman has presented a brief but fascinating chapter on the experience of doctoring (Kleinman 1988: chap. 14).

11. On the ideas of "appeal" and "response," I have in mind Gabriel Marcel's seminal work (1940; 1951, vol. 1).

12. Specifically in its strong emphasis on what for Edelstein is a "fusion" of two principal virtues: justice (*dike*) and disciplined restraint (*sophrosyne*) — which leads to the seminal ideas of confidentiality (vow of silence), protecting of patients (keeping them from "mischief"), and beneficence (Edelstein 1967:6–40, 326–47; Zaner 1988: chap. 8).

REFERENCES

Baron, Richard J. 1981. "Bridging Clinical Distance: An Empathetic Rediscovery of the Known." *Journal of Medicine and Philosophy* 6:5–23.

Buchanan, Scott M. 1938. *The Doctrine of Signatures: A Defence of Theory in Medicine.* London: K. Paul, Trench, Trubner.

Cassell, Eric J. [1972] 1985a. *Talking with Patients.* 2 vols. Cambridge: MIT Press.

———. 1985b. *The Healer's Art: A New Approach to the Doctor-Patient Relationship.* Cambridge: MIT Press.

Coene, Roger E. 1978. "Dialysis or Transplant: One Patient's Choice." *Hastings Center Report* 8:7.

Conetta, R., F. M. Tamarin, D. Wogalter, and R. D. Brandstetter. 1987. "Liqueur Lung." *New England Journal of Medicine* 316:348–49.

Edelstein, Ludwig. 1967. *Ancient Medicine.* Baltimore: Johns Hopkins University Press.

Engel, George. 1988. "How Much Longer Must Medicine's Science Be Bound by a Seventeenth-Century World View?" In *The Task of Medicine: Dia-*

logue at Wickenburg, ed. K. L. White, 113–36. Menlo Park, Calif.: Henry J. Kaiser Family Foundation.

Gorovitz, Samuel, and Alasdair MacIntyre. 1976. "Toward a Theory of Medical Fallibility." *Journal of Medicine and Philosophy* 1:51–71.

Gurwitsch, Aron. 1964. *Field of Consciousness.* Pittsburgh: Duquesne University Press.

Hardy, Robert C. 1978. *Sick: How People Feel about Being Sick and What They Think of Those Who Care for Them.* Chicago: Teach'Em.

Hauerwas, Stanley. 1986. *Suffering Presence.* Notre Dame, Ind.: University of Notre Dame Press.

Husserl, Edmund. [1950] 1960. *Cartesian Meditations.* The Hague: Martinus Nijhoff.

———. [1929] 1969. *Formal and Transcendental Logic.* The Hague: Martinus Nijhoff.

———. [1913] 1982. *Ideas Pertaining to a Pure Phenomenology and to a Phenomenological Philosophy,* Book One. The Hague: Martinus Nijhoff.

Kleinman, Arthur. 1988. *The Illness Narratives.* New York: Basic Books.

Lenrow, Peter B. 1982. "The Work of Helping Strangers." In *Things That Matter: Influences on Helping Relationships,* ed. H. Rubenstein and M. H. Bloch, 42–57. New York: Macmillan.

MacIntyre, Alasdair. 1981. *After Virtue.* Notre Dame, Ind.: University of Notre Dame Press.

Marcel, Gabriel. 1951. *Le Mystère de l'être.* Vol. 1. Paris: Éditions Montaigne.

———. 1940. *Du refus à l'invocation.* Paris: Gallimard.

May, William. 1984. "Parenting, Bonding, and Valuing the Retarded." In *Ethics and Mental Retardation,* ed. L. Kopelman and J. C. Moskop, 141–60. Dordrecht, Boston, Lancaster: D. Reidel.

Pellegrino, Edmund D. 1979. "The Anatomy of Clinical Judgments: Some Notes on Right Reason and Right Action." In *Clinical Judgment: A Critical Appraisal,* ed. H. T. Engelhardt, Jr., S. F. Spicker, and B. Towers, 169–94. Dordrecht, Boston, London: D. Reidel.

———. 1982. "Being Ill and Being Healed: Some Reflections on the Grounding of Medical Morality." In *The Humanity of the Ill: Phenomenological Perspectives,* ed. V. Kestenbaum, 157–66. Knoxville: University of Tennessee Press.

———. 1983. "The Healing Relationship: The Architectonics of Clinical Medicine." In *The Clinical Encounter: The Moral Fabric of the Physician-Patient Relationship,* ed. E. A. Shelp, 153–72. Boston, Dordrecht: D. Reidel.

Pellegrino, Edmund D., and David C. Thomasma. 1981. *A Philosophical Basis of Medical Practice.* New York and Oxford: Oxford University Press.

Rawlinson, Mary. 1982. "Medicine's Discourse and the Practice of Medicine." In *The Humanity of the Ill: Phenomenological Perspectives,* ed. V. Kestenbaum, 69–85. Knoxville: University of Tennessee Press.

Schutz, Alfred. 1967. *The Phenomenology of the Social World,* trans. George Walsh and Frederick Lehnert. Evanston, Ill.: Northwestern University Press.

Schutz, Alfred, and Thomas Luckmann. 1973, 1989. *Structures of the Life-World.* 2 vols. Evanston, Ill.: Northwestern University Press.

Spiegelberg, Herbert. 1986. *Steppingstones Toward an Ethics for Fellow Existers: Essays 1944–1983.* The Hague: Martinus Nijhoff.

Zaner, Richard M. 1970. *The Way of Phenomenology.* New York: Bobbs-Merrill.

———. 1973a. "Examples and Possibles: A Criticism of Husserl's Theory of Free-Phantasy Variation." *Research in Phenomenology* 3:29–43.

———. 1973b. "The Art of Free-Phantasy Variation in Rigorous Phenomenological Science." In *Phenomenology: Continuation and Criticism, Essays in Memory of Dorion Cairns,* ed. F. Kersten and R. Zaner, 192–219. The Hague: Martinus Nijhoff.

———. 1981a. *The Context of Self.* Athens: Ohio University Press.

———. 1981b. "The Disciplining of Reason's Cunning: Kurt Wolff's Surrender and Catch." *Human Studies* 4:365–89.

———. 1988. *Ethics and the Clinical Encounter.* Englewood Cliffs, N.J.: Prentice-Hall.

———. 1990. "Medicine and Dialogue." *Journal of Medicine and Philosophy* 15:303–25.

~ *10* ~

TOWARD A HERMENEUTICAL BIOETHICS

Drew Leder

Introduction

Hermeneutics is a fashionable term these days in academe, surfacing not only in literary criticism, but in diverse fields such as anthropology, sociology, theology, philosophy. At times it designates a specific discipline with its own historical development, canon of key texts, and contemporary debates. At other times, "hermeneutics" or "hermeneutical" more loosely characterizes a style of approach, a way of thinking, often contrasted with methodologies that are reductionist in nature, involved with "technological" mastery of a subject matter through a positivist and preformed logic.

The term first came into popular usage in the seventeenth and eighteenth centuries. Invoking Hermes, the Greek messenger of the Gods and mythical discoverer of language and writing, *hermeneutics* was initially used to refer to the principles of biblical interpretation.[1] Especially in the wake of the Protestant revolution, clergy needed manuals of interpretation to assist them in the exegesis of sacred scripture. Subsequently, the meaning of *hermeneutics* was broadened to refer to the interpretation of secular as well as sacred literature, thus dovetailing with the classical discipline of philology.

Through the work of Friedrich Schleiermacher (1768–1834) and Wilhelm Dilthey (1833–1911), hermeneutics took on yet more encompassing significance, as key to our understanding of human understanding itself. For Dilthey, the human sciences (*Geisteswissenschaften*) such as psychology, economics, literary criticism, and jurisprudence, involved with the subject matter of human beings, their activities and creations, employ a methodology distinct from that used in the natural sciences; through a hermeneutical process of "understanding" one enters into and comprehends living human experience, rather than simply "explaining" a scientific object.[2]

Heidegger, working within the tradition of twentieth-century phenomenology, goes even further; hermeneutics is not simply a regional enterprise but of ontological significance, for we interpretively construct and experience the world in all its dimensions (Heidegger 1962:188–95). The ubiquity of interpretation becomes evident on reflection. For example, I interpret a literary work as I draw sense, narrative structure, and personal pertinence from its black marks on paper; I interpret a visual field as I form it preconsciously into background and foreground, containing objects charged with cognitive and affective meaning; I interpret the significance of traces on an oscilloscope, and the scientific data that I accumulate over time; I interpret the facial expressions of a friend during our conversation; and on and on.[3] In a broad sense, we can say that each of these fields of meaning comprises a "text," defining the latter as any set of elements which constitutes a whole and takes on meaning through interpretation (Daniel 1986). Whether the text is literary or perceptual, scientific or interpersonal, it gives over its significance only through interpretive acts.

Hans-Georg Gadamer, a student of Heidegger, has done much to thematize the far-reaching import of hermeneutics in his influential work *Truth and Method*. Taking off from Heidegger's analysis of the "fore-structure" of understanding (Heidegger 1962:191–92), Gadamer suggests that all interpretation is necessarily "prejudiced" (Gadamer 1975:235–40). This term need not be understood pejoratively; it merely indicates that we come to any text with a set of prejudgments shaped by our personal and cultural history, and by the pragmatic interests which channel our reading. A contemporary individual seeking spiritual enlightenment cannot help reading the Bible differently from a fifteenth-century counterpart, or from a modern-day minister seeking proper counsel for a parishioner, a theologian gathering evidence for a scholarly paper, a widow coming to terms with her spouse's recent death, a skeptic attending to the sexism of biblical images. The text opens itself up differently depending upon the expectations and questions we bring to it. We can never find a "view from nowhere" (Nagel 1986), detached from the situatedness of human life.

This situatedness bears upon what has often been termed the "hermeneutic circle," addressed by a variety of thinkers from Schleiermacher to Gadamer. In reading a text, one makes sense of a part through anticipating the meaning of the whole in which it is embedded. One has certain expectations of the story's unfolding genre, plot, and significance, which shape one's reading at each moment. Yet one's understanding of the whole text is gradually constituted out of one's interpretation of its individual parts. This suggests the possibility of a vicious circle rendering interpretation unscientific and static, for one may find in the text only what one came looking for.

Heidegger and Gadamer reject this notion in favor of emphasizing the *productivity* of the hermeneutic circle. Though one must enter the circle through one's prejudgments and expectations, these always remain provisional and the text itself can extend, modify, or challenge them. A sensitive reader permits the interpretive object its otherness; such a reader does not merely subsume the text within preformed categories, but engages it as a partner in respectful dialogue (Heidegger 1962:194–95; Gadamer 1975:235–38, 258–67, 325–51).

The Hermeneutic Structure of a Bioethical Case

To speak of approaching bioethics hermeneutically is first to highlight and thematize the interpretive nature of the bioethical situation. A case in bioethics, no less than a literary work or a perceptual field, has meaning that only emerges through interpretation. The ideas discussed above can thus operate within bioethical inquiry. However, rather than simply referring to the universality of interpretation, one can also ask what distinguishes the hermeneutic structure of bioethics from that seen in other human activities. In bioethics, what is peculiar about the nature of the "text" being studied and the kinds of understanding brought to bear?

One difficulty presents itself immediately; bioethics reveals itself as a multileveled discourse unfolding through various modes of abstraction. For example, in the case of a woman deciding whether to proceed with surgery on her newborn who, due to congenital abnormalities, is severely and perhaps terminally deformed, we might have the mother trying to see her way to the proper ethical choice; the hospital committee attempting to reconcile legal precedent, moral principles, and the contingencies of this particular situation; an author of a piece in the *Hastings Center Report* responding many months later to a written document describing this case; a writer in a bioethics textbook delineating the abstract principles of personhood and social justice which should dictate our treatment of such newborns; etc. All are common forms of bioethical inquiry, each with its own textual and interpretive structure.

I choose, however, to focus initially on the living and unfolding case, for bioethical reflection only has meaning insofar as it originates from and returns to the life-world of actual individuals. Here a number of points emerge that help distinguish the interpretive structure commonly seen in bioethics from that of other disciplines and activities.

First, the unfolding case is written in a complex variety of discursive elements. In the situation described above, the deformity is imprinted on the child's body, its extent and consequences to be clinically interpreted. But then too there are the scans and lab values which elucidate the clinical picture, communications between the individuals involved, the medical charts in which a variety of findings and impressions are recorded, relevant legal statutes and decisions, standard procedures — whether written or secured by informal precedent — which are followed at the hospital, the physician's office, and so forth. The text which one is trying to interpret thus is not restricted to a single medium (for example, black marks on paper) but involves persons, bodies, pictures, numbers, speech, procedures, and the like.[4]

Furthermore, just as there are many textual elements, the bioethics case usually unfolds in the context of multiple and conflicting interpretations. In a modern clinical setting, not only the patient seeks to understand and resolve the dilemma but often the patient's family and friends, the primary physician, consulting specialists, the hospital ethics committee and lawyers, and sometimes even the courts or the voting populace. Moreover, each individual or group comes armed with a different set of prejudices, to use Gadamer's term. That is, the training, life-history, and pragmatic interests of these various participants can lead to widely diverging perspectives. The mother is concerned about the very real consequences — emotional, financial, existential — for herself and family members of different courses of action. The physician has been trained to look for and diagnose medical pathology, and whenever possible, bring to bear the clinical armamentarium. The lawyer wishes to protect the hospital from possible liability. Their manner of reading the case will necessarily diverge, shaped by the interpretive tools they have at their disposal, and the differing worlds of concern in which each person operates.

Moreover, that this case has emerged as one for bioethical reflection suggests that it provokes broad interpretive conflicts which other cases may not. If there is a clear social consensus about what is right in a given situation (for example, treat consenting bacterial pneumonia patients with the appropriate antibiotic), it becomes a simple clinical decision and not one for thematized moral consideration. Where consensus breaks down (for instance, should we allow pneumonia patients to refuse this simple treatment, in essence permitting their suicide on the ward? do we have an obligation to admit and provide such treatments to everyone regardless of their ability to pay?), then we have the beginnings of a recognized bioethical dilemma. Thus the hermeneutical complexity characteristic of a case in bioethics arises not simply from the complex discursive elements of the text, the sheer number of different interpreters reading it, and the widely divergent training and concerns they bring to bear. It arises also from the lack of clear *social* consensus about how events are to be interpreted. In the case mentioned above of mother and child, the question of what to do is bound up with one's reading of the story. Is this newborn a full-fledged person in danger of being subjected to the cruelest form of discrimination against the handicapped? Is this a dying child whose suffering may be needlessly prolonged by unnatural medical intervention? Is this not a "person" at all, and thus not guaranteed the safeguards provided to members of our moral community? There is no clear social consensus about just what we are witnessing, the nature and status of the main actors in this story, the unfolding plot line, or even to what narrative genre it belongs.

Given the profound disagreements that arise in many bioethical cases, and the significant impact of their resolution on the lives of individuals, we can say something further about the hermeneutics of bioethics: *praxis* is central to the unfolding interpretive work. That is, interpretation is not in service to free-floating theory but intimately bound up with practical consequences. Gadamer has suggested that questions of praxis and application are involved in all hermeneutical enterprises (Gadamer 1975:274–305). Taking as paradigmatic the juridical situation where one seeks to interpret a legal statute to see how it applies to a current case, Gadamer notes that even in literary hermeneutics, the reader relates the text to his or her present concerns and questions. Nevertheless, in bioethical interpretation, as in juridical, we see this element of pragmatic application heightened and brought to the fore. One seeks to understand the case in order to know *what to do*. The practical consequences are often of the utmost importance, sometimes dwarfing any other decision in the lives of the individuals involved.

Moreover, as the case involves living persons and is progressing in real time, its interpretation and the practical consequences that flow from it dynamically transform the text as it is unfolding. For example, an insurance company comes into conflict with a doctor and patient about whether to fund a bone-marrow transplant. Is it really a standard and medically indicated treatment for this cancer? While the parties laboriously debate the question, the cancer progresses until it is untreatable, the argument rendered moot. Clearly, the "text" would have evolved differently if interpretive consensus had been reached and treatment initiated.

We might see this as a special form of the "hermeneutic circle" discussed above. In any interpretation, there is a circular movement wherein the reader and text reflexively interact. While the text shapes and modifies the reader's interpretive structures, these structures also shape the text as he or she encounters it, highlighting certain elements and obscuring others. In a sense, the reader's expectations and interpretations *transform* the experienced text. However, this is true in the bioethical case in a way that goes beyond the literary text: that is, how the participants interpret events and consequently respond quite literally changes the "story line," as in the above cancer case. It is as if the reader(s) of the text is not only a character within the story but also an author constantly extending and redirecting the plot.

This temporal reading/writing is all but unavoidable. Since the case is progressing in time, even to do nothing is to do something. As the insurance company hesitates, the cancer multiplies and metastasizes. While the mother considers abortion, the fetus each moment is growing into maturity. As the debate continues whether to let a patient die, pain is prolonged, money is spent, clinical indicators rise and fall. A bioethics case (outside of the textbook) is not like a literary text handed down through generations for calm perusal, but a shifting, slippery, churning event, whose parameters might change radically from day to day. One never steps into exactly the same river, and each step, or step withheld, influences its course.

Heretofore my analysis has been merely descriptive, using notions drawn from hermeneutics to analyze the bioethical case. We have seen that such cases often are "written" in a complex variety of discursive elements, and subject to multiple conflicting interpretations, wherein questions of practical application are paramount. Subsequent interpretation and consequent praxis reflexively transform the unfolding text. However, this meta-analysis hovering above bioethics does little to clarify what would be a hermeneutic approach *within* bioethics; that is, how might one approach a case hermeneutically, as opposed to, for example, through a method driven by ethical theory?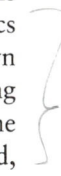

Truth-Telling: A Hermeneutical Analysis

To clarify a possible answer to this question, I will turn to a case example, one well-worn in the annals of bioethics. A patient is found to have a carcinoma which in all probability will prove fatal. The physician wonders whether to tell her patient the truth about his condition and prognosis or whether to conceal certain aspects.

Bioethicists have often approached such dilemmas through reference to grounding theoretical propositions and their application to the case at hand. A utilitarian calculus may be brought to bear, with concern for maximizing happiness and favorable outcome, while minimizing suffering. For example, the very word *cancer,* with its dire connotations, could plunge the patient into depression, sap his will to live, ruin what could be his last days, and cause other forms of turmoil and degeneration which might be avoided through strategic dissimulation. Conversely, and more commonly in contemporary bioethics, a deontological approach is favored. Whether the consequences are sanguine or not, bioethicists often view truth-telling as ethically mandated.

To lie to the patient by commission or significant omission is to violate Kant's categorical imperative on two grounds: it fails the test of universalizability, since the very possibility of effective discourse rests upon the assumption of truth-telling and, moreover, a lie fails to show respect for the other person and his rational autonomy (Kant 1969). In this case, if the doctor lies to the patient, she is manipulating him without his consent and depriving him of his ability to decide the course of his treatment and future life in relation to the facts of his condition. The doctor paternalistically abrogates his liberty in a pernicious way by the act of deception.

However, a hermeneutical analysis reveals much that this move to overarching theory conceals. As we have seen, hermeneutics as a discipline seeks to highlight the complexities of the interpretive situation. From the point of view taken by most contemporary hermeneutics, there is no such thing as unproblematic "truth-telling." For one thing, it is not clear how much the physician should reveal before we would agree that she has spoken the truth. Might she refer simply to a "troublesome growth" and leave it up to the patient to inquire, if he wishes, whether it is malignant? If she speaks that dread word, *cancer,* does she need to detail the stage, the type, the statistics concerning survival rates for this tumor? Moreover, since this communication is unfolding in time, how much need be told immediately? Can she reveal the facts gradually, carefully gearing her communication to the patient's cognitive and emotional state, and still tell the truth? The deontological mandate to "tell the truth" begins to dissolve into ambiguity upon inspection.

Moreover, inherent in the classical notion of truth is the idea that one can take up an objective standpoint from which reason can uncover *what is the case.* In contrast, contemporary hermeneutics has stressed the notion that interpretation is inescapably perspectival. We can only approach a text through the structure of our prejudices, to use Gadamer's term again, as personal and cultural history have shaped them.

The physician cannot avoid presenting what is occurring from her own interpretive standpoint. On the individual level, she has a fund of clinical experience, a set of values, a particular treatment perspective, that sets her off from other physicians. This may unavoidably structure her mode of presenting the case, and probably should — were she to strive for a standpoint of purified objectivity, all personal elements eradicated, the denuded communication that resulted might come no closer to "the truth." Moreover, in addition to what sets her apart, the physician shares with most other physicians a communal interpretive system built up through long years of training. In merely describing the patient's problem as a "cancerous tumor," she is actively reshaping the situation into a *medical* story, as opposed to one whose key terms are existential, religious, or belonging to some other genre.

Where before the patient experienced suffering, tried to make sense of it, reached out to others, reshaped plans, now he is being informed of cell types, stagings, statistical survival rates, surgical and radiological options. This is not simply "the truth" about what is here unfolding but the *truth-according-to-Western-medicine*. The medical interpretive system powerfully reveals and makes sense of certain aspects of the text but just as powerfully conceals others: hence the contemporary lament that medical readings of the "case" often obscure attention to the experience, suffering, and core humanity of the ill.

Thus at the very moment when the doctor thinks she is telling the truth, the patient may experience a profound failure of communication. We see an example of this in *The Death of Ivan Ilych:*

> To Ivan Ilych only one question was important: was his case serious or not? But the doctor ignored that inappropriate question. From his point of view it was not the one under consideration. The real question was to decide between a floating kidney, chronic catarrh, or appendicitis. It was not a question of Ivan Ilych's life or death, but one between a floating kidney and appendicitis. And that question the doctor solved brilliantly, as it seemed to Ivan Ilych.... All the way home [Ivan] was going over what the doctor had said, trying to translate those complicated, obscure, scientific phrases into plain language and find in them an answer to the question: "Is my condition bad? Is it very bad? Or is there as yet nothing much wrong?" (Tolstoy 1960:121–22)

Here the physician's language and concerns so greatly diverge from those of the patient that Ivan comes away in the dark about what to him is the most important matter. "Speaking the truth," then, is not simply a matter of producing words; it describes a complex communicative relationship between individuals, each with her or his own interpretations and pragmatic concerns.

Just as "truth-telling," viewed hermeneutically, is a far more ambiguous and rich phenomenon than that spied from the heights of deontological theory, so the notion of autonomy comes in for a reworking. As we ask if the doctor who "speaks the truth" is, in fact, doing so, so we can ask if this "truth" genuinely fosters personal autonomy, as suggested by Kantian-style theory.

Many authors have drawn attention to the importance of narrativity in making of one's life a coherent whole. For the most part, individuals learn values and meaning not from philosophical theory — applying, for example, the utilitarian calculus — but from the rich legacy of stories with which any culture is endowed (Alderman 1982:127–53). Stories of growing up, of journeys, physical or spiritual in nature; stories of heroes or religious figures and the exemplary way in which they live; stories of great loves and battles, or the challenges of everyday life; from these we learn how to see the world, how to find meaning in the twist and turn of events, and how to construct worthy responses.

Just as we preconsciously unify a visual field into figure and ground with Gestalt coherence, so we automatically seek the narrative coherence of our lives, and when this is broken, we experience a deep loss. Illness of a serious kind often constitutes such a fracturing: the logical progression of our lives is ruptured in what may seem an incoherent way. Career goals, family ties, all the dreams of the future, are now thrown into doubt by what? — a strange lump or a shadow on an X-ray. This shattering of our life's plot by something so unpredictable and absurd can bring about a sense of profound disempowerment. Our life no longer makes sense, we are no longer in control, and our responses seem as meaningless as this shocking occurrence.

Thus the reclamation of an experience of lived autonomy is often tied to a re-weaving of narrative structure. The patient seeks to "make sense" of events and to do what is best; autonomy as lived out is not just the exercise of an arbitrary power of choice but the attempt to choose *well* in the context of one's life-story, with its own plot, aims, and values.[5] The health care provider can play a crucial role in restoring autonomy by helping the ill person reconstruct meaning in the face of the threat posed by events. The life-story has taken a radically new turn, but it need not thereby cease to be a story; the illness might be read as a journey into the unknown, a battleground inviting heroism, a cross to bear with spiritual fortitude, or a call to increased intimacy with others.[6] It is not necessarily the job of the physician to supply this story in a paternalistic fashion; it will usually evolve from within the patient's own experience and intuition (Brody 1987:182–92). But the physician can listen to and support the healing story, tactfully question destructive elements (for example, an overemphasis on sin, guilt, punishment, and despair), and, in general, play the role of a respectful dialogue partner who hears and speaks to the patient's need for narrative.

However, the physician often reads the illness simply in medical terms — as a matter of neoplastic cells, metastases, and survival rates. When the physician presents this medical "truth" without sensitivity, it can further undermine the patient's search for meaning and genuine autonomy already threatened by the illness. The patient feels disempowered in the face of a foreign jargon, a strange story which, while it makes sense to the doctor, has little to do with the ground of the sufferer's own life. This medical story can tend to overwhelm the other narratives which help the person construct significance and life-enhancing responses.

One could reply that these medical truths are nonetheless empowering on the level of enabling real-life action. Regardless of their narrative poverty, these data allow the patient to make informed decisions in relation to the panoply of treatment options. In this sense, clinical truths restore "autonomy," etymologically meaning "self-rule," to the degree possible.

While, of course, much is correct about this perspective, it conceals other elements. A hermeneutic analysis is sensitive to the multiple contexts — historical, psychological, social, political — within which a story unfolds, and which provide frameworks for fuller interpretation.[7] Thus, to understand the story told to the patient and its pragmatic repercussions, one must attend to the broader contexts in which it is enacted. For example, the patient may receive "the truth" about his illness and treatment options but find himself constrained by economics. For many in our society, proper medical care is an unaffordable luxury, and questions of personal finances and insurance coverage, or lack thereof, deform and constrict the clinical context. Are medical truths empowering when we cannot act upon them?

Then too, social power-relations shape the communicative structure itself. The physician is often in a multiply determined position of power over the patient.[8] The doctor, after all, is the healthy one; the patient, sick. The doctor knows what is happening clinically, while the patient can only strive to understand. The doctor often has a higher-status and more lucrative career than that of the patient. Not unusually, race and gender distinctions reinforce this pattern: the doctor (unlike our imagined case) may be a white male, the patient, a minority or a woman.

Moreover, medical institutions are designed to empower the physician, not the patient; it is clear who is king of the private office or the hospital, while the patient sits meekly in the waiting room or lies prone in the hospital bed awaiting examination.

We might ask whether in such settings the patient can genuinely experience as empowering the "truths" articulated by the physician. The medical diagnosis pronounced, the esoteric terminology used, the treatment options presented, constitute a discourse which draws the patient ever deeper into the institutional context just described. Foucault has suggested that modern institutions enact power over individuals through a complex interweaving of languages and practices, all of which promise to be liberating — cooperate and you will be "cured," or "normal," or "forgiven," or "reformed" (Foucault 1980; 1979; 1975; 1973). So too, the "truths" of medicalese promise knowledge and power to the individual, but only by introducing him or her into a context which can be radically disempowering: the alienating hospital room with the medical residents who sweep in and out unexpectedly, the hospital gown half open in the back, the high-tech procedures and their staggering expense, the hundred other humiliating or dehumanizing details that adorn the world of modern medicine. Contemporary treatments often extend, rather than repair, the loss of autonomy inaugurated by illness.

Hermeneutics and Interpretive Complexity

The above case can be used to contrast a hermeneutical with a theory-driven approach to bioethics. It may seem that the issue chosen, that of truth-telling, is idiosyncratic in its focus on the communicative act, and therefore more slanted toward hermeneutic analysis than many others. There is some validity to this point: hermeneutics has long focused on the transmission of meaning through language, and so an issue where language is centrally at stake provides an inviting place to initiate hermeneutic reflection. We have seen, however, that interpretation comes into play at all levels of human understanding and decision making, such that we can approach every bioethical issue hermeneutically. Thus we can draw certain general points from this case.

The theory-driven approach, briefly presented above, promises a resolution to the dilemma of truth-telling. It makes use of clear distinctions (for example, telling the truth versus withholding or distorting it), and of rational principles such as "universalizability" and "respect for persons." An ahistorical logic claims to validate the answer arrived at.

Whether Kant's categorical imperative or Bentham's utilitarian calculus, it uses a principle to evaluate the objective rightness of an act independent of personal or social interpretive distortions.

Such an approach has significant strengths — hence its abiding popularity within bioethics. Ethical theories can help clarify the structure of a complex dilemma; provide guides and justifications for decisive action; embody values most of us share, such as happiness, equality, justice, and autonomy; and serve as powerful reminders of these values in contexts where they are neglected — for example, an institutional setting insensitive to suffering or deprivations of freedom.

Nonetheless, the above case exposes the partiality of such an approach. This "top-down" methodology, wherein one commences with high-level theory, can obscure the rich complexity of actual cases. Even the very schematic case presented above illustrates how attending to concrete detail is crucial in articulating the ethical dimensions of a situation. Modes of "truth" or "falsity," "coercion" or "autonomy," often come down to the words chosen and the words never said; the class, gender, and race of participants; the rooms in which communication takes place; the time-constraints placed on conversation and decision making. A hermeneutic approach, oriented toward the close reading of narratives, may better note the significance of such elements imperceptible from the heights of ethical theory.

Moreover, as discussed, a hermeneutic reading of the dense text presented by any case can refer to the wide variety of *contexts* — phenomenological, psychological, religious, linguistic, economic, institutional, and political — in which it unfolds. A recourse to an abstract and presumably ahistorical rationality tends to distract attention from these modes of concrete embeddedness. As we see above, notions of "truth" and "autonomy" are at best incompletely specified, at worst obscurantist and distorted, unless one articulates the modes of speech and action possible within the life-world of *these* participants and the vectors of force pressing on them from within and without. A hermeneutical approach can be more open to the many influences shaping a text and thus to the many interpretive strategies that can be brought to bear upon it.

Perhaps the greatest strength of the hermeneutic perspective, as I here understand it, is this openness to a variety of interpretive perspectives. A foundationalist ethics tends to valorize a single principle such as that of utility, or the categorical imperative. Even a more moderate principlism usually restricts itself to a limited number of principles brought to bear on any case — for example, Beauchamp and Childress's use of "respect for autonomy," "beneficence," "nonmaleficence," and "justice" (Beauchamp and Childress 1989). Though a specific mode of interpretation, such as that found within psychoanalysis or Marxism, may be similarly restrictive, the overall approach here designated as "hermeneutical" is open-ended. Twentieth-century hermeneutics tends to reject the notion that there is a single correct interpretation in favor of an acknowledgment that any text is susceptible to an indefinite variety of readings. This is not to say that each reading is equally significant or useful; however, one should not foreclose the possibility of multiple interpretations which overlap, supplement, clash, and converse with one another in ways that lead one to a deeper understanding of phenomena.

A multiplicity of interpretations can often first be found embodied in the case participants themselves. As discussed, the patient, family, physicians, nurses, hospital lawyers, chaplain, and others may all take divergent viewpoints on a case, representing their respective world of concerns. A hermeneutic approach would begin with an attempt to *listen* carefully to these voices of the characters within the drama.

However, we cannot rest only with what the characters speak. There may be interpretations of the case that, while highly significant, are inaccessible for various reasons to the participants. Ricoeur suggests that we have entered an age characterized by the "hermeneutics of suspicion": instructed by the work of Marx, Freud, and Nietzsche, we have learned to look beneath the surface text of individual and social self-awareness to uncover hidden forces that motivate events (Ricoeur 1970:32–36). Whether as a result of psychological repression, ideological distortion, the will to power, or simply the difficulty of distancing oneself from structures in which one is immersed, it is often impossible to fully satisfy the injunction to "know thyself." For example, in the above case of "truth-telling," neither patient nor doctor may become reflexively aware of the social contexts and power-relations that structure their communication. But this can and should become available to the hermeneut seeking a complex and comprehensive reading.

The standard textbook of bioethics frequently lacks this hermeneutic complexity. Therein we often find a canonical set of terms, theories, and principles explained in introductory sections and instantiated in the articles or case discussions judged worthy of inclusion. For example, now that the issue of surrogate motherhood has found its way into textbooks, authors often treat the subject in utilitarian or deontological terms. They consider the psychological effect upon the various participants or whether the context of "rent-a-womb" and "buy-a-baby" preserves respect for persons. While such concerns are highly significant and may ultimately be judged decisive, so much remains unconsidered or only tangentially addressed. For example: the market pressures and alienating labor-options that may lead women to become surrogate mothers; the fetishism of commodities described by Marx, and how this infiltrates our treatment of human beings; the way gender roles as conceived of within our society shape our notions of "motherhood"; the history of medicolegal doctrines concerning reproduction and the role such doctrines have played in supporting patriarchal power; the paradigm of body-as-machine ascendant since Descartes, and how it has structured our sense of the way bodies may be used. Such perspectives help illuminate morally significant dimensions of surrogate mothering, but one must often turn to works in sociology, law, feminism, history, political economics, and metaphysics — not to one's textbook of bioethics — to see them addressed.

It might appear that to introduce such perspectives would be to dismantle bioethics as a discipline. Where would be its autonomy, its methodology, its unique focus and contribution if it were to incorporate all these voices? Is this not in essence a prescription for the demise of bioethics?

This is true only if we identify bioethics with one particular view of its project. If we see bioethics as grounded in an ahistorical rationality, this influx of motley perspectives is indeed a threat. It introduces *heteronomy*, to use a Kantian term, laws foreign to its own *telos*.

However, a hermeneutical bioethics might conceive its project quite differently. It need not define itself primarily in opposition to other discourses but as home to all morally relevant interpretations and insights, whether they originate in psychoanalytic theory, historical analysis, political debate, or Kant. Nor must this mean the collapse of bioethics as an integral project. After all, bioethics is never simply identical to psychoanalysis, history, or politics; it is always mining the resources of these fields for the way in which they shed light on specifically *ethical* themes. The domain of moral inquiry remains intact; we are interested in what *should* be, not simply in what is, and thus with questions of freedom, responsibility, mutual obligation, duty, caring, virtue and vice, the good life, and social justice, as they play out in health care and the biological sciences. An adequate treatment of such issues opens onto the widest of terrains. A hermeneutical bioethics then is not just one approach as opposed to the others in this book — phenomenological, feminist, cross-cultural, and so on — but the very space wherein these perspectives are articulated and engage in dialogue. Whether this dialogue be congenial or clashing, it promises to enrich our bioethical reflection.

What Becomes of Decision Making and Truth?

Yet something crucial still seems to be missing from this style of reflection: a calculus for decision making. After all, we are not simply seeking rich readings but answers, guides for action in the clinical wards and halls of government. The physician or politician often turns to the bioethicist to *resolve* an issue, not just open it up for endless interpretation, and there are real needs — clinical, financial, temporal — for closure.

Moreover, what becomes of the notion of ethical truth? Is not this hermeneutic approach simply a sophisticated relativism, spinning out endless interpretations without criteria for preference? How can we tell a right interpretation from a wrong, a valuable "prejudice" from one that distorts and impairs our moral sense?

Such questions do indeed present difficulties for hermeneutics and may expose certain pragmatic and theoretical weaknesses. This style of doing bioethics is less suited to supplying quick answers on the ward and might not be as popular with doctors seeking the spot ethics consultation. Moreover, the issue of truth within hermeneutics continues to be a thorny one, given its contemporary abandonment of reference to an ahistorical guarantor. Once this secure foundation is gone, whether supplied by God or purified reason, it becomes difficult to provide guidelines for interpretive truth.

Hermeneutic thinkers respond that an abandonment of "objectivism" need not plunge us into relativism.[9] Though we cannot step outside our tradition to employ a purified logic, our tradition itself gives us bases for judgment. We have consensually validated standards of what constitutes a reasoned argument. Moreover, our dialogue with the text at hand, and with other interpreters, allows us to become aware of and move beyond the limits of our prejudices. Thus we no longer conceive of "rationality" as a disembodied faculty for apprehending pure truth but as a communal dialogue which progresses through revelatory give and take.

A full discussion of such points would take us well beyond the bounds of this paper. Suffice it to say that in the context of our deeply divided society, appeals to social consensus and communal progress remain problematic. A clarification of how interpretations are to be judged better or worse, revelatory or obscurantist, remains a central challenge for hermeneutic thought.

However, this hermeneutically reframed notion of rationality does suggest new and productive roles for the bioethicist. It has been tempting to view such a figure as the *answer person*, showing us what course of action moral reasoning mandates. But if hermeneutic thought undermines this notion, different roles are invited. For example, the bioethicist can become the *articulator* of the perspectives of case participants, allowing their voices and concerns to emerge more fully. He or she is then better able to act as a *facilitator* of dialogue between parties, fostering mutual understanding and respect. Whereas the standard textbook often portrays bioethics as a battle between "pro" and "con" perspectives, each attempting to attack and destroy the other, Gadamer stresses that hermeneutics begins with a spirit of dialogic openness; one approaches a text (or another person) with the sense that they have something to teach, a perspective capable of transcending, overturning, or revising one's own in a productive way (Gadamer 1975:261–62).

Moreover, as discussed, the hermeneut not only helps articulate, and facilitate dialogue between, the various positions of case participants but also acts as the *recaller* of contexts and perspectives which are systematically obscured. We are always, to a degree, blind to our own prejudices; we live in a tradition as a fish in water. However, the hermeneut, knowing prejudice is an inevitable constituent of understanding, is in a better position to become self-reflective about those structures — historical, political, metaphysical — that limit and channel our discourse. This awareness may allow revision of the canonical list of bioethics issues; for example, reflection on how the Western tradition has largely expelled nonhumans from the realm of moral concern[10] can and has helped sensitize us to questions raised by animal experimentation, and the importance of including these in our future textbooks. Moreover, we have seen how a sensitivity to forgotten contexts enriches even canonical issues such as "telling the truth" to patients. The bioethicist thus emerges more as a Socratic interlocutor than an "answer person." He or she is the *gadfly* who questions the settled presumptions of our discourse, dismantling premature claims to truth, closure, and virtue. Moreover, he or she is the instigator of cooperative dialogue from which all participants learn. If one does not arrive at absolute truth (which for Socrates always eluded those caught within the mortal frame), one may nonetheless evolve toward richer interpretations. That is, through careful reading of the text, self-reflection about one's prejudices, and openness to others, one can arrive at an understanding and course of action likely to be responsive to more features of the situation, and thus more nuanced and efficacious.

The individual who is "pro-life" vis-à-vis abortion, for example, might not change his or her basic stance as a result of hermeneutic reflection but might come to a formulation and plan of action that is more complex. He or she may see, in common with many "pro-choicers," the need to address forces of poverty, ignorance, racism, and social breakdown that lead to unwanted pregnancy; the sexism that has grounded a history of male control over female reproduction; the lack of public support, economic and psychological, for bringing an unintended pregnancy to term and then raising the child; the possible hypocrisy of being "pro-life" on this issue but leaving unchallenged militaristic policies from which thousands die, and which siphon off funds from needy mothers and children.[11] The abortion issue is thus reframed in a way that heightens awareness of the multiple contexts in which it is embedded, and allows for a multidimensional response.

Obviously, this process will not bring an end to moral conflict; different interpreters will continue to disagree. But no moral framework has resolved all differences, nor in our pluralistic society is there a single framework to which all consent. In such a world, hermeneutics does have a crucial role to play in fostering careful readings and respectful dialogue.

What of Religion?

In closing, it is appropriate within the context of this volume briefly to address the place of religion within a hermeneutic bioethics. On the one hand, contemporary hermeneutics tends to undercut religious absolutism. Truth is no longer unquestioningly secured by reference to divine authority and the validity of a Torah, Bible, or Koran. In this sense, twentieth-century hermeneutics conflicts directly with certain modes of religious thought.

On the other hand, a hermeneutical approach may prove far more friendly toward faith-based perspectives than a bioethics based on standard ethical theory. We remember that hermeneutics first developed as a set of methods to interpret the truths of sacred scripture. In the modern world, the very notion of "truth," at least in public discourse, has been largely detached from its religious origins, and identified with a community of experts — whether scientists, philosophers, technocrats, ethicists — who are seen as exercising a purified rationality. This pure rationality is no longer the province of theologians; on the contrary, religion takes the form of threat, potentially leading us from the light of shared reason into the darkness of dogmatic, private, and coercive belief. Hence, the relative absence of religiously based argumentation in contemporary bioethics of the sort canonized within textbooks. Even the religious thinker is often at pains to keep this perspective in the closet and to show that he or she can arrive at conclusions independent of any faith concerns.

While religious prejudices have had their pernicious side, hermeneutic reflection reveals that the expulsion of religion is itself a constricting prejudice of the modern age. In the lives of many (if not most) individuals, faith-based modes of understanding play a key role in experience. Especially in the situations examined by bioethics involving issues of birth and death, justice and equality, illness, risk, and existential crisis, individuals are likely to turn to religious resources for making sense of events and constructing moral responses. And why should they not? Faith-based perspectives can give rise to modes of interpretation and action which are complex, consistent, sensitive, and illuminating.

As earlier discussed, we tend to develop our moral sense not by studying theory but through the stories of moral heroes and failures transmitted by tradition. We find a rich representation of such stories in our religious heritage. Does the categorical imperative provide a worthier ground for ethical response than the parable of the Good Samaritan or the story of Job? Then too, religion is a source of its own articulated principles — the Ten Commandments, for example, or those presented in the Sermon on the Mount. Though not validated by pure reason, such rules find their own traditional and experiential supports. A hermeneutic bioethics, having no allegiance to the ideal of a purified rationality, need not reject these references. While religious thought is not permitted to trump all other participants, it is welcomed as a serious player at the table. Otherwise the public dialogue known as "bioethics" can become impoverished and irrelevant to the deepest concerns of many whose cases are under scrutiny.

NOTES

1. For an overview of the history and major figures of hermeneutics see Palmer 1969.

2. See, for example, Dilthey 1976:170–245.

3. On the hermeneutics of perception and scientific inquiry, see Heelan 1983.

4. This complicated textuality is also characteristic of clinical hermeneutics, wherein the health care practitioner interprets a wide variety of information in seeking to arrive at a diagnosis. See Leder 1990:9–24.

5. For an exploration of "actual" autonomy as experienced and lived out in the context of impairment, institutional settings, and health care, see Agich 1993 and Katz 1984.

6. On the stories which shape the lives and self-understanding of the chronically ill, see Kleinman 1988.

7. In arguing this, I am taking up Gadamer's position, contra Habermas,

that hermeneutics is not just concerned with surface discourse, but capable of, even suited to, exploring the various contexts that shape a social language and praxis in ways that may escape the society's own self-understanding. See Gadamer 1976:18–43; for a general discussion of the Habermas-Gadamer debate, see Warnke 1987:107–38.

8. On the asymmetrical relationship of doctor and patient, see Zaner 1988:84–86, 251–55.

9. See Bernstein 1983.

10. See, for example, Singer 1990.

11. For examples of such an analysis, see *Sojourners* (November 1980). For an example of a dialogical approach to the often acrimonious abortion debate, see Callahan and Callahan 1984.

REFERENCES

Agich, George. 1993. *Autonomy and Long-term Care.* New York: Oxford University Press.

Alderman, Harold. 1982. "By Virtue of a Virtue." *Review of Metaphysics* 36 (September): 127–53.

Beauchamp, Tom L., and James F. Childress. 1989. *Principles of Biomedical Ethics.* 3d ed. New York: Oxford University Press.

Bernstein, Richard J. 1983. *Beyond Objectivism and Relativism: Science, Hermeneutics and Praxis.* Philadelphia: University of Pennsylvania Press.

Brody, Howard. 1987. *Stories of Sickness.* New Haven: Yale University Press.

Callahan, Sidney, and Daniel Callahan. 1984. "Breaking Through Stereotypes." *Commonweal* (5 October): 520–23.

Daniel, Stephen L. 1986. "The Patient as Text: A Model of Clinical Hermeneutics." *Theoretical Medicine* 7:195–210.

Dilthey, Wilhelm. 1976. *Selected Works,* trans. and ed. H. P. Rickman. Cambridge: Cambridge University Press.

Foucault, Michel. 1980. *The History of Sexuality, Volume One: An Introduction,* trans. Robert Hurley. New York: Vintage Books.

———. 1979. *Discipline and Punish: The Birth of the Prison,* trans. Alan Sheridan. New York: Vintage Books.

———. 1975. *The Birth of the Clinic,* trans. A. M. Sheridan Smith. New York: Vintage Books.

———. 1973. *Madness and Civilization: A History of Insanity in the Age of Reason,* trans. Richard Howard. New York: Vintage Books.

Gadamer, Hans-Georg. 1975. *Truth and Method,* trans. and ed. Garrett Barden and John Cumming. New York: Seabury Press.

———. 1976. *Philosophical Hermeneutics,* ed. David E. Linge. Berkeley: University of California Press.

Heelan, Patrick A. 1983. *Space-perception and the Philosophy of Science.* Berkeley: University of California Press.

Heidegger, Martin. 1962. *Being and Time,* trans. John Macquarrie and Edward Robinson. New York: Harper and Row.

Kant, Immanuel. 1969. *Foundations of the Metaphysics of Morals*, trans. Lewis White Beck. Indianapolis: Bobbs-Merrill.

Katz, Jay. 1984. *The Silent World of Doctor and Patient*. New York: Free Press.

Kleinman, Arthur. 1988. *The Illness Narratives*. New York: Basic Books.

Leder, Drew. 1990. "Clinical Interpretation: The Hermeneutics of Medicine." *Theoretical Medicine* 11:9–24.

Nagel, Thomas. 1986. *A View from Nowhere*. New York: Oxford University Press.

Palmer, Richard E. 1969. *Hermeneutics*. Evanston, Ill.: Northwestern University Press.

Ricoeur, Paul. 1970. *Freud and Philosophy: An Essay on Interpretation*, trans. Denis Savage. New Haven: Yale University Press.

Singer, Peter. 1990. *Animal Liberation*. 2d ed. New York: New York Review of Books.

Tolstoy, Leo. 1960. *The Death of Ivan Ilych and Other Stories*. New York: New American Library.

Warnke, Georgia. 1987. *Gadamer: Hermeneutics, Tradition and Reason*. Stanford: Stanford University Press.

Zaner, Richard. 1988. *Ethics and the Clinical Encounter*. Englewood Cliffs, N.J.: Prentice-Hall.

~ *11* ~

NARRATIVE CONTRIBUTIONS TO MEDICAL ETHICS
RECOGNITION, FORMULATION, INTERPRETATION, AND VALIDATION IN THE PRACTICE OF THE ETHICIST

Rita Charon

[T]he moral law gives rise by an intrinsic necessity to storytelling.
... Without storytelling there is no theory of ethics.[1]

Introduction

As the field of medical ethics matures, the complexity of the cognitive, affective, and interpretive acts through which ethical decisions are constructed becomes clearer. Once understood primarily as a project of administering universally applicable principles and adjudicatory rules to health care conflicts, the practice of medical ethics increasingly has come to include the search for the meanings of singular human situations.[2] Narrative knowledge and practice, those modes of thought and action with which humans comprehend and respond to particularized human events to endow them with meaning, are being recognized as central features in considering and resolving biomedical ethical cases. This narratively grounded view of medical ethics solicits contributions from disciplines that recognize and interpret human situations, among them anthropology, history, linguistics, psychology, sociology, and literary criticism. With overlapping competencies in narrative studies, members of these disciplines can help to contextualize and particularize the conflicts faced in medical ethics, contributing methods with which to generate telling descriptions grounded in evidence, and then to choose trustworthy readings of those descriptions. Sometimes called narrative ethics, these activities are more appropriately conceptualized as the narrative contributions to the trustworthiness of medical ethics.[3]

To begin with, the ethics deliberation seeks to recognize the narrative coherence, however obscured, of the patient's life. In addition, the medical ethicist faces narrative tasks in identifying the multiple tellers of the patient's story, the several audiences to whom the story is told, and the interpretive community responsible for understanding it. The medical ethicist relies on narrative methods to examine contradictions among the story's multiple representations, conflicts among tellers and listeners, and ambiguities in the events themselves. Finally, all participants in an ethical deliberation — the medical ethicist, the health professionals, the patient, and the patient's family — require that which only narrative knowledge can give: the coherence, the resonance, and the singular meaning of particular human events.

Narrative competence can increase the effectiveness and accuracy of medical ethics deliberations throughout all stages of ethical decision making — the recognition of the ethical problem, the written or oral formulation of the problem, the interpretation of the ethical case, and the validation of the chosen interpretation as the most reasonable and helpful among the many alternative interpretations available. This essay will discuss several aspects of each of these four stages of ethical deliberation, suggesting specific questions or approaches that a narrative framework throws into relief.

Narrative studies suggest that individuals achieve identity and intimacy by telling and following stories, as cultures define their values and membership through the narrating of myth and epic. "We live," says Peter Brooks, "immersed in narrative, recounting and reassessing the meaning of our past actions, anticipating the outcome of our future projects, situating ourselves at the intersection of several stories not yet completed" (Brooks 1985:3). Through such narratives as fiction, journalism, history, and autobiography, human beings seek the meaning of their experiences, subscribe to a causality, and represent and configure the world so that it makes sense enough to act in it. Although narrative's form of knowing-in-telling may seem like second nature and undefinable — in Roland Barthes's words, "international transhistorical, transcultural, narrative is *there*, like life" — one can imagine its absence or its opposite, a state of affairs in which the facts cannot add up to a story (Barthes 1988:95).

Those actions, events, and interactions that occur under the medical gaze differ from those of ordinary life only in being more likely to involve bodies, illness, pain, or death.[4] Heightened by their proximity to death and therefore sometimes appearing atypical, the events that concern the biomedical ethicist otherwise share most characteristics of what Jerome Bruner describes as the "rich and messy domain of human interaction" (Bruner 1991:4). Rarely solitary and more commonly dyadic, collective, dialogic, interpersonal, at times intersubjective, the events of illness and health care unfold in sequences that, once configured by corporeal, emotional, social, and spiritual significance, reveal meaning to all who act — to the patient, the caregivers, and all who accompany them. Applied ethics has conferred some order upon the messy domain of illness by positing the centrality of a set of principles — beneficence/ nonmaleficence, autonomy, and justice — and by deriving such rules as informed consent, confidentiality, and truth-telling from those principles to guide action in quandary cases. A formalist sanitization of chaos, however, may not be sufficient for comprehending the significance of these events; the parties require a particularized (and usually affectively charged) grasp of their meaning. If, as Bruner suggests, "we organize our experience and our memory of human happenings mainly in the form of narrative — stories, excuses, myths, reasons for doing and not doing, and so on," then an understanding of biomedical ethical cases that is informed by the knowledge of narrative theory may offer the essence that is unobtainable using solely formalist methods (Bruner 1991:4).

Several things happen when someone recognizes that an ethical issue exists. First, the case is examined by the patient, health professionals, legal professionals, ethicists, family members, or hospital administrators — the examiners chosen by the context and content of the problem. Second, the examination results in a formulation of the case framed by its author's perspective, usually a written case but sometimes a bureaucratic form filled out with sketchy details or an oral tale told on rounds.

Third, the case as formulated is then submitted for interpretation. Not unlike a careful reading of a literary text, this interpretive step requires that the interpreter or reader pull together sequences of events into meaningful wholes, contextualize the narrative in multiple dimensions, adopt alien points of view, recognize metaphorical systems, grasp the allusions that widen the tale, tolerate ambiguity, recognize multiple contradictory meanings of a story, and hear the story to the end. That is, those who appreciate the ethics case act toward it as a good reader would act toward a tragedy by Shakespeare or a novel by Henry James — assuming that the story, however chaotic or mandarin, means something and that the careful reader will uncover ways to accommodate the contradictions and to judge the ambiguities. The interpretive community of the case may include all who sit on a hospital ethics committee, all doctors and students on a ward team, the primary doctor and the primary nurse, the family, the patient, or anyone else who encounters the case. Through many readings, they achieve an interpretation that most accurately reflects their beliefs and practices.

Fourth, this interpretation is submitted to validation testing. Agents in the case must be assured that the achieved interpretation is reasonable, is somehow better than alternative interpretations, depicts the facts and events of the case accurately and faithfully, and leads to defensible action. During validation testing, interpretations may be rejected because they are incomplete, biased, or in conflict with institutional values or practices. Once the interpretation has passed a test of validation, it may lead to action. But the one who must act may lend still another test of validation. For example, if the cardiac arrest resident walks rather than runs to initiate CPR, he or she has clearly rejected on appeal the interpretation leading to the choice to resuscitate.

Although described here as discrete steps, in practice they occur simultaneously and influence one another. To illustrate, here is an analogy: Medical students are sometimes baffled when watching the heart at work through echocardiography for the first time. They have carefully learned the sequential steps of the cardiac cycle: first the right atrium fills with deoxygenated blood; then it contracts and sends the blood through the tricuspid valve to the right ventricle, which then contracts to send the blood through the pulmonic valve to the pulmonary circulation. The oxygenated bloods returns to the left atrium, is passed through the mitral valve to the left ventricle, and in systole is pumped through the aortic valve to the systemic circulation. The echocardiogram, however, reveals that all these events happen at once; the student is dazed by the simultaneity and unable to recognize any discrete event. So, too, the recognition, formulation, interpretation, and validation of an ethical decision are inseparable, occurring simultaneously, and the facts of the case exist dialectically with their interpretation.

Literary critics recognize "the impossibility of establishing well-grounded distinctions between fact and interpretation, between what can be read in the text and what is read into it" (Culler 1982:75). Never absent from the messy domain of human interaction, the dualisms of narrative have implications for the methods of approaching problems in biomedical ethics. If the stages of recognition, formulation, interpretation, and validation are separated for heuristic purposes, they are recombined in the acts of ethical discernment. The following discussion will outline the narrative elements inherent in the accomplishment of these stages. No matter who — analytically trained philosopher, clinician-ethicist, or narrative ethicist — accomplishes them, narrative knowledge contributes to the accuracy and effectiveness of these processes as they reach toward reasonable understandings of complex human troubles.

Recognition

Little consensus exists on the constitution of an ethical problem. Robert Walker and his colleagues compared doctors' and nurses' perceptions of ethics problems on general medical services, finding intergroup discrepancies on the existence and the nature of the problems and suggesting that "differences in professional orientation lead physicians and nurses toward different views of what counts as an ethics problem" (Walker et al. 1991:428). The pattern of problem recognition can be different in otherwise similar hospitals — i.e., requests for consultation coming from nurses, social workers, patients, and house officers in one hospital and almost exclusively from attending physicians in the other. In addition, as Joel Frader laments, often "no one involved realizes that an ethical problem exists, much less one that might lend itself to consultative assistance" (Frader 1992:36). One can hope for a state of affairs in which all involved in the clinical encounter recognize that every physician-patient encounter involves a moral dimension.

Recognition of an ethical problem belongs to the cognitive category of surprise, "an extraordinarily useful phenomenon to students of mind, for it allows us to probe what people take for granted.... [S]urprise is a response to violated presupposition" (Bruner 1986:46). Only if surprised will a witness notice an event and acknowledge the dissimilarity between one case and others. In an enterprise like medicine, which is based on distinguishing the remarkable from the unremarkable and consigning the unremarkable to inattention, only the step of recognizing something as a problem elevates it to the plane of action. For example, a patient's acceptance of treatment is not noted with the vigor with which a patient's refusal of treatment is met, and yet the acceptance may be as ethically challenging as the refusal. Recognition of the ethical problems, that is, is stamped with the perspective of the person in the recognizing seat, usually the health professional and not the patient. What excites surprise or recognition in medicine reveals what is and is not taken for granted, the step of recognition affording information on the nature of the interpretive community.

For example, medical ethical problems may remain unrecognized because of gaps in clinicians' abilities to perceive the self within the body. In contrast, phenomenologists who study medicine describe the sick person and his or her experiences of illness "not so much as a specific breakdown in the mechanical functioning of the biological body, but more fundamentally as a . . . disintegration of self and world. . . . This is not surprising when one recognizes the *illness-as-lived* is a disruption of the *lived body*" (Toombs 1988:207). The care of the body is the care of the self, as a self does not *have* a body but *is* that body. The clinician, then, who fails to recognize self-within-body may easily mistake ethical concerns for technical concerns. An internist, for example, dismisses the concerns of a young mother with a congenital muscle disease who reports muscle twitches in her two-year-old daughter. The doctor schedules nerve conduction tests in the remote future instead of facing the complex ethical situation of the mother, guilty with the fear that her child has inherited her disease. Just as narrative within the medical discourse maintains the selfhood of the patient — or "conjures up another realm of events . . . in which the patient reappears as a person" — so too narrative rescues these ethical issues from the domain of nonmeaningful corporeal concerns (Young 1988:3).[5]

Hidden by inattention or by mistaken assignment of concerns to technical categories, ethical problems can also be hidden within the secrecy at the heart of a medical case. As readers of fiction know, no narrative tells all that it can to each reader. "[A]ll narratives are capable of darkness," reminds Frank Kermode, "so dark that special training, organized by an institution of considerable size, is required for [their] interpretation" (Kermode 1979:14). Narratives from scriptures to Shakespeare hide their secrets from all but the inside few, and complex multivoiced medical cases are no exception. "We glimpse the secrecy through the meshes of a text; this is divination, but what is divined is what is visible from our angle. It is a momentary radiance" (Kermode 1979:144).

William Carlos Williams, poet and physician, allows his physician-narrator in "The Girl with the Pimply Face" to recognize a self-preservative and substantial will behind the slouching truant's acned front and to act on that evidence by offering her a course of treatment. He adopts the nonjudgmental clinical imagination that enables him to perceive the deeper meaning of the actions of the truculent young girl. Similarly, the step of recognizing ethical problems requires professional competence of a very particular sort, not solely an intellectual expertise but more saliently a narrative sensitivity to the central secrecy of human situations: the existence of unresolved conflicts that, once recognized, can come to the light of day. Higher degrees of narrative sensitivity may well reveal ethical conflicts that require more subtle action than the grueling end-of-life decisions or right-to-refuse-treatment dilemmas, conflicts that require the ethical equivalent of care instead of cure — requiring, that is, not intervention toward a solution but human acknowledgment, clarity, and acceptance.

Formulation

Different from the telling of a folktale, a newspaper story, or an autobiography, but related in kind to these accounts, the telling of a medical ethics case requires the teller to adopt an implied author ("the second self created in the work" [Booth 1983:137]), to draw up a narrative contract with the listeners, to frame the relevant content of the account, and to infer such relationships as temporality and causality within the narrative. Unaware of the complexity of their acts, many tellers — including doctors who write medical case histories — view their acts of narration as impersonal reports that anyone could have written, that is, they believe that the writing of such documents as medical cases or ethical cases is universal and replicable and unproblematical. This is not the case.

Always an act of self-disclosure, writing reveals mental, ideological, and meaning-making properties of the writer. Agreeing with John Gardner's assertion that "moral fiction communicates meanings discovered by the process of the fiction's creation" (Gardner 1978:108), some would argue that a moral dimension exists in this self-disclosive aspect of writing. Taking pen to paper commits the writer to syntactical and semiotic declarations and slips, for language is unable to resist the mark of its maker. "The traces of the storyteller," writes Walter Benjamin, "cling to the story the way the handprints of the potter cling to the clay vessel" (Benjamin 1969:92). A declaration of loyalty to the ideology and epistemology of Western medicine, the act of taking pen to paper in a medical chart ropes the writer into forms of discourse founded on beliefs about professional authority and omniscience.[6]

In conceptualizing the literal writer (or teller) of the ethical case history as the author, I do not mean to deflect attention from the patient and family, those whose lives are being examined and to whom, ultimately, the story belongs. The patient, that is, remains the source of the story; the writer only renders it for his or her colleagues so that they can act. But to examine, for the present, the literal writer of the case — sometimes the ethics consultant, sometimes the nurse, the intern, the attending physician, or the social worker — allows an examination of the theoretically driven processes of editing, handling point of view, and narrative framing that contribute to the case's interpretation and outcome. The literal writer, that is, determines the perspective from which the case will be seen, chooses the traditions within which to locate the case, judges the elements that are contributory and noncontributory, and establishes the cognitive and affective maps with which readers will follow the narrative trail. For example, a nurse tries to limit the visiting hours of the wife of a demented patient because the wife interferes with treatment, removing intravenous catheters and attempting to feed the patient despite the presence of a feeding tube. The intern decides that a gastrostomy tube is needed for proper feeding, and when the wife refuses to allow the procedure, the intern discusses the issue with the patient's son. Both nurse and intern are viewing the case from their limited points of view, choosing actions that streamline their work but failing to address the possibility that the central issue is the wife's denial of her husband's serious illness.

In formulating the case, the writer or teller adopts narrative rather than logico-scientific modes of thought. In differentiating these two modes of cognitive functioning, Bruner notes that "the structure of a well-formed logical argument differs radically from that of a well-wrought story.... The term *then* functions differently in the logical proposition 'if x, then y' and in the narrative *recit* 'The king died, and then the queen died' " (Bruner 1986:11–12). Imbedded in human intentions and behaviors, the ethical case can be formulated only by adopting a narrative discourse; a logico-scientific discourse is unable to perform the requisite examination of beliefs, motives, and relationships of the case. In the words of J. Hillis Miller, "Even when it is defined as pure practical reason, ethics involves narrative, as its subversive accomplice. Storytelling is the impurity which is necessary in any discourse about the moral law as such, in spite of the law's austere indifference to persons, stories, and history. There is no theory of ethics, no theory of the moral law and of its irresistible, stringent imperative, its 'Thou shalt' and 'Thou shalt not,' without storytelling" (Miller 1987:23).

As lean and muscular a mode as the logico-scientific, narrative discourse respects its own rules and adopts its own epistemological assumptions about the world and those who act within it. To say that the writer of the ethics case adopts narrative discourse means that the writer accepts the power and constraints of storytelling, defined by Barbara Herrnstein Smith as structural and performative "verbal acts consisting of *someone telling someone else that something happened*" (Smith 1981:228). The narrative act presupposes and must identify such features as the motives of the teller and the audience, the shared conventions and traditions that form the background for the narrative act, the hierarchy of influence between teller and audience, and the reasons the story is told, keeping in mind the dictum that "the fact that something is true is never a sufficient reason for saying it" (Smith 1981:229, n. 24). In the case of the demented patient above, both nurse and intern were "telling" the case in order to justify their chosen actions. A full evaluation by an ethics consultant allowed the formulation to be widened to include the points of view of the wife, the son, the hospital attorney, and the neurologist. Rather than being viewed as obstructing care, the wife was found to have severe emotional problems of her own in view of the rapid deterioration of her husband and the less-than-optimal care he had received at other hospitals. By telling the case from the perspective of the wife and not solely the perspectives of the health professionals, the ethics consultant helped the ward team to develop a trusting relationship with the patient's wife, to offer her care for her own problems, and to desist in the plan to divide the family members.

Once having accepted the mode of narrative discourse, then, the writer of the ethics case chooses a narrative stance. Some ethicists interview patients and family members, examine patients and evaluate them medically, talk with the health care team, or read the chart, each action altering the stance of the narrator from patient advocate to health care team member to expert consultant (Frader 1992:41). The problems surrounding the narrative stance are reflected in the escalating division within medical ethics on questions of professional loyalty, identification with medicine, the value of the ethicist as "stranger" in the clinical setting, and mounting concern that "insider" status carries "the seeds for the collapse of critical distance" (Barnard 1992:15).[7] An act of some consequence, the ethicist's adoption of a narrative stance will influence the interpretation of the case and subsequent action and therefore requires explicit attention.

With discourse and stance in hand, the writer then decides what to tell. "Every morning brings us the news of the globe, and yet we are poor in noteworthy stories," writes Benjamin. "The value of information does not survive the moment in which it was new.... [N]arrative achieves an amplitude that information lacks" (Benjamin 1969:89–90). Recollecting William Carlos Williams's disdain of newspaper reports when compared with "the hunted news I get from some obscure patients' eyes," Benjamin's opposition of story and information clarifies the material of the case history (Williams 1967:360). Neither only story nor only information, the ethical case requires both an articulation of the radiant aspects of singular lives and a record of measurable, objective findings. Examination of an ethical case requires, that is, material obtainable through both narrative means and logico-scientific, or formalist, means.

Not new to scientific and intellectual inquiry, dualistic methods combining qualitative and quantitative elements (or narrative and logico-scientific) have been developed by such social scientists as ethnomethodologists, anthropologists, and sociolinguists. Clifford Geertz describes ethnographic work as inseparable from both the data-gathering field techniques of the investigator and reflection on the meaning of culture. The work of a social anthropologist in, say, the highlands of central Morocco is not unlike the work of the hospital ethicist in, say, the crash room of the neonatal intensive care unit. Like Geertz's ethnographer who accepts the task of making sense of conceptual structures "at once strange, irregular, and inexplicit...which he must contrive somehow first to grasp and then to render," the ethicist must somehow see clearly the moral dilemmas facing the patient and must engage in the grasping and the rendering, or the recognizing and the formulating, that require both the information and the story (Geertz 1973:10). The information that the patient's wife removed the intravenous needle from her husband's arm cannot by itself direct action. However, the combination of that information with the narrative dimensions of motivation and personal meanings attached to the action helped the ward team in its course of action.

Finally, all materials gathered, all interviews accomplished, the writer writes the formulation. Some ethics consultants feel "a need for a form that will facilitate the intake and analysis of such consultations" and, in response, have designed a thirty-one-line outline into which the consultant can fit all relevant information. This form reserves two lines for "Patient's Values and Beliefs" and one for "Family Dynamics" and appends a handy checklist of five potentially relevant principles (Doukas 1992:5, 13). In contrast, other consultants write notes in medical charts, much as does any consultant delivering an opinion, adopting the voice of the effaced omniscient narrator. Another group of consultants rely on the written notes of the medical staff as their primary texts, seemingly unaware that the implied authors of those texts are advancing multiple goals, not all of them congruent with the ethical goals of the team or the best interests of the patient. Finally, some have discovered the usefulness of writing detailed stories, not merely of the acute events leading to the current ethical dilemma, but of the biographical and cultural identity of the patient. The feature "Case Stories" in the journal *Second Opinion* reflects the desire of clinicians and ethicists to tell and to consider detailed and affect-laden stories about patients, their families, and their doctors and nurses (see Hunter and Miles 1990a). Nurses have also been developing methods of telling stories, not only about their patients but also about their own personal responses to the patients, toward goals of recognizing ethical problems and clarifying moral choices within an ethics of care.[8]

Methods of representing reality are saturated with ideological assumptions about its underlying structures. This is as true for the bioethicist choosing a formulation method as it is for the sociolinguist choosing a transcription method. Medical ethics consultants could with benefit heed Elliot Mishler's warning that all methods of linguistic transcription "reflect theoretical assumptions about relations between language and meaning, and between method and theory, and are consequential for what we report as findings as well as how we interpret and generalize from those findings" (Mishler 1991:277). Literary scholars are now giving deserved scrutiny to the ways in which the medical profession encodes ideological and hierarchical assumptions about patients into the technical materials of medical work, such as the medical case history. Medical ethicists too must inspect the implications and messages of the oral and written forms in which they represent reality, for their means of representation cannot help influencing their conclusions.

Interpretation

If formulation is by definition a narrative undertaking, interpretation of the formulation, too, engages the participant in activities based in narrative knowledge. Hayden White suggests that "interpretative discourse is governed by the same principles of 'configuration' as those used in narration to endow the events that comprise the 'story' being told with the structural coherency of a 'plot'" (White 1989:18). Relying on Paul Ricoeur's conception of configuration as the process that "transforms the succession of events into one meaningful whole ... which makes the story followable," White asserts that "interpretative discourse tells a story — a story in which the interpreter is both the protagonist and the narrator and whose characteristic themes are the processes of search, discovery, loss and retrieval of meaning, recognition and misrecognition, identification and misidentification, naming and misnaming, explanation and obfuscation, illumination and mystification, and so on" (Ricoeur 1985:67; White 1989:18).

The ethicist, then, engages in multiple narrative acts nested within one another and influencing one another, and the implied author of one stage becomes the protagonist of the next. For example, in the act of collecting information on a patient with lung cancer who has refused radiotherapy, the ethics consultant learns that the radiologist, if his lungs were in the same condition as the patient's, would also refuse treatment. Furthermore, the ethicist cannot help being reminded of his own brother, a heavy smoker who has recently lost thirty pounds. The life experiences of the multiple tellers of the story, then, influence the interpretation of the patient's actions. To interpret the events in an accurate and helpful way the consultant must recognize not only the sources of "bias" in the logico-scientific information but also the sources of meaning in his own narrative conclusions. He must be able on scrutiny to separate his search for meaning from the patient's.

Not an unfamiliar notion in literary studies, the dual roles of author as source and as interpreter of a story lend depth and accuracy to the act of writing. In the preface to *Princess Casamassima*, Henry James writes, "The teller of a story is primarily, none the less, the listener to it, the reader of it too" (James 1908:viii). As the case is being formulated, the work of interpreting has already begun: one moment of the dialectic between formulating and interpreting (or writing and reading) is the setting down, the other the taking up. Although an uncommon reading situation because the writer of it *is* the reader (the formulation and interpretation accomplished by literally the same person or mutual members of a small interpretive community), interpreting an ethics case nonetheless shares features with other acts of reading.

As Wolfgang Iser says of the act of reading a literary text, "it owes its presence in our minds to our own reactions, and it is these that make us animate the meaning of the text as a reality" (Iser 1978:129). Interpreting the ethical case, then, brings into play the interpreter's cognitive and metaphorical skills as he or she orders events, recognizes similarities to and differences from other cases, and pulls together all that is read, at the same time universal and particular, into an understandable whole. Although its influence is not identical from reader to reader, the text "activates our faculties, enabling us to recreate the world it presents. The product of this creative activity is what we might call the virtual dimensions of the text. . . . [It is] not the text itself, nor is it the imagination of the reader: it is the coming together of text and imagination" (Iser 1974:279). Even though the ethics case reports actual events and not fictional ones, the interpreters of these events have no choice but to adopt the power and constraints of language, calling into play all the connotative and affective dimensions of words. No intravenous medication circumvents the liver, and no reading circumvents the associative language-borne system of making meaning of human perceptions and stories.

Like the biblical scholar who engages in Nicholas of Lyra's four levels of interpretation — *litera, moralis, allegoria,* and *anagogia* (literal, ethical, historical, and mystical), the reader of the ethics case perceives and integrates multiple, simultaneous interpretations. In addition to involving a multiplicity of interpretive levels, "[t]he ethics of narrative is a peculiarly *reflexive* study," as the reader participates fully in the search for the meaning of the text (Booth 1988:40). In the stage of interpretation, the object of interpretation and the preexisting theories of the interpreters meet. Either "the object may succumb to the interpretive intentions of the interpreter...or...the object may reveal to the interpreter the unknown of this theory and permit the constitution of a new theory" (Kristeva 1983:86). Meaning "to be mutually indebted," to interpret is to allow the possibility of change for both reader and read; the process is potentially a spiral toward greater clarity rather than a repetitive cycle of nondiscovery (Kristeva 1983:86).

Accustomed to reading ethical cases to arrive at universal and replicable decisions through the application of principles and the rules derived from them, some ethicists may balk at notions of virtual texts, multileveled interpretations, and reflexivity. On inspection, however, the conventional process of choosing an interpretation relies on just such interpretive practices. Ethical issues are often recognized *because* a conflict exists between two health providers or between the patient and the family members. In an inpatient medical survey of 185 ethical problems, the most frequently seen contextual feature was interstaff conflict (Walker et al. 1991:426). Without the existence of more than one compelling interpretation, many ethical issues would not come to light. These problems come to attention, then, precisely because neither party is willing to cede his or her understanding of the issue and choice of action.

In the most extreme cases of conflict among interpretations, the court — or more specifically the judge — is asked to choose among conflicting readings; one person's discernment then resolves the case. Based on an accumulation of practice and precedent, the judge's ruling nonetheless is an individual reading, accepted on the grounds of alignment with state and federal law and the authority vested in the judge by the system of jurisprudence. The locus of authority rests in the tradition of legal findings, much as the locus of an authority for interpretation of literary texts rests in the traditions of criticism, either to be accepted or contested. But neither the ethical, the legal, nor the literary case is ever read ahistorically or apolitically; all interpretation is related to prior and future kindred readings and, at the same time, contributes to and derives from semiotic and cultural systems that attribute meaning to events.

Properties of individual readers can predictably influence their readings. Says Annette Kolodny, "whether we speak of poets and critics 'reading' texts or writers 'reading' (and thereby recording for us) the world, we are calling attention to interpretive strategies that are learned, historically determined, and thereby necessarily gender-inflected" (Kolodny 1985:46). When college teachers assign stories to their students, they know that the women will respond in predictably different ways from the men. When graduate students read narratives (oddly, the reading of lyrical poetry seems not to be influenced by gender), they will split along gender lines in their capacity to enter the narrative worlds held forth by the novel.[9] Readings of ethics cases also are likely to be influenced by the gender, culture, and class of the reader and need to be critiqued for such influence.[10] Additionally, the power hierarchies within a medical center can influence readings, ruling some interpretations unacceptable not on the basis of legitimacy but on the basis of institutional needs and professional dominance.

If, as J. Hillis Miller argues, any act of reading includes an ethical dimension, the reading of an ethics case does so doubly. "The ethical moment in the act of reading, then, if there is one, faces in two directions. On the one hand it is a response to something, responsible to it, responsive to it, respectful of it.... On the other hand, the ethical moment in reading leads to an act" (Miller 1987:4). In reading a literary text, the reading leads to such actions as writing criticism or teaching in class. In reading an ethical case, the reader acts much more specifically *in the world* as a consequence of the reading, recommending this or that resolution of the case. Before leading to action, however, the interpretation must undergo a process of validation.

Validation

The step of seeking validation is critically important to the ethicist and to the subject of ethical inquiry. A false interpretation of a literary text, in a manner of speaking, hurts no one; a faulty ethical interpretation has profound consequences for patients and for the whole enterprise of medical ethics. Unlike interpretations in clinical medicine, natural sciences, or literary studies, interpretations in medical ethics cannot be held to conventional processes of validation. The clinician, for example, can judge interventions with outcome studies, the natural scientist can assess findings with the criterion of replicability, the literary critic can look for such attributes as internal coherence, correspondence, and comprehensiveness. Although by no means unproblematical in these other fields, validation in medical ethics rests on particularly unclear ground. In fact, the ethicist has little ground, save for the formally legal, upon which to call a decision a good one.[11]

Other "inquiry-guided" practices, like ethnographic or socio-linguistic studies, that "explicitly acknowledge and rely on the dialectic interplay of theory, methods, and findings over the course of a study" have had to develop alternative validation methods (Mishler 1990:416, n. 1). Mishler has reformulated the concept of validation on the grounds of trustworthiness, defined as "the degree to which we can rely on the concepts, methods, and inferences of a study, or tradition of inquiry, as the basis for our own theorizing and empirical research" (Mishler 1990:419). Recognizing the interpretive community as the source of validation, Mishler's reformulation locates the authority for judging a conclusion's rightness of fit on its acceptability to others doing similar work, acknowledging the form of knowledge-in-practice that obtains in any discipline, like biomedical ethics, that requires mentored apprentice-ship and clinical training.[12] "[F]ocusing on trustworthiness rather than truth displaces validation from its traditional location in a presumably objective, nonreactive, and neutral reality, and moves it to the social world — a world constructed in and through our discourse and actions, through praxis" (Mishler 1990:420).

As a method of systematizing validation processes, Mishler proposes Thomas Kuhn's concept of the exemplar, that is, a particular instance drawn from practice in which an investigator reaches (and demon-strates the manner of having reached) widely accepted conclusions that appear to the interpretive community as reasonable. "Exemplars con-tain within themselves the criteria and procedures for evaluating the 'trustworthiness' of studies and serve as testaments to the internal his-tory of validation within particular domains of inquiry...together they constitute normal practice — the ordinary, taken-for-granted and trust-worthy concepts and methods for solving puzzles and problems within a particular area of work" (Mishler 1990:422–23).

The increasing interest in a casuistic practice of ethical inquiry may herald a shift toward the exemplar as a means of achieving valida-tion in biomedical ethics. Modern casuistry is marked by "first, reliance on paradigm cases, second, reference to broad consensus, and, finally, acceptance of 'probable' certitude" through a process of "continual self-correction that follow[s] criticism" (Jonsen 1986:71, 70). "Ethics and clinical medicine," writes Stephen Toulmin, "are both prime examples of...fields in which we should, above all, strive to be *reasonable* rather than insisting on a kind of *exactness* that 'the nature to be the case' does not allow" (Toulmin 1982:742). Struggling with the issues of validity or validation, medical ethics joins other fields of interpretive inquiry in probing the nature of certitude, not only in theoretical discourse but in practical, performative verbal and moral acts.[13]

Medical ethicists who adopt such practices of validation encounter two complicated tasks. The first is deciding who, in fact, belongs to the interpretive community, assessing the place of patients, families, nurses, doctors, social workers, community members, and pastoral care professionals in the ranks of interpreters. Although one could have assumed that the hospital ethics committee was just such an interpretive community, these committees have recently begun to shift away from case review to policy formation and thus their helpfulness as validation loci is in doubt (Blake 1992; Ross 1989; Cohen 1988). The second narratively based task facing biomedical ethics in a multicultural and religiously pluralistic society is the identification of the means by which ethicists can reasonably and responsibly arrive at a full and unbiased reading of the cases that come before them.

Finally, because medical ethics exists in both discursive realms and realms of action, some interpretations may well be validated through longitudinal studies of the outcomes of ethical decisions. For example, clinicians study the effects of their interventions, not only on the immediate resolution of the treated problem but on such long-term outcomes as patients' functional status and mortality. Through prospectively following outcomes of decisions for patients or their survivors, bioethicists may review the contexts and sequelae of their practice and thus achieve some rigor in distinguishing effective from ineffective approaches to making decisions.

Coda

The place of narrative knowledge and narrative theory within biomedical ethics is a matter of concern to those who practice such ethics and to those whose meaningful lives depend on methods of finding reasonable and fitting solutions to medical ethics problems. Excluding no one, then, the interest in narrative in ethics has emerged with both a theoretical and a practical dimension. Since narrative practices are involved in all stages of recognizing, formulating, interpreting, and validating ethical decisions, narrative competence is among the required capacities of any biomedical ethicist.

An appreciation of narrative knowledge and practice by ethicists leads to particular methods of work. Those, like Ron Carson, who espouse "thick description" in medical ethics rely on an accumulation of particulars about a patient and his or her culture to convey personal, grounded evidence that can point toward right actions. Practiced interpretation, or discernment in Carson's terms, is the method adopted by the ethicist to "detect, discriminate, and decide.... It is to recognize, especially to perceive both distinctiveness (salience) and connectedness (pertinence)" (Carson 1990:55). Closely related to hermeneutics, casuistry, practical reason, and thick description, discernment is "characterized by being personal, responsive, satisfied with probable certainty, and morally engaged with the commonplaces of communities of experience to ascertain what befits the case at hand in the community in question — what is the right thing *for us* to do?" (Carson 1990:58–59).

Carson also calls attention to the spiritual relationships within health care as appropriate concerns of the ethicist, thus incorporating realms of faith and religious meaning in the domain of ethical discernment. The allusive myths and beliefs of a patient's theology may deepen his or her story. In the face of worsening diabetes, for example, an observant Orthodox Jew refused to take insulin on the Sabbath. His internist recognized biblical diction in the patient's description of his life — he spoke of being a witness to cruelty and of being an exile away from his Eastern European neighborhood. In grappling with his deteriorating physical status, the patient was rendering his life as an exodus from the promised land of polity and health. The internist respected his wishes to avoid the use of syringes on the Sabbath, aware that the theological dimensions of the patient's autobiography explained his otherwise irrational decision about his health care. The theological content of ordinary lives can pressure health care decisions, not only in such spectacular ways as the refusal of blood products by Jehovah's Witnesses or the withholding of treatment from an infant with acute leukemia by Christian Scientist parents but also in the routine ways in which individuals make sense of their past and make choices for their future. The narratively competent ethicist will include the religious themes and stories as serious determinants of behavior and guidelines worthy of respect.

More universally, faith-based concerns permeate all ethical deliberations. If, in fact, narrative sensitivity uncovers ethical issues that require not action but acknowledgment, then the ethicist is striving to understand and to articulate the ways in which a patient places himself or herself in the world to achieve personal meaning. Rather than acting as an instrumental enterprise seeking the most highly sanctioned action, a narratively competent ethicist will uncover ways in which the caregiver can accompany a sick person and his or her family through the painful, boring, disruptive events of illness. Narrative competence endows the ethicist or health provider with the means and the motives to see clearly what the illness produces for those whose lives are changed by it, to adopt the perspectives of those who suffer, and to serve them by recognizing and articulating the coherent human acts within the chaos of physical sickness. When viewed from this perspective, the practice of ethics is related to the empathic practice of medicine or nursing in which practitioners strive for diagnostic accuracy and therapeutic effectiveness as well as personal witness and compassion for the person who suffers.

Those, like Steven Miles and Kathryn Hunter, who locate ethical meaning within the story of a patient's life would have the ethicist be concerned with "the narrative coherence [that] must be constructed from a person's history of moral choices and relationships with others" (Miles and Hunter 1990b:63). Rather than an intervention accomplished during an acute hospitalization by a stranger, Miles and Hunter's model transposes ethical inquiry into the longitudinal relationships between health professionals and patients, allowing the grounds of moral choices to become clear over the course of lived-through intersubjective experiences of health and disease. "Narrative ethics sees health care as a part of life which must be engaged on its own terms rather than as a special time outside of history and culture to be analyzed with professionalized (and then popularized) ways of thinking about life choices" (Miles and Hunter 1990b:63). Their radical proposal reconfigures the work of medical ethics from a specialized competency to an integrated responsibility fulfilled by all who are sick and all who care for sick people. Of course, not all patients are accompanied through wellness and illness by trusted primary-care health professionals who can bring a knowledge of the patients' life choices and traditions to bear on serious decisions regarding treatment and its limits. Still, the narrative ethics proposal challenges not only medical ethics but all of clinical medicine to center the moral dimension of health care within view of all participants and to acknowledge that such issues are omnipresent elements of lives as they are being lived.

Although not an independent method that promises to replace all existing efforts in the field of medical ethics, a narrative approach can make existing methods work more accurately and effectively. The principlist methods of ethical inquiry remain as the structure for clarifying and adjudicating conflicts among patients, health providers, and family members at the juncture of quandary. The principles upon which bioethics decisions have been based — patient autonomy, beneficence, nonmaleficence, and justice — continue to guide ethical action within health care. Narrative competencies, however, have the power to particularize such decisions, to increase involvement of both patients and providers in clarifying ethical choices, and to take timely longitudinal steps toward ethical recognition that will obviate quandary ethics. The recognition of the narrative components in the actions of all bioethicists potentially can remove sources of bias, can assure a conceptual understanding of the personal contributions to ethical decision making, and can favor a practice that respects the singular aspects of each clinical situation without raising relativistic or unduly situational fears.

Students and practitioners in the health professions and medical ethics can learn to clarify the narrative elements of biomedical ethical deliberations. By now, literary scholars often teach both narrative theory and literature in medical centers, and research in medical topics often adopts narrative methods.[14] Consciousness of the importance of narrative concerns has been raised within the medical community, leading to such formulations as the following from a case story in the journal *Second Opinion:* "As authors, presenting a story that was not ours, we faced questions of ethics and responsibility" (Warshaw and Poirier 1991:60). Not only, that is, have ethical concerns aroused narrative interests, but narrative concerns have aroused ethical interests. The sophistication of the medical literature in terms of narrative theory and practice has increased appreciably in the years since the discipline of literature and medicine was established. This growth is reflected not only in journals devoted to its study but also in publications addressing specifically narrative questions in health care (for example, Kleinman 1989; Brody 1987; Coles 1989).

Narrative knowledge, then, has already contributed substantially to the trustworthiness of biomedical ethics. It has helped make explicit the narrative elements of the processes of any biomedical ethics deliberation. Next, it has singled out aspects of medical ethical work — like the identification of narrative stance — that cannot be absent from the enterprise. Moreover, it has recommended changes in medical and ethical training to better equip practitioners with narrative competence. And, finally, it has advanced proposals for change rooted in the recognition of the centrality of storytelling in medical ethics. One reads of people "doing ethics" or "doing casuistry." But one does not "do narrative," a phrase that seems to suggest that one can choose *not* to. Rather, narrative forms of knowing, telling, and reflecting are inborn parts of being human and are central aspects of making difficult choices in troubling human situations, no more elective than the systole and diastole of that baffling heartbeat.

NOTES

1. Miller 1987:2, 3.

2. For evidence of this global shift toward the particular, contextualized, or spiritual considerations in medical ethics, see Burrell and Hauerwas 1977; Coles 1970; MacIntyre 1981; Gustafson 1981; and May 1983. See also the "Case Stories" feature of the journal *Second Opinion*.

3. Narrative theory, it must be emphasized, is a concern of many intellectual disciplines and can be approached with the methods of any of several fields. Written by one trained in literary criticism, this discussion offers predominantly the views from literary studies, though by no means discounting the contributions of narrative cousins in other fields.

4. This is not to suggest that the medical gaze, as described by Michel Foucault in *Birth of the Clinic*, is ordinary: "Doctor and patient are caught up in an ever-greater proximity, bound together, the doctor by an ever-more attentive, more insistent, more penetrating gaze, the patient by all the silent, irreplaceable qualities that, in him, betray — that is, reveal and conceal — the clearly ordered forms of the disease.... [T]o look in order to know, to show in order to teach, is not this a tacit form of violence, all the more abusive for its silence, upon a sick body that demands to be comforted, not displayed?" (1973:15–16, 84). A matter of rescue, the events that can be trapped and transformed by that medical gaze require a different kind of vision, one that perhaps may be offered by the ethicist with narrative competence.

5. See Zaner's essay in this volume for an articulation of the phenomenological basis of biomedical ethics decision making.

6. See Banks and Hawkins 1992 for essays deconstructing the medical case history, demonstrating the influence that genre exerts over thought and practice.

7. When medical sociologists write about insider status, they mean alongside the patients: "An inside perspective focuses directly and explicitly on the subjective experiences of living with and in spite of illness" (Gerhardt 1990:1149). That "insider" for the biomedical ethicist has come to mean close to the doctor and not close to the patient may be a matter of some concern for all involved. See Larry Churchill 1978 and David Rothman 1991 for discussions of strangerliness at the bedside.

8. See Parker 1990; Benner 1991; and Cooper 1991 for discussions of nursing's turn toward stories to capture the relational dimensions of an ethics of care.

9. As an introduction to the field of gender and reading, see Flynn and Schweickart 1986. See especially the essays by David Bleich, Elizabeth Flynn, and Patrocinio Schweickart in the anthology.

10. See *Second Opinion* 17, no. 2 (October 1991) for a collection of essays on feminism and biomedical ethics. See also Gudorf's essay in this volume.

11. An urgent concern of natural scientists, literary scholars, historians, and sociologists as well as medical ethicists, the politics of interpretation and the very nature of validation of interpretations are the subjects of active scholarship. See Mitchell 1983, especially essays by Stephen Toulmin and Hayden White as well as the essay of Mishler cited above.

12. Conceptualizing medical ethics as a craft or practice helps to situate the required skills within the framework of tacit knowledge, reflective practice, and a community of practitioners. See Polanyi 1983 and Schön 1984.

13. See also Jonsen and Toulmin 1988 and the essay by Stephen Toulmin in this volume.

14. See Hunter 1991 for a defense of the teaching of literature and narrative theory to medical students and practitioners to increase the effectiveness of their work.

REFERENCES

Banks, Joanne Trautmann, and Anne Hunsaker Hawkins, eds. 1992. "The Art of the Case History." *Literature and Medicine* 11.

Barnard, David. 1992. "Reflections of a Reluctant Clinical Ethicist: Ethics Consultation and the Collapse of Critical Distance." *Theoretical Medicine* 13 (March): 15–22.

Barthes, Roland. 1988. "Introduction to the Structural Analysis of Narratives." In *The Semiotic Challenge,* trans. Richard Howard. New York: Farrar, Straus and Giroux.

Benjamin, Walter. 1969. *Illuminations,* ed. Hannah Arendt, trans. Harry Zohn. New York: Schocken Books.

Benner, Patricia. 1991. "The Role of Experience, Narrative, and Community in Skilled Ethical Comportment." *Advances in Nursing Science* 14:1–21.

Blake, David. 1992. "The Hospital Ethics Committee: Health Care's Moral Conscience or White Elephant?" *Hastings Center Report* 22:6–11.

Booth, Wayne. 1983. *The Rhetoric of Fiction.* Chicago: University of Chicago Press.

————. 1988. *The Company We Keep: An Ethics of Fiction.* Berkeley: University of California Press.

Brody, Howard. 1987. *Stories of Sickness.* New Haven: Yale University Press.

Brooks, Peter. 1985. *Reading for the Plot: Design and Intention in Narrative.* New York: Vintage Books.

Bruner, Jerome. 1991. "The Narrative Construction of Reality." *Critical Inquiry* 18:1–21.

————. 1986. *Actual Minds, Possible Worlds.* Cambridge: Harvard University Press.

Burrell, David, and Stanley Hauerwas. 1977. "From System to Story: An Alternative Pattern for Rationality in Ethics." In *Knowledge, Value and Belief,* vol. 2 of *The Foundations of Ethics and Its Relationship to Science,* ed. H. T. Engelhardt, Jr., and Daniel Callahan, 111–52. Hastings-on-Hudson, N.Y.: Hastings Center.

Carson, Ronald. 1990. "Interpretive Bioethics: The Way of Discernment." *Theoretical Medicine* 11:51–59.

Churchill, Larry. 1978. "The Ethicist in Professional Education: The Role of the Stranger." *Hastings Center Report* 8:13–15.

Cohen, Cynthia. 1988. "Is Case Consultation in Retreat?" *Hastings Center Report* 18:23.

Coles, Robert. 1989. *The Call of Stories: Teaching and the Moral Imagination.* Boston: Houghton Mifflin.

———. 1970. "Medical Ethics and Living a Life." *New England Journal of Medicine* 301:444–46.

Cooper, Mary Carolyn. 1991. "Principle-oriented Ethics and the Ethic of Care: A Creative Tension." *Advances in Nursing Science* 14:22–31.

Culler, Jonathan. 1982. *One Deconstruction: Theory and Criticism after Structuralism.* Ithaca: Cornell University Press.

Doukas, David. 1992. "The Design and Use of the Bioethics Consultation Form." *Theoretical Medicine* 13:5–14.

Flynn, Elizabeth, and Patrocinio Schweickart, eds. 1986. *Gender and Reading Essays on Readers, Texts, and Contexts.* Baltimore: Johns Hopkins University Press.

Foucault, Michel. 1973. *The Birth of the Clinic: An Archaeology of Medical Perception.* New York: Vintage Books.

Frader, Joel. 1992. "Political and Interpersonal Aspects of Ethics Consultation." *Theoretical Medicine* 13:31–44.

Gardner, John. 1978. *On Moral Fiction.* New York: Basic Books.

Geertz, Clifford. 1973. *The Interpretation of Cultures.* New York: Basic Books.

Gerhardt, Uta. 1990. "Qualitative Research on Chronic Illness: The Issue and the Story." *Social Science and Medicine* 30:1149–59.

Gustafson, James. 1981. *Ethics from a Theocentric Perspective.* Chicago: University of Chicago Press.

Hunter, Kathryn Montgomery. 1991. *Doctors' Stories: The Narrative Structure of Medical Knowledge.* Princeton: Princeton University Press.

Iser, Wolfgang. 1978. *The Act of Reading: A Theory of Aesthetic Response.* Baltimore: Johns Hopkins University Press.

———. 1974. *The Implied Reader: Patterns of Communication in Prose Fiction from Bunyan to Beckett.* Baltimore: Johns Hopkins University Press.

James, Henry. 1908. *The Novels and Tales of Henry James.* The New York Edition, vol. 5, *Princess Casamassima.* New York: Charles Scribner's Sons.

Jonsen, Albert. 1986. "Casuistry and Clinical Ethics." *Theoretical Medicine* 7:65–74.

Jonsen, Albert, and Stephen Toulmin. 1988. *The Abuse of Casuistry: A History of Moral Reasoning.* Berkeley: University of California Press.

Kermode, Frank. 1979. *The Genesis of Secrecy: On the Interpretation of Narrative.* Cambridge: Harvard University Press.

Kleinman, Arthur. 1989. *The Illness Narratives: Suffering, Healing, and the Human Condition.* New York: Basic Books.

Kolodny, Annette. 1985. "A Map for Rereading: Gender and the Interpretation of Literary Texts." In *The New Feminist Criticism: Essays on Women, Literature, and Theory,* ed. Elaine Showalter, 46–62. New York: Pantheon.

Kristeva, Julia. 1983. "Psychoanalysis and the Polis." In *The Politics of Interpretation,* ed. W. J. T. Mitchell, 83–98. Chicago: University of Chicago Press.

MacIntyre, Alasdair. 1981. *After Virtue*. Notre Dame, Ind.: Notre Dame University Press.

May, William F. 1983. *The Physician's Covenant: Images of the Healer in Medical Ethics*. Philadelphia: Westminster Press.

Miles, Steven, and Kathryn Montgomery Hunter, eds. 1990a. "Case Stories: A Series." *Second Opinion* 15 (November): 54.

———. 1990b. "Commentary." *Second Opinion* 15 (November): 60–63.

Miller, J. Hillis. 1987. *The Ethics of Reading: Kant, deMan, Eliot, Trollope, James, and Benjamin*. New York: Columbia University Press.

Mishler, Elliot. 1991. "Representing Discourse: The Rhetoric of Transcription." *Journal of Narrative and Life History* 1:225–80.

———. 1990. "Validation in Inquiry-guided Research: The Role of Exemplars in Narrative Studies." *Harvard Educational Review* 60:415–42.

Mitchell, W. J. T., ed. 1983. *The Politics of Interpretation*. Chicago: University of Chicago Press.

Parker, Randy Spreen. 1990. "Nurses' Stories: The Search for a Relational Ethic of Care." *Advances in Nursing Science* 13:31–40.

Polanyi, Michael. 1983. *The Tacit Dimension*. Gloucester, Mass.: Peter Smith.

Ricoeur, Paul. 1985. *Time and Narrative*, trans. Kathleen McLaughlin and David Pellauer. Chicago: University of Chicago Press.

Ross, Judith Wilson. 1989. "Why Cases Sometimes Go Wrong." *Hastings Center Report* 19:22–23.

Rothman, David. 1991. *Strangers at the Bedside: A History of How Law and Bioethics Transformed Medical Decision Making*. New York: Basic Books.

Schön, Donald. 1984. *The Reflective Practitioner*. New York: Harper and Row.

Smith, Barbara Herrnstein. 1981. "Narrative Versions, Narrative Theories." In *On Narrative*, ed. W. J. T. Mitchell, 209–32. Chicago: University of Chicago Press.

Toombs, S. Kay. 1988. "Illness and the Paradigm of Lived Body." *Theoretical Medicine* 9:201–226.

Toulmin, Stephen. 1982. "How Medicine Saved the Life of Ethics. *Perspectives in Biology and Medicine* 25:736–50.

———. 1983. "The Construal of Reality: Criticism in Modern and Postmodern Science." In *The Politics of Interpretation*, ed. W. T. J. Mitchell, 99–117. Chicago: University of Chicago Press.

Walker, Robert, Steven Miles, Carol Stocking, and Mark Siegler. 1991. "Physicians' and Nurses' Perceptions of Ethics Problems on General Medical Services." *Journal of General Internal Medicine* 6:424–29.

Warshaw, Carole, and Suzanne Poirier. 1991. "Case and Commentary: Hidden Stories of Women." *Second Opinion* 17, no. 2 (October): 48–61.

White, Hayden. 1983. "The Politics of Historical Interpretation: Discipline and De-sublimation." In *The Politics of Interpretation*, ed. W. J. T. Mitchell. Chicago: University of Chicago Press.

———. 1989. "The Rhetoric of Interpretation." In *The Rhetoric of Interpretation and the Interpretation of Rhetoric*, ed. Paul Hernadi, 1–22. Durham: Duke University Press.

Williams, William Carlos. 1967. *The Autobiography of William Carlos Williams*. New York: New Directions Books.
Young, Katherine. 1988. "Narrative Embodiments: Enclaves of the Self in the Realm of Medicine." In *Texts of Identity*, ed. John Shotter and Kenneth Gergen. London: Sage.

~ 12 ~

CHARACTER AND THE MORAL LIFE
A VIRTUE APPROACH TO BIOMEDICAL ETHICS

James F. Drane

Perhaps it would be appropriate to begin an essay on character and virtue with a story. Story and character belong together, and both are rare in mainstream North American biomedical ethics. This particular story was told by a prominent Christian ethicist, James M. Gustafson, who made a case for the place of character and virtue in Christian ethics in his book *Can Ethics Be Christian?* The central character in the story is not a physician but easily could serve as a model for the character and virtues of a good physician.

> In the mid-1950's on a hot summer night a colleague and I had worked past midnight on a report marking the termination of a brief but intensive interdisciplinary study. We left our workroom in a midtown Manhattan hotel to go to the bar for some refreshment. Near us was seated a rather drunken young soldier, who proceeded to order another drink. He paid for it with a twenty-dollar bill, but my observing colleague noticed that the bartender gave him change for a five. My colleague insisted that the soldier receive the rest of his change. The bartender protested that the soldier had given him a five, and not a twenty-dollar bill. An argument ensued, and finally the bartender gave the soldier fifteen dollars, asserting that he was doing it only to keep peace in the establishment.
>
> The soldier's inebriation progressed to the point where it was clear that he would soon "pass out." Certainly he was rapidly losing control of his speech and his muscles. My colleague talked to him as best one could in these circumstances and finally took the

soldier's wallet from his pocket. There was identification indicating that the young man lived at a Long Island address. We took ten dollars from the wallet, and my colleague wrote a note indicating that we had done so, that we were putting him in a cab and giving the cab driver the ten dollars to take him home. He [my colleague] also gave our names and professions, and the telephone number of the hotel in which we were quartered by the corporation for whom we were doing the study. Thus the soldier or his family could make contact with us if they desired any further explanation.

We more or less dragged the soldier onto Lexington Avenue, where we hailed a taxi. My colleague gave the driver the ten-dollar bill and the address. He also took the driver's name and license number and indicated that we had the young man's name and address. Thus the driver knew that it would be possible to check out whether the drunken soldier had been delivered home. My colleague also informed the driver that we knew how much money was left in the wallet.

When the taxi drove off, we returned to the bar. (1985:1–2)

Stories and character considerations are rare in mainstream U.S. biomedical ethics because in North America, this discipline plays on only a small section of the ethical turf. It is focused mainly on quandaries and dilemmas generated by discrete acts: abortion, euthanasia, genetic engineering, withdrawal of nutritional technologies, experimentation, transplants, and so forth. Mainstream U.S. biomedical ethics is highly individualistic, focused on rights, and rationalistic in its discourse: in effect the farthest thing imaginable from stories and parables about good persons who can serve as models for others. U.S. biomedical ethics works at finding appropriate abstract principles and rules to apply to particular quandaries, and then finding a compromise between contradictory claims that individuals with different visions of life can agree to. Following set methodologies for handling each dilemma is important, and, ideally, intermediate practical rules can be developed to help decision makers handle similar problems when they occur. U.S. biomedical ethicists tend to be the physician's ally as he or she struggles to make the right decision and do the right thing in a conflict situation. It is the dominant biomedical ethics in the U.S. because it works in this culture. And yet it also has serious limitations.

Mainstream U.S. biomedical ethics is sometimes referred to as "the principles approach" because it centers around abstract ethical standards like autonomy and beneficence and justice, which presumably bind every person no matter what that person's particular background or perspective. The principles approach claims to be universal, and the principles bind each rational person in the same way and to the same degree. Differences in beliefs about life presumably do not interfere with rationalistic ethical reflection about problem cases. The abstract principles, rightly applied, help define the right action. Getting to agreement about right action requires rationalistic skills and logical argument, which presumably stand over and above the many different beliefs about life that characterize today's pluralistic professional population. Mainstream U.S. biomedical ethics presumably is independent of institutional loyalties because pure reason rather than socioculturally contaminated thinking operates in clinical deliberations. The only authority is the authority of rational discourse, which grapples with the contradictory claims that create moral dilemmas (Kohlberg 1981).

To suggest that character and virtue have a place in contemporary medical ethics comes across as strange to most U.S. ethicists. At one seminar where I spoke about this topic, a colleague asked what sense it makes even to discuss such topics "because nothing objective is connoted by these terms." He was partially right. Character and virtue, which refer to the inner being of persons, are nowhere nearly as objective and analyzable as discrete medical acts or rules of behavior. And yet we do see something about right and wrong from reading the above story. Rules and principles and methodologies and rights play no part at all in this little parable, and yet something very obviously right comes through in the narrative. The story points to a different type of ethics or, better, a different area of the field of ethics. It illustrates what one means when one speaks about a good person as distinct from a right act.

The ethics illustrated in the story is about style, a type of personality, and yes, a form of excellence. Probably no one would deny that what the professor did was right, yet from all appearances, he acted without referring to any of the concepts and categories central to mainstream U.S. biomedical ethics. Rather, his action was the expression of a well-formed character. He did what he did "naturally," without giving it much thought. We see here an example of personalist ethics in response to another person: an ethics of responsibility, or a relational ethics that seems obviously appropriate to medicine, where everything starts and finishes with a doctor-patient relationship and where most of the doctor-patient contacts have nothing to do with quandaries or dilemmas or conflict of rights.

Physicians, however, do procedures. They take action, and they decide on alternative options. For all these reasons, mainstream U.S. biomedical ethics is practical, despite the fact that it covers only a certain area of medical practice. On the other hand, doctors are in a special relationship with every patient. They profess to be helpers of people in need and in the very act of establishing a relationship assume obligations to address needs. Patient dependency creates a situation that some doctors respond to well and others do not, no matter how much exposure they have to rationalistic argumentation, rules, and ethical principles. The way Jim Gustafson's friend responded to the helpless drunk is similar to the way good doctors everywhere respond to a very ill patient.

No doubt, objective ethical rules could be teased out of the story, and it could be argued that Jim's friend was applying principles and defending rights and weighing consequences. But these categories alone are not adequate to the whole experience. There were no moral rules that told the professor what he should do in that situation, just as no moral rules could tell doctors what to do in most of the situations they face. And no ethical rule either abstract or concrete could be found that would require a person to take the subtle and delicate steps this professor took to achieve that final excellent result. Doing the excellent thing was a matter of intuiting what was appropriate by a person who had developed a certain way of being that included a sensitivity for persons in need and an ease with human relatedness. He didn't need to reflect a great deal, because the actions were habits formed by previous experiences and sustained within communities by moral beliefs, images, and ideals. The story illustrates better than any argument that character and virtue in many situations are more important than methodologies of moral reasoning, rules, principles, rights, and the like.

Why Character and Virtue Considerations Dropped Out of the Mainstream

When my colleague at that seminar questioned even a mention of *character* and *virtue* because the words sound so subjective and strange, he was reflecting an absence of attention to these categories in mainstream U.S. biomedical ethics literature, as well as a gap that has developed between ethics and psychiatry. In the latter discipline, character and character traits are key categories, which are not considered purely subjective. Major psychiatric theorists, for example, have well-worked-out definitions and finely nuanced descriptions of character types — both normal and pathological. Paranoid, cyclothymic, schizoid, explosive, obsessive-compulsive, hysterical, asthenic, antisocial, passive-aggressive, narcissistic, borderline: these are some of the well-defined flawed character types. Karl Jaspers is just one prominent psychiatrist-philosopher whose important work centers around the concept of character, which he describes as

> the particular way an individual expresses himself, in the way he moves, how he experiences and reacts to situations, how he loves, grows jealous, how he conducts his life in general, what needs he has, what are his longings and aims, what are his ideals and how he shapes them, what values guide him and what he does, what he creates and how he acts. In short, personality is the term we give to the *individually differing and characteristic totality of meaningful connections* in any one psychic life. (1968:428)

U.S. and European psychological theorists both secular and religious have outlined stages through which character grows toward moral maturity (Piaget et al. 1965; MacIntyre 1981; Fowler 1981; Gilligan 1982). This literature pays some attention both to character formation and to recognizable character traits or virtues. The influences on both are traced to events in personal histories. To think that character and virtues are too subjective to be useful is simply not true. Character configurations can be judged good and bad, better and worse. The configurations may not be perfect unities, but they are sufficiently recognizable, especially in their deficient forms. More and more frequently, emotionally disturbed U.S. patients are diagnosed with character disorders, and their treatment takes the form of character education.[1] Morally deficient character formations provide information about the concept of character and character traits at large.

Although one sees little about character and virtue in contemporary U.S. biomedical ethics literature, these considerations never entirely disappeared even in the literature of northern European thinkers. Schopenhauer's work provides an obvious example of character-based ethics (1961). Heidegger (1962) is another good example. Even some of the early English philosophers who inspired the North American concern with act-ethics continued to talk about character.[2] But there is no doubt that a shift occurred away from character and virtue considerations, especially among northern European utilitarians and deontologists. And these two ethical traditions are the major influences on North American-style biomedical ethics.

One explanation for this shift is related to language. Heidegger (1962) made the point again and again that the translations of key Greek philosophical terms into Latin frequently obscured their original meaning. This certainly happened with the Greek word for ethics, ἠθικα, from ἠθος, *ethos,* which had two meanings. The oldest meaning was residence, home, place where one resided. This word was used first to refer to the place where animals reside, later to human habitations, and finally to the inner place or inner dwelling of human beings. In this last sense, ἦθοσ (*êthos*) is the ground of *praxis,* the source of actions. In a second and slightly different sense, *éthos* meant not the source or root of acts and habits but rather the acts and habits themselves. This second sense of *éthos* made external acts, habits, and customs primary. Ethics even for Aristotle and certainly since then has focused more on *éthos* in the sense of external acts, habits, customs and less on *êthos* as the inner wellspring of human action.

The translation of the Greek word *éthos,* with its two senses, by the Latin word *mos-moris* contributed to the loss of the older sense of the word as inner source of external acts. *Mos,* from which we get the word *moral[s],* especially in its plural form, *mores,* means something external rather than internal: ways, customs, behaviors. The notion of ethics as acquired character or inner source of acts (*êthos*) gave way to the emphasis on external behaviors and customs (*éthos*). If one spoke of ethics in the sense of inner self, it was more likely to be understood as the result of acts and habits rather than their source or root. Acts and habits gradually become primary.[3]

St. Thomas Aquinas was aware of the two original senses of the Greek word for ethics and talked about comparable meanings of the Latin word *mos,*[4] but he was not able to stop the slide toward the common meaning of *mos-moris* as external custom and external behavior. Since Latin lacked a word that purely and simply meant what *êthos* originally meant, the latter was lost except to the most philologically disposed philosophers or theologians.

Etymology, however, is not the only explanation for the loss of the focus in ethics on inner being. Character may in fact be the source and root of acts and behaviors, but the latter are much more visible, easier to identify and evaluate. Character is also more ambiguous. Certainly it does not lend itself to the Anglo-Saxon pragmatic concerns with ethics as related to law.[5] External acts and behaviors can be made subject to law, but not inner being or character. Not every Anglo-Saxon ethicist is as interested in legal reform as Mill and Bentham were, but most are concerned about specific acts and pragmatic norms.

Anglo-Saxon ethical tradition clearly has had a major influence on North American biomedical ethics, but Medieval Catholic theology has also been influential. Catholic theology, without totally abandoning character considerations, has also focused on acts for very practical reasons. Priests had to judge discrete acts that people revealed in the confessional. The confessor, like the doctor, didn't have all day to think about a case; he had to make a quick and defensible judgment about certain acts. The confessional drove theological ethics more and more toward the analysis of acts. American biomedical ethics, with its own pragmatic objectives, followed naturally in the same direction.

Mainstream U.S. biomedical ethics ignores both the psychological and psychiatric literature that addresses character and the rich theological literature on the subject. The Catholic tradition, following classical Greek philosophical influences, gave a prominent place to character and virtue in ascetic theology. Despite the linguistic problems referred to above and the focus on acts rather than character created by the confessional, *ascetic* theology and spirituality focused primarily on character and virtue. Here religion influences ethics primarily in the changes it effects in persons. Recently, some Protestant thinkers have called for greater attention to this emphasis and tradition (Hauerwas 1974, 1975). The absence of attention to character and virtue in mainstream U.S. biomedical ethics reflects its strong secular preferences as much as its inattention to psychology and psychiatry.

Catholic spirituality was strongly focused on inner disposition and attitudes that were influenced by religious stories, rituals, and symbols. Religion and religious experience aim at creating a certain inner way of being rather than specifying particular acts. Believers whose relationship with God is based on total trust and loyalty and love, for example, become certain types of persons. For Christians, the imitation of Christ is an imitation of his inner attitudes and his ways of relating to others. For all these reasons, religion and theology generated an ethics of character and virtue. Sincere religious belief creates a way of being, which becomes a way of seeing, and finally becomes a way of responding to reality.

We see mainstream U.S. biomedical ethics clearly expressed in the goals established for an ethics curriculum in medical schools, set out by the influential De Camp Report published in the *New England Journal of Medicine.*

> Before presenting our recommendation for a basic curriculum, we want to make explicit certain beliefs we hold about the teaching of medical ethics. First of all, we believe that the basic moral character of medical students has been formed by the time they enter medical school. A medical-ethics curriculum is designed not to improve the moral character of future physicians but to provide those of sound moral character with the intellectual tools and interactional skills to give that moral character its best behavioral expression. (Culver et al. 1985:253–55)

Even this statement suggests that the character and virtues of physicians are important. But do we know enough about professional character formation and its traits to make the concept of character-based ethics a reasonable one for modern biomedical ethics to work with? Is it possible that character and virtue considerations simply would not be helpful in actually doing medical ethics? I think not. Character is a perceptible reality, not just the product of actions but also a source. Certain spontaneous acts show a person's character, sum it up, and define it. Character is not as visible as an action, but neither is it invisible or undefinable. Character refers to personality structure, with special emphasis on its ethical components. It refers to the kind of person who makes a decision or acts in a certain way. It directs our attention to inner realities: motives, dispositions, intentions, and attitudes. It is a designation for the inner being of a person: a constellation of distinctive personal traits (virtues and vices). Obviously these inner realities are connected to acts and decisions, and yet external acts can conceptually be separated from the acting person. Just as external acts can be ethically evaluated, so too can internal moral traits and qualities of being. It makes sense to speak about persons as good and bad, kind and unkind, caring and uncaring, faithful and unfaithful, just and unjust, selfish and unselfish, prudent and imprudent, and so forth. One task of this essay is to try to provide an outline of the character traits that belong to a good doctor. After describing what character and virtue mean, we will move to the normative task of justifying a certain content to the self of a good doctor.

Subjective Dimension of Character and Virtue

Character and virtue have to do with stable attitudes called "dispositions" that can rather easily be identified. Some people, for example, are obviously cynical. No matter what comes up, they always respond with the same attitude. When confronted by examples of basic human goodness, they respond with disbelief, sneering, and sarcasm. In the face of life and creativity, they stand for death and destruction. Their response to belief is disbelief. They exude not happiness and joy but pessimism and gloom. Rather than liking other people and being drawn toward them, the cynic is disposed to dislike and to aversion. We find the noun *cynic* and its adjective form *cynical* in all modern languages because these words refer to recognizable character types. Their persistent dispositions have everything to do with ethics because they define what cynical persons have created of themselves, and their personal creation has everything to do with their decisions and acts.

To talk of character and virtues is to suggest consistency and regularity not just of inner dispositions but of corresponding external actions as well. Even cynical people may on occasion be kind and thoughtful, but ordinarily they are not. Kind and thoughtful persons, on the other hand, are regularly kind and thoughtful. In situation after situation, they respond in the same way; they repeat a certain pattern of behavior over and over. We can say that we know the moral quality of such persons because from their dispositions flow repeated and consistent behaviors that we call virtues or vices. Virtues and vices are the habitual patterns of moral behaviors which make possible the claim of "knowing the way some people are." Virtues and vices flow from dispositions and attitudes. They make certain behaviors "natural," "almost automatic," as we saw in the example of the professor and the drunk. An ethics of virtue and character ends not in specific, discrete acts required by codes or rules and decided upon after careful consideration of alternatives, but in behaviors that are nearly spontaneous. Rather than figuring out what is the right thing to do, the right thing comes "naturally" and flows "automatically" from persons for whom ethics has primarily meant development of their character.

Dispositions and attitudes are linked with basic beliefs and visions of life by way of will and commitment. Only when religion is sincerely held belief does it have an ethical influence on the believer's inner dispositions and perceptions. The same is true of any philosophical vision. Once-and-for-all commitments to a vision, belief system, or even to a professional ideal like medicine have a major influence on the formation of the inner reality we call character. Such commitments involve values and ideals, dispositions, and ways of acting. Consistent behaviors in turn over a long period are external expressions of character-forming commitments as well as reinforcers of that inner formation. Irreversible decisions and life commitments give both breadth and depth to character. Without life commitments to someone or something beyond the self, human beings live superficially: only in the present and for whatever present satisfactions are available. What a person decides to do with his or her life "once and for all," however, gives both a form and depth to character. Something stable is created at such times that admittedly can be undermined but not dissipated in every little change or slip. Character, then, refers to this transtemporal inner personal being, formed by personal effort rather than given by nature, from which flows distinct forms of doing.

Besides commitment and transcendence, character and virtue also involve emotion. Dispositions and attitudes, perceptions and intentions, commitments to a religious or philosophical or professional ideal, all these have a strong emotional dimension. A person who is hostile, for example, can know about kindness, but has no emotional investment in it. An ethics professor may know a lot about truth, but may consistently behave dishonestly because of pleasure he or she derives from that behavior. A just person delights in doing justice, and unjust behavior sickens him. What drives a personality to choose moral values and disvalues, thereby creating character, are strong feeling states. In turn, engaging in the behaviors which flow from a formed character structure provide emotional satisfaction. People love doing what is "second nature."

Affect, either positive (satisfaction) or negative (repulsion), linked to chosen values contributes to the stable elements of a character. We cannot understand a person's character without understanding his or her conscious commitment to values, goods, and visions, but the affect the person invests in these counts equally. Identifying what a person "loves" and gains satisfaction from provides insight into that person's character.[6] The virtuous person not only has a "feel" for certain values embedded in situations, but could be said to have a "taste" for them and a "touch" for them as well. States of affect connected to values rivet character traits into place and make them part of one's self. They explain the disposition of a virtuous person to do the right thing as well as the opposite disposition in the case of vice. They explain what we perceive as permanent and stable dimensions of character and virtue.

Søren Kierkegaard (1954:89–132; 1959) best explained the relationship between a certain type of moral self and absolute commitment in the sense of once-and-for-all decisions.[7] To decide to become a doctor, or a judge, or a priest, means that the decision maker has chosen himself or herself as doctor, judge, or priest, including all the moral values associated with the chosen profession. Alasdair MacIntyre (1981) expanded on this connection by making a distinction between the values internal or essential to a profession and values external to it. The roles or tasks or work one chooses, like the religions or philosophies in which a person believes, have built-in moral values that have everything to do with character and virtue development.

Once-and-for-all commitments and affect linked to the values inherent in a certain professional practice combine to weave personality elements into character traits, either virtues or vices. If a doctor is committed to medicine and takes delight in meeting the needs of sick people, virtuous acts and behaviors involving patients will come naturally. Will is central to character formation, but formed character and virtuous behavior also bring with them a cognitive advantage. A good doctor will insightfully assess the moral values embedded in doctor-patient relationships.

The affect associated with character can be both positive and negative. Aversion and disgust would be associated with acts which violate a professional commitment to patients. For a physician with positive character and virtue, hearing about the misuse of patients for research or profit or power or sexual pleasure would cause disgust. The absence of negative affect in the perpetrator of such behaviors is indicative of vice and character deformation. To suggest that medical ethics is just about acts and rules is severely to limit that reality. A fuller medical ethics explicates something much richer.

An ethics that restricts itself to conceptual analyses of cases, acts, procedures, and rules is admittedly more tidy. And we cannot ignore the fact that northern European philosophers, besides having a preference for act ethics, were suspicious of emotion, which plays so prominent a role in character and virtue. Kant was clear about this suspicion. He held that moral feeling "is superficial, since those who cannot think expect help from feeling" (1959:61). He wanted ethics to be a strictly cognitive discipline, and he has many followers among American medical ethicists.

Similarly identifying and quantifying the consequences of discrete acts or particular rules has a certain rigor about it that brings ethics closer to science. Tracing the history and definitions of the principles makes it possible to apply them to problematic cases and come up with defensible policies. All this can be done without any reference to feelings or to the character and virtues of acting persons. Yet the impressive tools of contemporary U.S. biomedical ethics in the hands of cold, selfish, uncaring persons are obviously inadequate to the ethical task facing medical practitioners. Something more than carefully defined acts, tidy rules, and calculated consequences is needed.

A case is not being made here for an exclusive ethics of virtue and character, but more modestly for consideration of these other elements. In some circumstances they may play a marginal role; for example, when a doctor must decide whether to withhold intrusive life-saving technologies from an elderly incompetent patient in crisis whom no one knows. In such a situation, a calculating, cognitive mind may be more important than a virtuous character. And yet, whether physicians and U.S. bioethicists like it or not, they have developed moral characters replete with virtues and vices. These may not play a crucial role in everything they do, but they play a larger role in their supposedly purely rational decisions than they might admit. If medical ethics is so rationalistic and deductive from agreed-upon ethical principles, then why is there so much disagreement, even among ethicists who are members of the same utilitarian or deontological "congregation"?

Character, then, is something we can identify and understand. And most will agree with the classical thinkers that it is not something we find ourselves with, but something we construct over a lifetime. *Ethos* for us as for Aristotle, is a human creation:

> By doing the acts that we do in our transactions with other men we become just or unjust, and by doing the acts that we do in the presence of danger, and being habituated to feel fear or confidence, we become brave or cowardly.... Thus, in one word, states of character arise out of like activities.[8]

What we do and the values we commit ourselves to gradually make us certain types of persons. Character, then, is the word we use for the someone we create by our acts and omissions. A given disposition or direction (*passio*), our cultural environments, and our institutions all influence the moral character we develop. But most of us are aware of the difference between influences on us and our acceptance or rejection of them on a personal level. Most of us recognize the moral direction of our personality to be something we had a hand in creating. And yet to concentrate on the inner or subjective elements in character and virtue leaves the picture only half drawn. Now we turn to the social and cultural components of character and virtue.

The Social Dimension of Character and Virtue

Mainstream U.S. biomedical ethics shows little awareness of just how much it reflects U.S. culture. If character and virtue played a larger role in U.S. biomedical ethics, it would not be as blinded to cultural influences, because in character and virtue ethics, the sociocultural connection is so obvious. Character-creating commitments take place in social settings.

The character-society relationship goes both ways. Once formed, character has a big influence on the social environment. Character traits contribute to surrounding social groups, big and small, and give them a moral content. The idea that institutions or societies are good or bad depending on whether they have the right or wrong rules is an oversimplification. Norms, laws, policies (the objective moral elements) are critical for a good society but so too are virtuous people. Inner selves are both fashioned by and fashion a particular social world.

The lack of attention that staff in medical schools and medical facilities pay to character issues explains a corresponding inattention to their own social environments. The character of young doctors is strongly influenced by the social setting of medical schools: their symbols, beliefs, styles of communication, stories, histories, schedules, teaching techniques, and models. The whole medical world is full of objects that carry meaning, and students immersed in this social world internalize these meanings. The medical student internalizes a world of symbols, images, and models by making surrounding meaning-bearing realities his or her own. Without attending to character formation, the social surrounding forms character either well or badly. The student follows a once-and-for-all choice of the medical profession by moving through institutions, situations, and experiences with already assigned meanings and values. As the student internalizes these, his or her inner self is formed. Gradually social influences fashion the way a young doctor sees the world, thinks about it, and responds to it. In effect, they shape his or her character.

All this happens without overt attention to the moral dimension of what is happening. In a survey conducted by a young Israeli physician, a large percentage of medical students thought that their professors did not provide edifying moral example.[9] Students repeatedly referred to the need for more personal ethical input from their professors. Their teachers, they complained, did not practice medicine according to what they had understood to be professional ethical standards. The Israeli students at least recognized a deficiency. Some students, however, don't recognize it, and neither do those responsible for the social environment in medical institutions. Forming character is more like cultivating a garden than engineering a product, but it cannot happen without giving some attention to social "ground."

It may require some subtlety to make character development an explicit concern in medical institutions, but it is not impossible. First, the topic of character could be explicitly addressed in formal and informal settings. Courses in humanities or ethics could address the issue so that students realize that medical ethics is more than principles and analysis of acts. Stories about professional tragedies associated with defective character formation could be provided so students would know that their attitudes and dispositions are important and require attention. Biographies of great physicians could be presented as examples of either positive or negative character models. Faculty persons could be chosen with the idea of providing students with both proper academic training and sound ethical modeling.

The institutional environment of the medical school can be evaluated as to how it can influence the development of desired character traits. A school can develop a spirit in the sense of a moral environment. Even after graduation, hospital environments and physician associations could be concerned with more than flagrantly unethical acts. Exploitative, manipulative, narcissistic, and aggressive character types can be discouraged, or at least not rewarded by medical associations or institutions. Once character and virtue considerations are returned to medical ethics, they can have practical payoffs at a time when more and more examples of ethical problems originating in character flaws are brought to public attention.

Moral character can never be reduced to social influences. Individuals choose to accept or reject conditioning social forces. And neither moral conduct nor moral character is ever provided ready made in every detail. Individual human beings make their own characters and form their own virtues and vices but never without influence either from the larger society or from smaller social units in which human life is nourished. Both larger and smaller societies are essentially ethical entities in themselves and major influences on individual persons.

An Identifiable Medical Character

The idea of including considerations of character and virtue in mainstream U.S. biomedical ethics, however, meets with yet another problem: which character type or list of virtues from among the many possibilities are appropriate for physicians? Different cultures and different visions of life within a single cultural tradition can generate different and perhaps incompatible ideas about appropriate physician character and virtues. A Mormon community, for example, may form a more priestly physician, while an urban hospital community may form a more secular character type. But, we are not talking here about engineering rigid characters or virtues or photocopied personalities. The idea is to cultivate respect for the sacredness of human life, while at the same time trying to cultivate certain character traits that respond to the nearly universal similarities in the way human beings become ill and seek help from healers. The character and virtues of a good doctor derive from the needs of patients. Character and virtues, as we have seen, are closely linked to beliefs about life, and yet the near-universal beliefs about what it means to be ill and to seek medical help provide a near-universal model of what a good doctor is like.

Healing or doctoring takes place in every society. Although background assumptions about disease may differ, doctoring everywhere involves medical acts that help the sick person, and every society is concerned that healers act in an ethically appropriate way. Medical ethics in this sense is universal. Doctoring then has an ethical component both in its internal structure and in its sociocultural expression. Being a doctor involves meeting standards related to medical acts themselves as well as standards set by society. Violation of either one diminishes both the profession and the practitioner.

Standards of clinical behavior, for example, precede the medical practitioner, and he or she must repeat them until they become habits. But medical standards are too often thought of solely in terms of scientific or technological competencies; they include ethical competencies as well. It is not a coincidence that the first Western physicians, the Hippocratics, made ethical behaviors one of their distinguishing characteristics. Certain virtues and character traits distinguished the "real" doctors and separated them from quacks and fakes who treated sick people for their own personal gain. The Hippocratic Oath makes repeated reference to the virtues of a good doctor, and some of these have not lost their applicability 2,500 years later.

We turn now to a consideration of some of the character traits inconsistent with caring for sick people (vices), as well as those internal to medical practice (virtues), thereby constructing our picture of the good doctor.

Identifiable Medical Vices

A doctor who is committed to making money above all else lacks commitment to the sacredness of human life. He or she will not do what is best for patients when patient welfare does not generate income. Such doctors will multiply diagnostic tests and therapeutic interventions for their economic benefits. Even though this doctor's specific decisions and clinical actions might not violate a particular ethical rule, neither will they ordinarily serve a patient's best interest. Rather, the physician's best (monetary) interest will be served, and the core value of medicine will be undermined. Character traits that undermine core medical values are medical vices.

For some modern scientific physicians, the patient is an object, albeit a scientific object, exhibiting certain pathological features. Physicians who are disposed toward dominating pathological objects and demonstrating their technical expertise may become competent medical professionals, but they lack the personal qualities required for good medical practice. They do not treat patients with respect.

In cases of chronic illness, for example, the scientifically competent physician's commitments and loves tend to make him cold and aloof. A cold or impersonal style makes the doctor inattentive to the broader dimensions of a patient's personal life. An impersonal character type, in effect, does not meet the needs of patients. He or she may do well in an acute emergency or as a pathologist but not where personal relationship between doctor and patient is called for. When narrow scientific perspective and reliance on high technology fail to generate proof of pathology, impersonal doctors tend to leave patients untreated and uncared for. The technically and scientifically correct response to a patient often violates values at the core of a good doctor.

If a patient reaches the point biologically where medicine can provide no effective intervention, the doctor with an impersonal character would be inclined to abandon the patient. At that particularly difficult time, when the doctor may be the only person who could provide needed help to a chronically ill patient, the impersonal doctor delivers only hurt and disappointment. This particular internal disposition undermines what medicine is about and most likely does so without offending any specific ethical rule or norm.

Physicians who are drawn to medicine because of the power doctors exercise frequently hurt rather than help sick people. Physicians who love exercising power over other people will do little or nothing to empower patients to understand and manage their problems. The physician whose character is defined by love of holding power over others may, for example, provide disclosure that fulfills the legal requirements of informed consent but nevertheless leaves the patient ignorant, confused, and powerless.

For patients to become empowered, more than a legally correct communication is called for. Personal communication that takes place over time is what patients need. This, however, will not come from a doctor whose character is formed by commitment to and a love of power, anymore than it will come from the doctor whose character is formed by a commitment to money. Persons committed to power and money do not provide for patient needs.

Physicians who are committed to power and who love exercising power will also not be good colleagues. For them the health-care-team concept will be a fiction. They will prefer to exercise power alone and to do so over other professionals (for example, nurses) as well as over patients. Other physicians who might be colleagues are perceived as threats and treated as such. This type of character and its unvirtuous traits leave patient needs unmet and undermine a society's interest in efficient health care delivery.

Physicians who love power and money inordinately may also love themselves inordinately. Such physicians may choose to practice medicine for ego gratification. Self-centeredness and narcissism may not interfere with proper treatment of patients in acute care medicine, but a self-centered character will undermine any treatment over time. The doctor who loves to have his or her ego massaged cannot provide for the ego needs of sick and threatened persons.

A character formed by commitment to self-enhancement threatens more than patient benefit. Truth is very likely to be sacrificed as well. Anything that provides ego gratification is prized, and if truth does not provide enough gratification, then truth will be sacrificed. Truth and commitment to truth rarely coincide with love of self and commitment to self-enhancement. What enhances power and inflates ego may very likely not be the truth.

The patient's rights to make decisions will only threaten the character committed to power and self-enhancement. Historically, the informed-consent concept was driven by the goal of empowering patients. A physician whose character is formed by commitment to power and who takes satisfaction in narcissistic exercises will not be respectful of a patient's right because this diminishes the doctor's power.

Respect (from *respicere* — to look at, to give attention to) involves keeping a certain distance from the other. It means not to intrude into private areas, to be restrained, and not to manipulate. Power-dominated and narcissistic characters, however, gain satisfaction from intrusiveness, manipulation, and similar violations of respect. Since doctors know so much more than patients, they can communicate with patients in such a way as to puff themselves up and to get patients to do whatever they want.

In effect, because of such a character deficiency, patients will not be provided with a balanced truth but with a communication that while not overtly untrue, serves the physician's rather than the patient's needs. And instead of an equalization of power, the doctor will maintain power and exercise it paternalistically for the ego gratification it provides. The really narcissistic doctor goes beyond using the patient for ego gratification and may try to turn patients into disciples or sex objects. If a physician takes advantage of the patient sexually, then one of the worst ethical failures occurs. Here, character failure does coincide with the violation of ethical rules and laws.

If certain character traits undermine the essential ethical structure of medicine, others enhance and promote this structure. What character traits are internal to medicine? What states of inner being must healers bring to their relationships with the sick people who ask them for help? These states are, simply put, the virtues required to carry out the public promise to address sick persons' needs.

Specific Physician Virtues

The internal structure of medical practice, or the structure of the healer-patient relationship, suggests a fairly explicit list of virtues. These may not be expressed the same way in every culture. Any analysis of medicine's structural dimension, however, will include reference to the virtues identified below. People of all ages and cultures expect their healers to be gentle, caring, and concerned primarily for them. Because sick people everywhere bring fears and needs along with their symptoms, they expect the physician to respond to them in a personal way, not unlike a gentle parent. In the same vein, doctors are expected not only to provide medical information but also to be honest. Furthermore, patients' needs and the structure of the doctor-patient relationship require unselfishness on the doctor's part. Also, patients require that a physician be friendly.

Real caring always requires some exposure to danger on the part of the physician. Different cultures will make different assessments of how much risk a healer is required to assume. For example, nowhere will the healer be expected to expose himself or herself to certain death, but good doctors must always develop some degree of courage. A cowardly character is incompatible with the structural requirements of medical practice. If physicians are cowards, who will treat patients with AIDS and all the other infectious diseases? Rules and principles cannot define this courage component, but virtue and character ethics can reveal this aspect of proper medical practice.

Another virtue required by the internal structure of medical practice is prudence. Prudence has to do with the habit of discernment and careful appraisal. This virtue requires both experience and a capacity to learn from it. It requires training in looking ahead and anticipating what a patient has to face down the road.

Historically, practitioners of medicine have always enjoyed social privilege, legal immunity, and considerable authority. Doctors, until recently, were often thought of as priestly, and the character traits expected of them were similar to those demanded of religious figures. Confidentiality, for example, is a fancy term for the virtue of keeping secrets, which binds both doctors and priests. The Hippocratic Oath has the physician promising to make his life as well as his art "pure and holy." The sexual restraint required of a physician was similar to the purity required of the priest. The thinking was that if physicians were to have access to the private inner dimensions of a patient's life, they must have more excellent character traits than what are expected of other people. And if physicians exercise authority over people's lives, they must be not only pure but humble. Physicians learn from sick people and receive all the benefits associated with medicine from them. Since the authority they inevitably exercise over the sick can easily inflate their estimation of their own importance, they especially need humility.

Finally, the relationship between physician and patient requires a virtue of hope. Every serious illness forces the reality of death into consciousness, and, consequently, patients are afraid. Besides technical medical help, patients need help in facing the most threatening of life's possibilities. Whether in psychiatric or physical medicine, one of the most important contributions a doctor can make to patients is to provide some hope. For believers in Jesus Christ, loss and negativity are not final, not even the ultimate loss and negativity of death, and yet even the deeply religious person suffers from the threat of death. Because patients need hope when facing most medical problems, the good doctor is one who can provide it "naturally," as an expression of the person he or she is. Doctors cannot be expected to be priests in societies where these roles are separate, and yet an aspect of priestliness is still expected and appropriate in the modern physician. For the nonreligious patient who is critically ill, the only possible hope is that death will come without unnecessary pain, and the good doctor can and should have a natural ability to provide this hope.

Different virtues and character formations will be required for different professions, but there will also be shared moral traits. Respect, truthfulness, friendliness, and caring are required by the internal structure of any relationship between a trained professional publicly committed to do what is best for another in need. The medical virtues, however, will have their own particular forms and content. Some failures of virtue and character will be more devastating in medicine than in other professions. Since medicine serves ends and goals necessary to individual persons and to societies, good doctors with well-formed characters and appropriate virtues do good for society, for patients, and for themselves.

The virtues most characteristic of medical practice do undergo change over time. Different social, cultural, political, and economic situations have an impact on the doctor-patient relationship and require adjustments in medical ethics. Socialized medicine, for example, requires somewhat different virtues from capitalistically organized medical practice. Today's doctors are part of a history and need to be aware of its ethical dimensions. Ignorance of medicine's ethical traditions and history diminishes contemporary medical ethics and makes some physicians and some ethicists prone to sacrifice long-standing ethical accomplishments for some slight temporary convenience.[10] It took time to work out an ethics of virtue and character based on the sacredness of human life and the unique dimensions of a doctor-patient relationship. This ethics commands respect. Contemporary medical ethics should not ignore it.

Religion and Character Formation

Historically the relationship between religion and the character of physicians was particularly strong. Hippocratic physicians adopted an ethical code that assumed the development of character with the attributes of respect for life; benevolence (acting for the good of patients rather than the self); confidentiality (keeping patients' secrets); and even priestliness (keeping one's life and medical art "pure and holy"). Such high personal ethical standards presumably were influenced by Pythagorean religion. Besides the Hippocratic code, many other Hippocratic texts testify to religious influence on what can only be described as priestly virtue and character standards for physicians. *The Law*, a text for physician education, ends with these words: "things, however, that are holy are revealed only to men who are holy."

Later on, during the Christian era, there is no doubt about the strong religious influence on a medical ethics dominated by virtue and character considerations. Physicians in the medieval university were educated with priests in a social setting something like a pre-Vatican II Catholic seminary. The same high ethical ideals were expected of priests and doctors. Both medicine and priesthood were considered "vocations" (divine callings) and both professionals committed their lives to the service of others. A great deal of physician education, like priest education, had to do with ethics in the sense of self or character development. Through the nineteenth century, physicians, like priests, were exempt from taxes and enjoyed immunity from court testimony because of their personal obligations to secrecy. Even payment for physician services was called a "stipend" or "honorarium" — terms used for payments made for priestly services.

The first American Medical Association ethical code, in 1847, and revisions in 1903, 1912, 1947, 1955 were replete with references to "character and virtue." Standards by which physicians would determine the "propriety of their conduct" were meaningless without virtuous character. The Hippocratic ethical tradition was explicitly mentioned, and specific character traits were listed. The physician "should be modest, sober, patient, prompt to do his whole duty without anxiety; pious without going so far as superstition, conducting himself with propriety in his profession and in all the actions of his life." Section 2 of the 1847 code read, "in their relationships with patients, with colleagues and with the public, [physicians are expected] to maintain under God, as they have down the ages, the most inflexible standards of personal honor."

These references sound old-fashioned to modern physicians but this same character and virtue ethics is found in ethical treaties throughout medical history (*Percival's Medical Code* in 1803, *Medicus Politicus* from the Renaissance, *Epistulae and Admonita* in the Middle Ages). Historically, medical ethics has been a character and virtue ethics thoroughly influenced by religion and encouraging priestly traits. A radical revision of the AMA Ethical Declarations in 1980 rather precipitously set aside, but did not erase, this deep tradition. Most physicians today continue to think of themselves as decent, virtuous people serving the sick and the needy. And certainly many patients continue to expect a high personal ethics from their physician. Even secular patients are scandalized by the physician who abandons all priestly pretense of serving others to become just another businessman with a product to sell.

Little doubt exists that character failures constitute the most flagrant medical ethical failures today. Instances of physicians taking advantage of patients both financially and sexually are instances of character failures more than rule violations. An increase in character failures among physicians might be explained by the sudden official abandonment of character considerations either in official Medical Association Declarations or in medical school training. Secularization certainly has had an effect on physician character styles. Religion, either through its presence in society at large or through particular church communities, influenced personal ethical formation. Moral ideals and vital projects derived from religion were meant to be interiorized. Lived religion involves efforts not just to act in certain ways but to become certain persons through the development of moral attitudes and dispositions. Religion does not guarantee character and virtue, but the loss of religion can explain a perceived loss of character and virtue considerations in contemporary professional life.

Secular persons do not escape the ethical challenge of becoming good persons by rejecting religiously based morality. And secular physicians do not escape the project of becoming helpful, caring, respectful, and courageous professionals by setting aside traditional medical ethics. Some may rely on willpower guided by the anemic requirements of the current AMA Ethical Declarations to guide their personal development, but not many. And no one seriously believes that becoming a virtuous doctor will come naturally or effortlessly. The ageless wisdom of philosophy and religion support the idea that moral will alone does not produce the virtuous or even the decent person. Moral will alone is more likely to create persons suffering from moral delusion. The religiously informed moral will is at least less likely to ignore its own weakness and inadequacies, sins, and guilt. Besides providing ample opportunities for reflection on how a personal moral self is developed and constant encouragement to reach for personal ethical ideals, religion also makes a place for forgiveness and the new starts so critical to character development. Secular cultures, even humanistic ones, do not provide similar opportunities for character and virtue development, and it shows.

Secular physicians who understand ethics as rules and act analysis go along making their clinical judgments and creating an inner ethical self out of attitudes, social influences, and critical life choices. No one escapes the task of making him or herself ethically. Each person starts with certain "givens," biological and social. These constitute the raw material out of which ethical inner selves are made. As important as they are, however, they determine neither character nor virtue. Humans are always at a certain distance even from biology and social environment; they can choose either to go along or to oppose and change. Religion may be accepted as an influence or rejected. But even if religion is not related to the ongoing project of ethical self-creation, inevitably it becomes related when a vital project hits the wall of failure. Inevitably human beings have to choose their lives either as loss and despair or as gift and hope. In either case ethical self-creation inevitably involves religion in the sense of a life choice based on faith. There is no way of avoiding character-creating choices, and character ethics will always be religious in the sense of involving an act of faith about the ultimate meaning of life.

Conclusion

The worst of all ethical failures in medicine point up by contrast what might be the key virtue in medicine, friendship. This may sound strange to U.S. readers. How can medical friendship be the key ethical characteristic in medicine when we never hear anything about it in the literature of medical ethics? What does medical friendship mean? What does a capacity for friendship have to do with the practice of good medicine or becoming a good doctor?

Character and virtues are important today because they have everything to do with the quality of a doctor-patient relationship. Nothing is more important to a patient than this relationship, and yet attention to it has dropped out of both mainstream medicine and medical ethics. To talk about medical friendship is to reintroduce the concept of a bond that is threatened in contemporary medicine. The technical mentality today, like the magical mentality in prehistorical medicine, does away with a doctor-patient relationship. Both mentalities physically separate doctor and patient by making diagnosis and therapy depend either on a machine or a formula; a piece of technology or a ritual. In neither case is a personal relationship between healer and patient necessary. Consequently, the whole idea of a character trait or virtue which makes that personal relationship possible also slips from consideration.

But patients have neither abandoned an expectation of friendship with their physician nor agreed to adjust to impersonal technical medicine no matter how impressive its claims. The most common reasons for malpractice claims are disappointments not about technical outcomes, but about impersonal physician attitudes, that is, unfriendliness. The virtue of friendliness and the vice of unfriendliness may be at the heart of an all-important personal doctor-patient relationship.

Friendship and friendliness are important in life and especially important in medicine. Patients need a special kind of affection and love from a physician. Many patients feel alone, vulnerable, and frightened and look to the doctor much as a child does to a parent. When neither love nor friendship is forthcoming, patients feel disappointed. If they are treated with indifference or hostility, their disappointment becomes anger.

Unfriendliness is a medical vice — a core medical deficiency — because it undermines the all-important personal relationship between doctor and patient. The doctor's character is the first medicine a doctor provides, and if it is unfriendly, then the patient's condition could be worsened. Even if the physician provides powerful drugs, their effect can be diminished if unfriendliness has undermined the doctor-patient relationship. Separateness and hostility between doctor and patient are untherapeutic in the extreme. Friendliness toward a patient on the other hand is the personal ground from which comes caring concern and a desire to help. All the virtues inherent in medical practice as well as all the vices that undermine its inherent ethical structure can be seen as grounded on this one character trait. Difficult as it is in modern medical care delivery, friendliness toward patients remains a fundamental good that deserves attention in ethics. And the fundamental vice of unfriendliness that is easily formed in today's impersonal training programs and health care institutions explains why patients are treated as things, organs, or disease categories rather than as persons.

Freud recognized the strong affect that is likely to develop between patient and physician. In the case of psychiatric therapy, the affect can reach the point of great intensity and great potential either for insight or for exploitation. Between the doctor and patient in nonpsychiatric medical practice, affect on the part of a patient who is being attended and helped is real and sets up an expectation of response that is possible only when the doctor has developed the virtue of friendliness. Only then does real trust develop, with all its therapeutic benefits. For this reason, sexual violation of an overly affectionate patient is so immoral. It demonstrates a character deficiency that makes the practice of effective medicine impossible. Increases in the incidence of sexual relations between doctors and patients cannot be addressed with another set of rules. The solution lies in attention to character formation in medical training and a refocusing of attention on the many-sided doctor-patient relationship.

Ending with the notion of friendliness as a dimension of ethical medicine sums up the strange idea of refocusing attention in mainstream biomedical ethics on character and virtue. Doing so will considerably broaden the ethical playing field beyond what the mainstream principles approach identifies as biomedical ethics. Integrating the inner being of the doctor into a biomedical ethics of acts and rules will enhance it as a form of applied philosophy without diminishing any of the power of the mainstream principles approach.

NOTES

1. Character types associated with cultural influences we find in much of the critical commentary on twentieth-century America (see Lasch 1979). Another instance of contemporary interest in character, but not confined to pathological character types, is the work of Harvard psychiatrist Robert Coles (1977–80; 1990). His many books on children seek insight into the nature of character through direct contact and anecdotal reports on children whom he interviews. Coles's latest book related to children and morality is 1990.

2. Actions are assessed as "signs or indications of certain principles (origins) in the mind and tempers" (Hume 1973:477). Virtuous or vicious action "must depend upon durable 'principles' of the mind which extend over the whole conduct and enter into the personal character" (1973:575).

3. Etymological reflections on philosophical terms is characteristic of many continental philosophers. The analysis provided here comes from the work of several Spanish philosophers; see, for instance, Aranguren 1983:22.

4. *Mos* autem duo significat. Quadoque enim significat consuetudinem...; quandoque vero significat inclinationem quandam naturalem, vel quasi naturalem, ad aliquid agendum: unde et etiam brutorum animalium dicuntur alique *mores*...Et haec quidem duas significationes in nullo distinguuntur: nam ethos quod apud nos *morem* significat, quandoque habet primam longam, et scribitur per η graecam litteram; quandoque habet primam correptam, et scribitur per ε. Dicitur autem virtus moralis a *more*, secundum quod *mos*

significat quandam inclinationem naturalem, vel quasi naturalem ad aliquid agendum. Et huic significationi moris propinqua est alia significatio, quae significat consuetudinem; nam consuetudo quodammodo vertitur in naturam, et facit inclinationem similem naturali.

In order to answer this inquiry clearly, the meaning of the Latin word *mos* needs to be examined. For this will tell us what moral virtue is. Its meaning is twofold. Sometimes it means custom...; sometimes a natural or quasi-natural bent toward doing something, in which sense brute animals are said to have *mores*....Both these meanings are not verbally differentiated in Latin: but in Greek there is a distinct word for each, for the word *éthos* which means the same as the Latin *mos* is written sometimes with a long η (eta) and sometimes with a short ε (epsilon)....Now *mos* means moral virtue in the sense of a natural inclination to do some particular action. The other meaning is akin, because custom sometimes becomes natural and produces an inclination similar to a natural one (Aquinas 1955:I-II, q. 58, art. 1; my translation).

St. Thomas Aquinas continued to make a distinction between what we call "character" in the sense of forged inner being and custom or external habits which may contribute to forging an inner nature. He uses the same word, *mos, moris,* for both. Later on, the original meaning of *éthos* (the natural inclination) was lost.

5. Utilitarian theory as developed by Bentham and Mill was focused on reform of the English legal system. This style of doing ethics still is most effective in areas of policy testing and development. For the connection between utilitarian ethical theory and its concern with legal reform, see Mill 1897:26–8.

6. Aristotle made the point about the relationships between virtue and satisfaction in several places. For example, *Nichomachean Ethics*, bk. II, chap. 3; *Nichomachean Ethics,* bk. VII, chap. 12. Thomas Aquinas following Aristotle also links delight and satisfaction with virtue and character development. Thomas Aquinas, *Summa Theologica.* "Quando constituitur res in proria operatione connaturali et non expedita, sequitur delectatio" (Aquinas 1955:I-II, q. 31 A. 1, ad. 1).

7. Kierkegaard's theory of the self and development of ethical character is worked out in *Either/Or: A Fragment of Life* (1959).

8. *Nichomachean Ethics*, bk. II, chap. 1, 1103b, 14–21.

9. Jesse Lachter, a sixth-year student at Israel Institute of Technology Faculty of Medicine, conducted the survey with assistance from a professor at Haifa University. It was reported at the Fourth International Bioethics Congress in Jerusalem, October 1991.

10. Those who are so willing to change the long historical proscriptions against aiding in suicide are an example of this. If they showed some awareness of what medicine was before the Hippocratic proscription, one might not be so distressed by their readiness to conform to today's cultural demands.

REFERENCES

Aquinas, Thomas. 1955. *Summa Theologica,* I–II. Chicago: Encyclopedia Britannica.

Aranguren, Jose Luis. 1983. *Etica.* Madrid: Editorial Alianza.

Coles, Robert. 1977–80. *Children in Crisis.* 5 vols. Boston: Little, Brown.

———. 1990. *The Spiritual Life of Children.* Boston: Houghton Mifflin.

Culver, Charles et al. 1985. "Basic Curricular Goals in Medical Ethics." *New England Journal of Medicine* 312, no. 4 (24 January): 253–55.

Fowler, James W. 1981. *Stages of Faith: The Psychology of Human Development and the Quest for Meaning.* San Francisco: Harper and Row.

Gilligan, Carol. 1982. *In a Different Voice: Psychological Theory and Women's Development.* Cambridge: Harvard University Press.

Gustafson, James M. 1985. *Can Ethics Be Christian?* Chicago: University of Chicago Press.

Hauerwas, Stanley. 1974. *Vision and Virtue.* Notre Dame, Ind.: Fides.

———. 1975. *Character and the Christian Life: A Study in Theological Ethics.* San Antonio: Trinity University Press.

Heidegger, Martin. 1962. *Being and Time.* New York: Harper.

Hume, David. 1973. *A Treatise of Human Nature.* Oxford: Oxford University Press.

Jaspers, Karl. 1968. *General Psychopathology,* trans. J. Hoenig and Marian W. Hamilton. Chicago: University of Chicago Press.

Kant, Immanuel. 1959. *Foundations of the Metaphysics of Morals,* trans. Lewis White Beck. New York: Liberal Arts Press.

Kierkegaard, Søren. 1954. *Fear and Trembling.* New York: Doubleday, Anchor Book Edition.

———. 1959. *Either/Or: A Fragment of Life.* Vol. 1, trans. David and Lillian Swanson; vol. 2, trans. Walter Lowrie. New York: Anchor.

Kohlberg, Lawrence. 1981. *The Philosophy of Moral Development: Moral Stages and the Idea of Justice.* San Francisco: Harper and Row.

Lasch, Christopher. 1979. *The Culture of Narcissism: American Life in an Age of Diminishing Expectations.* New York: W. W. Norton.

MacIntyre, Alasdair. 1981. *After Virtue.* Notre Dame, Ind.: University of Notre Dame Press.

Mill, John Stuart. 1897. *Utilitarianism.* London: Longmans, Green.

Piaget, Jean, et al. 1965. *The Moral Judgment of the Child,* trans. Marjorie Gabain. New York: Free Press.

Schopenhauer, Arthur. [1844] 1961. *The World as Will and Idea,* trans. R. B. Haldane and J. Kamp. Garden City, N.Y.: Doubleday.

~ *13* ~

CASUISTRY AND CLINICAL ETHICS

Stephen Toulmin

In recent years, discussions of medical ethics in American hospitals and among American physicians have been marked by a new emphasis on the need to deal directly and concretely with the moral problems that arise out of the condition of individual patients — in the emergency room, at the bedside, or in the intensive care unit. In this debate the term *casuistry* is used to refer to the direct analysis of particular cases in clinical medicine. This approach to the issues of medical ethics, indeed, has by now achieved institutional status: the University of Chicago School of Medicine has a Center for Clinical Medical Ethics; the *Journal of Clinical Ethics* is by now well established; the *Hastings Center Report* prints discussions of particular problematic cases; and so on. This being so, the Park Ridge Center's symposium on new directions in U.S. bioethics naturally takes a look at medical casuistry. Yet those of us who are associated with this strand in the debate would insist that medical casuistry is *not* just one more "new direction" in the evolution of bioethics. Rather the desire to keep the examination of moral cases on a clinical, pedestrian level is explicitly meant to stand aside from the academic, theoretical debates that characterize American bioethics in general.

Some writers (e.g., Alasdair MacIntyre) classify medical ethics as an "application" of ethics, in which the resolutions of particular medical cases are measured against the demands of general moral theory. Casuists reverse the relationship between theory and practice. Clinical medical ethics is not a new approach to *theoretical* issues *about* the morality of medical practice, competing with other approaches to theoretical bioethics. Rather, medical casuistry deals directly with *practical* issues *within* clinical medicine. Nor does our ability to resolve such questions depend on commitment to a previously well-established ethical theory. Rather (I will argue) the key issues that arise within the moral analysis of actual cases in clinical medicine are *pre*theoretical. This is so in two respects:

(1) the moral terminology in which such questions are stated is neutral, as between philosophical, theological, sociological, and other theoretical constructs;

(2) the ways in which we resolve issues in clinical ethics does not, typically, turn on the choice of one theoretical construct rather than another.

This claim that in clinical medical ethics, as in clinical medicine generally, our preoccupation is with the detailed circumstances of particular cases is not especially original. So understood, appeals to theory — whether in neurophysiology or molecular biochemistry, philosophical ethics or moral theology — are helpful only to the extent that they throw incidental light on particular cases. The argument for seeing this approach as typical of activities like medicine and navigation was stated more than two thousand years ago, in Aristotle's *Nicomachean Ethics*.

When a steersman decides how close to take his boat in to shore, before changing tack, he relies on accumulated experience of similar particular decisions in the past more than on any resort to mathematical calculation: the timeliness of his change of tack is a matter of judgment, based on his perception of how the coast shoals, of the momentary changes in the wind, and the like. Likewise, in medicine, a doctor decides how long to persevere with a particular antibiotic as the treatment for a patient's present state by a similar exercise of judgment: the decision when to conclude that another treatment is needed rests on observation of the patient's progress, and its interpretation depends on the doctor's experience as much as on any theoretical foundation in biochemistry or physiology.

We can return to Aristotle later. For the moment, let us remark only that, in analysis of particular cases, the moral and technical aspects of a decision are on a par. All judgments in clinical medicine have both technical and moral aspects; and, in each respect alike, the demands of timeliness and particularity limit the extent to which our judgments can safely be generalized.

The Moral Vocabulary of Clinical Medicine

In explaining why the arguments on which a "casuistical" clinical ethics relies are independent of any bioethical theory — are, indeed, *pre*theoretical — we can usefully spell out one more preliminary point.

For a long time, a supposed need to respect and conform to what was called the *fact/value* distinction shaped philosophical discussions of the relation of ethics to the sciences, not least the social sciences. But — it turns out — clinical medicine is a field of inquiry in which insisting on this distinction does more harm than good. In natural science, we may legitimately assume that a straightforward observation of a particular state of affairs — e.g., the present position of the planet Mercury — is just *factual*. It is the astronomer's business to record how things in fact are at the time of observation and not let that observation be influenced by "value" considerations concerning the state of affairs he or she considers desirable. In planetary astronomy, e.g., the question of what is in fact the case at any given time is not only *distinct* but *separable* from the question of what we would like that state of affairs to be, or what state of affairs we would seek to bring about if we had the chance.

This said, we must recall that what can be *distinguished* cannot necessarily — or always — be *separated*. Historically, the success of Newton's natural philosophy in the seventeenth and eighteenth centuries was due, not least, to the availability of the planetary system as a natural "laboratory" in which his theoretical calculations could be checked. Ever since ancient Babylon, human beings had viewed the movements of the planets as far distant and imposing: the idea that human intervention could manipulate or modify them, even to the slightest degree, was unimaginable. (Even today, plans to intercept and destroy asteroids approaching the Earth seem fanciful to all except the Promethean advocates of the High Frontier.) Before too long, however, the success of the new natural science brought it to a point at which any attempt to separate "facts" from "values" had to be qualified, if not abandoned. The eighteenth-century development of chemistry did not immediately challenge this separation; but the early-nineteenth-century development of a scientific physiology called it into question. Not for nothing, Claude Bernard referred to his new *homeostatic* theories of physiological function as contributing to "experimental medicine." From the beginning, then, the science of physiology was organized, at its core, around the distinction between *function* and *dysfunction* — between bodily organs operating in a desired mode, and the same organs operating in ways that doctors would seek to correct.

With the best will in the world, then, scientific medicine is never a purely *natural* science in which the separation of facts and values holds at all points. On the contrary, the conceptual skeleton of theoretical physiology is still implicitly value laden, not value neutral. And, if this is true of physiological theory, it is even truer of clinical medicine. Anybody who sits in on clinical discussions of problematic cases, and reflects on the terms in which a patient's condition is reported, recognizes that the language of medical recording is not as "value neutral" as rigorous conformity to the "fact"/"value" separation would demand. The central facts of clinical reporting are as much *moral* as *technical*. The very fact that someone is *sick* or *ill* creates a moral claim on the doctor's attention: the condition cries out for diagnosis and treatment. Nor, at this preliminary stage, is anything theoretical involved in our recognition that the individual in question is "ill" — i.e., that he or she complains of an illness. In exceptional cases, we may suspect that the complainant does not really have anything to complain about: that, as the saying goes, he or she is *malingering*. But then, the term *malingering* is itself one more term in the *practical* vocabulary of medicine, with which physicians were familiar long before there existed a science of physiology or biochemistry. Historically and pragmatically alike, that is, the basic conceptual vocabulary of clinical medicine is — and always has been — *pretheoretical.*

If this is true of the general vocabulary of clinical medicine, it is true even more if we become specific. Terms like "wound" and "pain," "fevered" and "unconscious" are familiar and intelligible to nurses and physicians, without their having to subscribe to a larger theory about the nature of trauma, the mechanism of fever, or the cause of fever. As they stand, all these basic "illness" terms serve to name *disabilities;* and the need to remedy them, in each case, goes without saying. We need no Portia to remind us that a human in pain needs relief (and is entitled to ask others for it) simply on that account. Nor does it take a philosopher — a Jeremy Bentham or a Thomas Aquinas, an Immanuel Kant or a John Rawls — to explain *why* relief is called for. Recognizing that this is the case is a general human insight, which operates on a level more basic than that of any theoretical axiom or principle.

When moral argument reaches the level of these insights, in clinical medicine or in everyday human relations, we deal with the familiar considerations that serve as a final locus of moral appeal: what Aristotle calls *ta eschata*, or "the ultimates." We recognize such ultimates — e.g., cruelty — when we see them, Aristotle tells us, in the way that we recognize basic geometrical figures — e.g., the triangle — when we see them; and we do not need to tell anyone, in addition, "By the way, cruelty also happens to be *wrong.*" To see an action as cruel is to recognize it as wrong *in this way* — as distinct from *lying* or *disloyal*, and as contrasted with *kind*. Similarly, we recognize someone who is *in pain* with the same basic clarity we do Aristotle's other ultimates, and we do not need to tell anyone, in addition, "By the way, pain also happens to be *bad.*"

For MacIntyre, all judgments in medical ethics — *being* "applied" — rely for their soundness on the validity of the broader system of ethical theory to which the medical practitioner subscribes. Does this mean that a physician's ability to see that a patient is in pain requires him to decide, in advance, that he is a Thomist rather than a Kantian or a utilitarian? That is a paradoxical conclusion, from which there are two ways of escape. On the one hand, we can reclassify the occurrence of pain as a physical fact, which is "value neutral" and so devoid of moral significance: taking that route, you are free to reject Aristotle's repeated warnings and treat all ethics as fundamentally *theoretical*. (This seems to be MacIntyre's choice.) On the other hand, you can acknowledge the moral ultimacy of such maxims as "pain demands relief" — recognizing that the "fact" and "value" aspects of *pain*, while distinct, are inseparable.

The casuist's approach to moral problems in clinical medicine takes the second of these routes. From this point of view, all the most fundamental issues in medical ethics were already settled at a *pretheoretical* level, in advance of particular problematic cases. The problems that divide physicians in clinical practice rarely arise because they are in disagreement about "personal values" — let alone, about matters of philosophical theory. They typically arise because the details of the particular situations that confront them in, e.g., cases of terminal illness *either* embody conflicts between two or more coexisting demands, about whose moral "value" we basically agree; *or else* arise at the margin of application of ideas (e.g., "autonomy") about which there would have been no problem, if the case in question had been paradigmatic — central, and free of ambiguity. The task of the medical casuist is, then, to refer difficult cases arising in marginal or ambiguous situations to simpler, more nearly paradigmatic examples and to consider how far the simpler examples can guide us in resolving the conflicts and ambiguities that awaken our moral perplexity.

The Certitude of Practice

At this point, we may return to Aristotle's reasons for accepting *experience* as having priority over *theory* in ethics generally, and more specifically in such fields as medicine and navigation. His classic example of this point may not go unchallenged today, but it is easy to find up-to-date illustrations of the same point.

"We *know that* chicken is good to eat," Aristotle says, "with more confidence than we have in any theory that claims to *explain why* it is good to eat." The practical experience behind the knowledge that chicken is light textured, and so particularly good to eat, has a familiarity and practical certainty that outstrip any confidence we may have in the explanations of dietitians or nutritionists. Another familiar example makes the same point with equal clarity: "We *know that* aspirin relieves headaches," we may say, "with more confidence than we have in any theory that claims to *explain why* it does." Physicians would be happy to have a satisfactory explanation of the therapeutic efficacy of aspirin — electrophysiological, biochemical, or whatever; but, absent such an account, it is unreasonable to see this as a reason for refusing to rely on aspirin as an analgesic.

What is true of "practical" knowledge in technical cases is true in moral ones also. We know that, within the limits of the possible, lost consciousness needs to be restored and pain cries out for relief; and these items of moral knowledge are more certain than any theory in philosophical ethics that may claim to account for, or justify, such beliefs. Again, this insight is not original, and need elicit no surprise. In *The Methods of Ethics*, for instance, Henry Sidgwick carefully avoided implying that philosophers better than other humans know what is right or wrong in practical situations: the philosopher's task (he says) is to describe the shared moral "intuitions" of their fellow human beings and fashion theories capable of doing general intellectual justice to those particular, intuitive judgments.

So the moral experience we acquire in the clinical practice of medicine reinforces a confidence that was already open to us, in advance of entering the field of medicine. Behind the special moral problems of medical practice, there lie certain basic families of moral claims and obligations, and a shared familiarity with what is or is not virtuous in the conduct of laypeople, or physicians. The concerns expressed in such obligations are close to the "ultimates" in Aristotle's account. A physician may be kind or cruel, trustworthy or unreliable, or conscientious or sloppy, and may speak truly or tell lies. The particular ways in which merit and fault are displayed in medical contexts reflect technical features and complexities "proper to" the practice of medicine, as distinct from shopkeeping or schoolteaching, being a loyal son, a good father, an upstanding citizen, or a conscientious judge. In a sense that is by now clear, these basic families of claims and obligations are *prior to* all theoretical issues in moral philosophy: not least those that go by the name of *bioethics*. So, in medicine as in law and other aspects of life, the goal of case analysis is not to explain, justify, or "do intellectual justice to" these basic insights; rather, it is to sort them, tell them apart, classify them into a practical taxonomy, and bring our understanding of paradigmatic cases to bear on other, harder cases, which are conflicted or marginal and so problematic.

The resulting taxonomy is the fabric of that part of "case ethics" that is special to medicine. For several reasons, it also overlaps the "case law" of medical practice. Some of these reasons are historical: the taxonomies of case ethics and case law have a common ancestry. The scholars of the medieval Christian Church did not distinguish law from ethics at all sharply, any more than Judaism does today. The categories of natural law were rooted in moral theology; and the classical discussions of problem cases — some inherited from Cicero's *de Officiis*, others developed in the Christian era — were understood as having both moral and legal relevance.

Alan Donagan made this point by arguing that "common morality" is a tradition that closely parallels, and even overlaps, the more familiar tradition of "common law." At the present time, indeed, the most perceptive contributions to medical casuistry often come in judicial decisions. However much we sometimes need to separate judgments of the morality of medical acts from their legal permissibility, in other situations the law and morality of medicine are very close. In the sequence of law cases that arise about the medical misfortunes of comatose patients, from Quinlan to Cruzan, the rulings of the courts can be used as texts for discussing the *morality* of continuing life support for irremediable patients. To that extent, the Supreme Courts of New Jersey and California have provided a moral as well as a legal analysis of life support for the comatose. Their analyses, differentiating particular kinds of cases in ever more discriminating ways, can be of great service to the moral practice of clinical medicine. It is not that they add any explanation or justification to our shared understanding of the points of issue: it is just that they give us practical criteria — "rules of thumb" — that can be relevant and helpful in handling similar problems in subsequent cases.

Summary and Conclusion

In presenting their aims as purely practical, medical casuists insist on the modesty of their claims. As in all diagnosis, they wish to treat patients *justly:* handling alike patients whose circumstances are similar in all relevant respects, and treating apart those whose circumstances display relevant moral differences. This modesty of aim is only one side of a coin. On the other side, they argue that the relevance of bioethics to clinical practice is overrated: its claims to depth are misleading, and they distract us from the practical needs of medicine. No doubt, intellectual contests between different bioethical theories are free to continue in academia; and, down the road, the theoretical points so established may have some practical implications for diagnosis and treatment. (Genetic counseling, for instance, was made possible by improved understanding of molecular biochemistry, risk assessment, and scientific genetics itself.) Still, it would be an error to assume, without more ado, that the intellectual results arrived at in bioethics help us resolve the moral problems facing us at the bedsides of particular patients. The primary classification of cases and circumstances is made on a casuistical basis: the relevance of theoretical points, whether biochemical or bioethical, needs to be shown subsequently, and independently.

By now, of course, the actual methods of "case reasoning" in clinical medicine have come a long way since the mid-1970s and the National Commission for the Protection of Human Subjects of Biomedical and Behavioral Research. After the commission's work ended, I shared with Albert Jonsen (himself a commissioner) the intellectual adventure of collaborating on a book about case ethics, with the title *The Abuse of Casuistry: A History of Moral Reasoning* (1988). Since then the literature on case reasoning in clinical medicine has grown continuously. The handbook *Clinical Ethics,* by Albert Jonsen, Mark Siegler, and William Winslade (1986), develops a taxonomy of "type cases" designed to map the whole field of clinical medicine; the subject is explored from a variety of different angles in other recent articles in the journals (see, for example, Jonsen 1991, 1990).

One final comment is in order. Looking back at the development of case ethics in the Middle Ages and the Renaissance, two points attract our attention. The institutional framework for these analyses was an *ecclesiastical* one, and the illustrations offered to support their taxonomy were often biblical or theological. The same is still true today. When the bishops of the American Episcopal or Catholic church publish statements on the morality of nuclear war, or the American economic system, they often support the substance of these opinions by quotations from the Bible, the Early Fathers, or other religious texts. In clinical medicine, as elsewhere, casuistry is therefore affiliated with religion, both as a matter of history and in the present day.

However, these religious and theological quotations do not *prove,* or *justify,* the moral distinctions they are used to illustrate. Rather, they clarify those distinctions and help give them a more vivid force. Whether in the Middle Ages or now, many classic examples in moral casuistry have come from outside religion. For medieval scholars, we noted, Cicero was no less learned and no less powerful an authority than Augustine. To claim *exclusive* correctness for the moral teachings of any one religious tradition, thus, is to display a historically uninformed dogmatism.

At the most basic level, the human considerations on which moral discernment operates are broader in scope than the teachings of any one religion. Judaism includes its Noachic Code, listing moral obligations that hold among Gentiles as well as Jews; Thomas Aquinas found the deepest roots of morality not in Christian doctrine but in a *ratio naturalis* ("natural reason") that in his view all human beings alike share. Each religious tradition, no doubt, uses its own repertory of parables and stories as a way of presenting the central human insights of morality in terms that carry conviction with the faithful in its own congregations. But, in this respect, religion provides an environment for moral thought, more than it does the foundations of moral practice. For us, as for Aristotle long ago, the roots of moral conduct remain practical rather than theoretical, familiar rather than arcane. As such, they are best understood if we clear our minds of theoretical cant and stay close to the particular insights we accumulate in the course of our pedestrian, concrete practical experience.

REFERENCES

Jonsen, Albert R. 1990. "Case Analysis in Clinical Ethics." *Journal of Clinical Ethics* 1, no. 1: 63–65.

———. 1991. "Casuistry as Methodology in Clinical Ethics." *Theoretical Medicine* 12:295–307.

Jonsen, Albert R., Mark Siegler, and William J. Winslade. 1986. *Clinical Ethics: A Practical Approach to Ethical Decisions in Clinical Medicine.* 2d ed. New York: Macmillan.

Jonsen, Albert R., and Stephen Toulmin. 1988. *The Abuse of Casuistry: A History of Moral Reasoning.* Los Angeles: University of California Press.

~ *Part Four* ~

Horizons in U.S. Biomedical Ethics

~ 14 ~

Rejecting Principlism, Affirming Principles

A Philosopher Reflects on the Ferment in U.S. Bioethics

Larry R. Churchill

The idea that bioethics simply involves the application of antecedently known principles to the novel conundrums of modern biomedicine forms the polemical context for this volume. I will refer to this idea as *principlism* and use this term to designate a popular approach to bioethics. This use of *principlism* is consistent with that of other authors in this volume except Childress, who defends "principle-oriented" approaches under the name *principlism*. (In other respects, the spirit of Childress's essay is similar to this one.) The essays here collected offer various testimonials to the poverty of principlism. Collectively they represent an irresistible critique and convincing evidence of the ferment both in bioethics and in the humanities more generally.

Some readers may be tempted to take this volume as an effort to find the new, correct approach. If principlism is mistaken or inadequate, should we not now turn to casuistry, hermeneutical theory, narrative, or feminist ethics? But we should resist such an interpretation, for it would simply mean replacing one dogma with another. The lasting value of this collection is in its exhibition of the irreducible pluralism of moral thought and the naivete of assumptions about theoretical hegemony in ethics. In this sense the problem is not principles per se but a tendency toward an exhaustive reliance on principles. Principles have frequently been asked to do too much work in bioethics, and have buckled under the strain. They have been saddled with moral functions that are better achieved through custom, habit, sentiment, and judgment. In addition, a deductivism in the name of principles has too often displaced more discursive and analogical modes of reasoning. It is no wonder that principles have fallen on hard times and are often reduced to the principlism that we all seem ready to reject.

In contrast to the substitutionary interpretation of these essays (one theory replacing another), I believe we should read them as midcourse corrections, as ways to rearticulate and reaffirm the power of principles in ethics without becoming captivated by them. In this sense, casuistry, hermeneutics, and phenomenology present their own sets of assets and liabilities as ethical modes of thought. If we can learn from these alternative approaches, affirming them but avoiding the urge to canonize them as the new truth, we will have achieved a great deal.

Just why we seem to search for single approaches in ethics in hopes of finding the final, or ultimately correct, theory and why principles are often involved in this search are matters I will discuss later. For now I want to rehearse briefly a few of the many important themes and points in these essays. Then I will offer suggestions on how bioethics is enriched if we can embrace principles without being seduced by principlism.

Some Challenges to Principlism

The basic and pervasive theme of most, if not all, of the essays is well stated by Henk ten Have. Bioethics as principlism — that is, as the application of antecedently derived principles to problem cases — is mistaken. The idea of applied ethics itself, he claims, should be seen as a particular cultural phenomenon, not acritically accepted as a timeless norm for the field. His attitude is not hostile to principles, but to principlism — namely, the dogma that all other approaches are inferior and tainted with the parochialism of local communities of belief or practice and, thereby, intellectually indefensible. In fact, the idea that a neutral moral language of principles bypasses the limitations of sentiment, custom, or tradition is itself an example of cultural parochialism. Ten Have's essay presents a systematic call for new theoretical perspectives and a new, larger, and more robust vision of bioethics.

But principlism not only embodies a view of ethics; it bespeaks a view of the moral self. Courtney Campbell speaks for many of the authors when he argues that the tendency toward "detached reflection," encouraged by excessive reliance on principles, marginalizes other views of the self. Campbell is specifically concerned about the spiritual dimensions of the self, but much the same thesis applies to Christine Gudorf's concern for the marginalization of women, James Drane's concern with the neglect of the virtues, and Renée Fox's concern about the peripheral status of the social self. (Special recognition should go to Fox, who has been the most persistent and one of the most insightful critics of bioethics over the past decade.) These critics advocate a less hierarchical, and more eclectic, culturally textured, socially sensitive way of going about the business of bioethics.

A far more radical and challenging thesis is presented in the essay by Márcio Fabri dos Anjos. He would have us ask, of principled approaches (or any approach), how bioethics has helped the poor and disenfranchised. "For whom," he asks, "does one do bioethics? Who benefits?" He charges that bioethics has separated itself from social ethics and from the concerns of justice. He warns that the hospital bioethicist can become a "domesticated prisoner . . . co-opted by an anti-ethical system." Finally, he suggests that bioethics must have a "mystique," by which he means a vision that informs its work, a horizon of meaning in which its work is anchored. This is not an argument against pragmatism and practicality or a suggestion that bioethics move away from concrete problems. Rather it is a recognition that bioethics must not only be intellectually rigorous but also socially purposeful. It must stand for something besides the professional self-interest of bioethicists. Without a vision, to paraphrase Abraham Lincoln, bioethics (and bioethicists) will perish.

In an ingenious essay, Richard Zaner eschews the frontal assault on principles and simply puts on exhibit — in good phenomenological fashion — a way of doing ethics in which principles are never mentioned. His richly textured account of an experience of illness and its moral implications is a powerful argument that does not *say* but *shows* that principles are not everything, sometimes not even terribly important in the lived world.

Stephen Toulmin, speaking for the tradition of casuistry, presents the greatest intellectual challenge to the principled approach. He seeks not simply to expand the conceptual repertoire of bioethics but to reverse the customary relationship between ethical theory and practice. This is not just another assertion that the applied ethics model may be parochial. Casuistry begins and remains much closer to the ground; it is "pretheoretical." By this, Toulmin means at least two things: that the moral terminology of the problems of clinical bioethics is neutral, or not privileged by, any theoretical construct; and that the resolution of these problems does not turn on the choice of one theory over another. So it matters not whether one is Kantian, utilitarian, or whatever, for the purposes of problem solving. Answers do not have to be justified by theoretical sponsorship. For Toulmin, the great mistake is to think that ethics must be theoretical. Bioethics, understood in the casuistic tradition, does not seek to explain or justify but to sort out, distinguish, and classify problems and insights into a "practical taxonomy... and so bring our understandings about paradigmatic cases to bear on other more difficult cases."

Space will not permit the cataloging and assessment of all the essays presented in this volume, nor would it provide a useful service to the reader to do so. The aim, after all, is not some new systematization. The value of these essays is in honing our critical thinking and disabusing us of the desire for a final, overarching, theoretical construct in bioethics. In what follows, I add my own critical remarks to those already offered. But with a difference. No doubt we should reject principlism and be clear about why we reject it. But we must also reflect on why principlism (or something like it) is an enduring temptation. Moreover, we must separate the abuses of principlism from the enduring value of principled thinking in ethics. The remainder of the essay is devoted to these tasks.

The Enduring Temptation of Principlism

Bioethics is a creature of the times. Principlism pervades bioethics because in ethics generally, principles represent the zenith of moral sensibility, and appealing to principles is the central move of ethical reasoning.

Much of our ordinary moral language reflects this view. We often talk of "acting on principle" or of someone being "a person of principle" as if this were the ultimate manifestation of morality, beyond which there can be no recourse. Or, in a more self-serving mode, we often claim regarding our own behavior that we have acted "on principle," meaning that we acted with consistency and integrity, while others were swayed to make compromises.

Because principles are often thought to reside at the pinnacle of the moral hierarchy, they are especially prone to overuse. The flaw lies not in principles themselves but in how we use them and in theories that encourage this overextension. So what concerns me is not only principlism but the appetite that principlism serves — the human need for moral assurance and certainty in an uncertain world.[1] In other words, it is precisely the importance of principles in ethical judgments, combined with our moral anxiety, that leads to the overextensions and distortions of principlism.

One such distortion is based on the belief that while moral customs are culture bound and subjective, principles transcend particular societies and historical circumstances and are, thereby, more objective. But this is true only so long as we isolate principles from actual events and separate them from the thinking of some moral agent. Only as concepts do principles seem to lack cultural contingency and context; their *use* is profoundly tied to time and context. Some principles, of course, do have normative force across cultural boundaries. But I am making a more practical point. Even granting a general normative status for a principle, this principle will have different applications and meanings in differing situations of use. Only as categorical abstractions (under theoretical sponsorships) can principles be thought of as independent truths whose appeal is to a universal human rationality. In their interpretation, principles become part of the histories and traditions of individuals and communities.

The principle of autonomy, for example, is highly prized by many in modern North American society, but not always in the same way and not by everyone. Autonomy seems self-evidently right as a guiding norm for those who draw their moral sense of self primarily from figures like J. S. Mill or John Locke; it is less so in communities influenced by Reformed Protestant traditions, such as Calvinism. And autonomy plays a negligible role in the moral reasoning of Jehovah's Witnesses. The key moral experience for Witnesses seems to be not autonomy but authority, of Scripture and God, and the chief norm is obedience to these authorities. The *meaning* of autonomy also shifts from one moral tradition to another. In Mill's thinking, autonomy means chiefly the absence of political and social restraint, whereas Calvinism tends to see autonomy as a matter of freedom of conscience.

Even within a cultural tradition, principles are situation-specific, in the sense that they are appropriate at some times and in some settings, but not in others. For example, patient self-determination is an important ideal in the care of chronically ill adults, but it has a greatly diminished role in emergency care involving children.

The idea that principles are always more firm and objective than moral customs, transcending particulars of time and place, has led many to think of them as antecedent criteria for morality. When they take on this role, principles not only become the zenith of moral reasoning, they become ends in themselves. This hampers their proper use. Principles cannot be put to work when they are deferred to as the high judge of our moral sensibilities. When a principle becomes a static shrine, it creates a distorted ethic — one that displaces persons from the center of our concerns and puts adherence to the principle in their place.

For example, in the midst of the furor over the Baby Doe regulations, then–Surgeon General C. Everett Koop once remarked, "We're not just fighting for this baby, but for the principle that every life is sacred" (*New York Times,* 13 November 1983). The implication was that fighting for an individual life was insufficient to explain his actions, and fighting for principle constituted an even higher form of moral undertaking than advocating for a person. When fighting *for* principles, it becomes impossible to *use* them as guides to direct our action. In such a scheme, principles take on intrinsic value, as things to be protected, rather than the means to respect and protect persons. Koop's enshrinement of the principle of sacrality, his appeal to transcendent leverage in judgment, relegated to the background precisely those persons in whose name this principle was invoked.

Another distortion of principles relates to their perceived role as adjudicatory standards in a quasi-legal process. In this context, principles are frequently thought to provide a common basis for resolving differences. The basic task here is seen as finding principles upon which we can all agree, then refining the skills of their application so as to arrive at resolution. This process will, in turn, reduce conflict and ambiguity but will also forestall the tendency for doctors or parents to rely exclusively on their private intuitions or apply provincial standards. Principles are seen, then, as the means by which decision makers can ensure consistency and strive for universalizability in actions, a norm that has dominated ethics since Kant.

Although consistency is generally a desirable characteristic of judgments, it is not the only, or even the first, measure of ethical decisions. Consistency can be a slippery criterion, since every case is unique in some respects. The need for consistency may obscure morally relevant differences, and a preoccupation with consistency can, at its worst, excuse us from looking closely and attending patiently to individuals. Seeking consistency above all else will cause us to focus on superficial aspects of troublesome situations, making the world seem more neat and manageable than it is.

My criticism of these distorted uses of principles should not be taken as criticism of principles per se. Principles are doubtless important in any scheme of ethics. My point is that their role must be carefully circumscribed. In principlism, their role is too large and preemptive of other aspects of moral life and moral judgments. Moreover, important aspects of principles are ignored by overemphasis on their justifying and consistency-seeking functions. When these functions are valued over all else, the result is a hierarchy that detaches principles entirely from moral traditions and in some cases even places principles over persons.

When this occurs, both persons and principles are abused. Persons are abused by being displaced from the central focus of deliberations, while principles, such as the sacrality of human life, are abused by blind subservience to them. This use of principles is destructive to moral reasoning and to our sense of ourselves as moral agents, since it encourages us to replace thoughtful, ethical deliberation with moral dogma.

In other words, devotion to principles involves an especially detrimental form of displacement — displacement of the central concern in ethics away from human judgments and toward propositional truths, algorithmic formulae, and automated processes. Principles, when used in this dogmatic way, keep us from attending to the similarities and differences between cases and encourage an all-or-none sense of morality engendered by allegiance to a monolithic ideal. George Eliot, describing the plight of Maggie Tulliver in *The Mill on the Floss*, put it well: "moral judgments must remain false and hollow unless they are checked and enlightened by a perpetual reference to the special circumstances that mark the individual lot" (1979:628).

Principles, then, should be seen as instruments for interpreting the moral facets of situations and as guides to action. Abuse of principles occurs when we shape (and frequently distort) circumstances to fit the favored principle. This abuse comes of thinking *from* a principle, rather than using a principle to think *with*. For example, sacrality of life can be made to gather and lump situations from a first-trimester abortion to withholding treatment or nutrition from those in chronic vegetative states. These situations may all represent, in some sense, violations of the sacrality of life.[2] But in what sense? Upholding the sacrality of life can take many forms. When the demands of care are beyond technical resources or human powers of endurance, sacrality of life can be acknowledged by letting life go. The alternative of prolonging dying, or sustaining a life devoid of potential, would in fact be disrespectful of life. Thinking *from* principles, then, means entering situations of choice having determined in advance which principles to use and how to use them. This would be like approaching each carpentry task determined to use only a hammer. The resulting damage to both tools and the task is similar in each case.

By contrast, using a principle as one instrument among others, to think *with*, is like coming to the task with a toolbox, prepared to survey the work and ready to employ what the job requires. When viewed in this way, principles are relieved of being the measure of decisions and can become instruments of exploration in the larger tasks of formulating the problem, delineating the values, and assessing competing interests. Principles by themselves never have the force of a proof, as in mathematics, but skillfully used, they can persuasively guide choices. Principles, therefore, should be seen less as forms of post facto justification and more as means of exploration and illumination.

Principles not only serve as instruments of thinking, they also suggest a particular understanding of the world in which certain choices appear as self-evidently right, or good. Principles shape and alter our perception of the world in which we choose, including who we understand ourselves to be and what alternatives are appropriate to us. Principles are like paintbrushes in the hands of moral artists; the artist should use them to portray the moral landscape and set the contours of our choices, altering the world we see and in which we will act.[3] For example, moral artists could use the Golden Rule to portray a world in which one's own self-regard and self-interest become yardsticks for imagining what the desires of another might be.

Thus, choosing a principle on which to act is also choosing a way to think and a way to describe the context of action. Monolithic principles that aspire to universal validity are self-fulfilling. They value the world as they portray it, without regard for alternative visions. Moral agents who rely on a single principle, applied indiscriminately at a distance from the situation of choice, are likely to be oblivious to critical factors. To accept their judgments as normative would be like designing a chromatic chart using the perceptions of the colorblind.

Thus it is possible to hold and use sound ethical principles in unsound ways. For example, to reiterate a previous point, the principle of the sacrality of life seems to function for many in our society as a free-floating omnibus norm, unanchored and thereby unresponsive to the specifics of any concrete situation. It therefore becomes less useful even in those situations for which it could have persuasive power.

Principles as ways of seeing can both enable and obscure. Espousal of single principles will distort the moral landscape and impede our ability to see alternatives. Only recourse to the lives of real people, in their concrete circumstance, will correct the oversimplified view of our moral resources that typifies principlism. Only the effort to live out and embody principles will demonstrate their proper range of application. Again, the answer to principlism is not a better theory but proper use of the ones we have.

I have used two similes to elucidate the proper role of principles: carpentry tools and paintbrushes. Tools and brushes are instruments to accomplish a task, but each can also be used inappropriately, for the wrong job, or in too wholesale a manner. Instruments always imply skillful use. So substituting these terms for those of the formula, or the deductive proof, will not by itself resolve the difficulty that concerns me. But recognizing the instrumental character of principles does point to the heart of the matter — namely, how we understand ourselves as moral agents and why we are subsequently tempted to make principles absolute.

The desire for objective and universal principles in ethics, for the security and certainty of principlism, is part of the human need to think that we are good people who can know and do the right thing — that is, to think of ourselves as righteous in a morally ambiguous world. It is precisely this need that tempts us to oversimplify situations of choice and to espouse clear and singular action guides. Our need for security makes us vulnerable to absolutes and to manipulation by moral slogans, including the moral slogans of ethical theorists. Adopting these theories and their dogmas will keep us hovering above the action like a god, parsing principles with great agility but in a way that is irrelevant to ethics as lived experience.

Conclusion

Principlism has many attractions. First, it is easy to know where one stands; ambiguity is reduced or eliminated. Moreover, principlism can be extremely efficient: novel situations can easily be assumed to be like previous ones; particulars and context do not have to be taken into account. Perhaps most important, embracing principles in this uncritical way makes us feel good about ourselves; it protects and confirms our self-image as good people.

Yet ironically, the possession of such universally valid principles, were it possible, would not make us better people, but nonhuman. An inherent tension in the human situation results from the temporal structure of moral judgments themselves. Such judgments are time-laden and thereby incur the same sort of partial, systematic opacity that characterizes our knowledge of any human activity. What Merleau-Ponty said of understanding our own history is also true of understanding our moral judgments.

> My hold on the past and the future is precarious, and my possession of my own time is always postponed until a stage when I may fully understand it, yet this stage can never be reached, since it would be one more moment, bounded by the horizon of its future, and regaining in its turn further developments in order to be understood. (1962:246)

The ambiguity and lack of certainty occasioned by our temporal situation is what makes the human condition human (rather than godlike), and our recognition of this is what makes ethical reflection both possible and important. Hence, the answer is not different or better principles, or the pretense of universally valid judgments, or even an assertion that our longing for moral certainty is not genuine, for it is. Rather what we need is an acknowledgment that even our most cherished principles have limits.

My aim here has been to indicate a refined role for principles as tools in the service of bioethics. Tools imply skillful users and appropriate contexts of use — dimensions I cannot discuss in detail here. My main thesis is that we cannot escape recognition of our agency by trying to replace judgments with principles. The ongoing critique of principlism attempts to recapture moral agency, and with it, a more robust cultural context. To emphasize that principles are tools is to see that they are always and only *our* tools. We cannot make up for using them poorly by claiming that they have some special status in and of themselves.

The skeptical disdain we should feel for principlism has been well expressed by Thomas Nagel in *The View from Nowhere*. Nagel insists that we are at a primitive stage in our moral development. "The idea that the basic principles of morality are *known*, and that the problems all come in their interpretation and application, is one of the most fantastic conceits to which our conceited species has been drawn. (The idea that if we cannot easily know it, there is no truth here is no less conceited)" (1986:186).

Yet for Nagel, hope also tempers this skeptical disdain. He continues, "the possibility of moral progress is an essential condition of moral progress. None of it is inevitable" (1986:186). The contributors to this volume are evidence of this hope in bioethics.

NOTES

Support for the writing of this essay was provided through a Charles E. Culpepper Scholarship in Medical Humanities.

1. An earlier version of this argument was developed in an essay coauthored with Jose Siman, "Principles and the Search for Moral Certainty" (1986).

2. 'Sacrality' is too complex a theological concept to be discussed here fully. However, Protestants typically believe that strong claims for the sacrality of human life run the risk of idolatry, since the relativity of all rights and values is part of the monotheistic affirmation that only God is of absolute and enduring value. See, for example, Niebuhr 1943.

3. As Hauerwas writes, "the moral life is best understood like an artist engaged in his skill than a critic making a judgment about the complete work" (1974:157).

REFERENCES

Churchill, Larry R., and Jose Siman. 1986. "Principles and the Search for Moral Certainty." *Social Science and Medicine* 23, no. 5: 461–68.

Eliot, George. 1979. *The Mill on the Floss.* New York: Penguin Books.

Hauerwas, Stanley. 1974. *Vision and Virtue.* Notre Dame, Ind.: Fides/Claretian.

Kant, Immanuel. 1949. *Foundations of the Metaphysics of Morals*, trans. A. W. Beck. Chicago: University of Chicago Press.

Merleau-Ponty, Maurice. 1962. *Phenomenology of Perception*, trans. Colin Smith. London: Routledge and Kegan Paul.

Nagel, Thomas. 1986. *The View from Nowhere.* New York: Oxford University Press.

Niebuhr, H. R. 1943. *Radical Monotheism and Western Culture.* New York: Harper and Row.

~ 15 ~

CLINICAL MEDICINE AND
BIOMEDICAL ETHICS IN THE 1990s
A PHYSICIAN REFLECTS

Christine K. Cassel

To reflect as a physician on the substantial scope of theoretical terrain covered by bioethics since its inception requires (and, equally, allows) me to remember the field as I encountered it in 1976 — the beginning of my professional life in medicine and the year the New Jersey Supreme Court handed down its decision in the Karen Ann Quinlan case. I was beginning my internship in internal medicine in San Francisco, aware distantly of the Quinlan case the way the rest of America was, through articles in popular magazine and newspaper reports. This landmark decision, the first of scores to follow that affirmed the legal acceptability of allowing a patient to die by discontinuing some form of life-sustaining treatment, is cited by many people as a turning point in U.S. bioethics.

Equally important, 1976 was the year the California legislature passed the Death with Dignity Act, the first state law establishing the legal validity of what we now call advance directives. This was an extremely controversial issue at the time (Glick 1992). It's hard in retrospect to imagine how controversial such a limited "living will" could have been, but it truly incited the same kind of dire predictions that we have heard more recently concerning potential legislation (also in California, among other places) to legalize physician-assisted suicide. It would lead to abuses comparable to those of Nazi Germany; it would undermine the integrity of the medical profession and its Hippocratic tradition; patients could no longer trust their doctors; and these patients, particularly the most vulnerable ones, such as those who are disabled, poor, and otherwise socially disadvantaged, would be deprived of rights and access to care.

We now know that the California Natural Death Act of 1976 did not lead to any of these threatened outcomes. It did lead to similar, and stronger, legislation in almost every state by 1993 (Hill and Shirley 1992). But we still don't fully understand the impact of advance-directive legislation as it has swept the nation over the past seventeen years. Most analysts believe the effect has not been as great as hoped for or as feared. In the midst of the rapid changes in the policy world and in the theoretical world of bioethics, this paper attempts a "midstream" analysis.

The year 1976 was also the time when doctors were beginning to discuss the possibility of writing "do not resuscitate" orders. Before, if doctors gave such orders at all, they did so in an erasable pencil on the nurses' notes, erasable chalk on the board in the interns' conference room, or in one particularly notorious case, by removable purple dots on the patient's chart. Rather than decide not to resuscitate patients, doctors more commonly dealt with the futility of attempting to prevent death in patients with terminal illness or extreme frailty by using the now infamous and, I hope, mercifully extinct "slow code." Clinicians like me went through the motions of cardiopulmonary resuscitation but without the alacrity and intensity necessary to offer any hope of success. This embarrassing and distasteful charade, practiced by thousands of health professionals, created a visceral, existential self-awareness and generated a constituency who wanted change.

Another major development in the mid-seventies was the beginning of the hospice movement in the United States. A few remarkable pioneering physicians took the lessons from St. Christopher's hospice in London and set up places to provide comfort care for dying patients, at first in California and Connecticut, and then gradually throughout the country. This was extremely controversial twenty years ago, and again, it is hard to imagine how much professionals resisted frank and open discussion of the care of dying patients. For those involved in pushing these frontiers, it was just as exhilarating as it was frightening to those who still tried to hide from the reality of human mortality in the ever-expansive promise of medical technology.

Reflections from the beginning of my involvement with medical ethics in the clinical setting thus inevitably devolve on death. It seems that the issues around death and dying were the major frontier of clinical ethics at that time. Perhaps in some important way those issues remain at the frontier, still unresolved (Callahan 1991; Cassel 1987).

Many other issues were being addressed by the ethicists of the time, including the moral quandaries of abortion, scientific responsibility in genetic engineering and recombinant DNA research, human experimentation, and the rationing of specific scarce resources, most notably renal dialysis. These areas were of journalistic interest to the public but probably of much less visibility to practicing physicians. Most physicians didn't do abortions or genetics research, and even the rationing of health care at that time was considered morally off limits to practicing physicians and properly kept within the boundary of policymakers. Science policy or philosophy of science was not as immediate for clinicians as the questions around death and saving life, whether those questions occurred at the very beginning of life in premature infants or later among elderly people or those afflicted with widespread and unstoppable malignancies.

After *Roe v. Wade,* abortion became more of an academic issue, and fewer articles on the moral questions around abortion appeared in the ethics literature. This topic was replaced, in a way, with analyses of new reproductive technologies, which raised many similar issues of conflicts between maternal, paternal, and fetal interests. Now it appears the moral problems of abortion and justice are even more vividly present for clinicians again . . . or perhaps, still. In issues of abortion and reproductive technologies, as well as in the issues concerning end-of-life care, physicians face daily decisions about their own patients and also find themselves inextricably bound to the public-policy debate. No longer are we secure within the boundaries of the bedside. Clinical care occurs in a public arena, and physicians now need to forge their professional role in that public arena. Although they hold diverse attitudes, not all physicians are full of vigor and enthusiasm for this new role. Resisting it, however, ends in cynicism and frustration.

For those of us interested in ethics in those early days, a major struggle ensued in trying to convince our colleagues not just of the importance but of the actual possibility of discussing moral questions in a clinical sense. For many people, morality was inexplicable and inarticulate. It was something you learned at your mother's knee. Ethics was something not to be discussed and not to be argued, and it was certainly neither probable nor admirable that one would change one's mind on a moral issue. One indication of a moral problem on the wards of a hospital in 1976 was the physician throwing up his hands in a gesture meaning "Well, this is a moral problem. We can't discuss this. Let's go on to the next patient."

Principles Are Useful

The emergence of principlism and its success over the past decade and a half relates in major part to its adoption, or at least the recognition of its validity, by the clinical world. Principlism gave clinicians the vocabulary with which to discuss the previously inchoate moral gut feelings. It presented categories and differentiations that could be understood. It provided a framework not too different from differential diagnosis or the algorithms of clinical decision making like those posted on the wall of the cardiac care unit related to the treatment of potentially fatal arrhythmias. And once language, data, and logic could be employed, then moral people could change their minds, and thus discussion could lead to resolution of moral uncertainty or conflict in a given case. This realization, that language, data, and reason were relevant to ethics, paved the way for ethics committees and ethics consultation.

Ethics also, although with some greater resistance, gave physicians a way of understanding, talking about, and eventually appropriating the attacks from the public on their own preeminent status. For the seventies, as has been pointed out by many people including Renée Fox, was also the decade in which the strong consumer voice in medical care emerged. This emergence has been traced to a number of trends, not the least of which was the growing commercialism of health care. But certainly no one can deny that the shift from "patient" to "consumer" had major influence on the clinician and on clinical medical ethics. The concept of autonomy underscored and (we thought) explained why physicians no longer could or should (or would have to) take the enormous burden of responsibility in making decisions where clinical uncertainty existed. The concept of informed consent required us to inform the patient of the options and ask the patient for his or her decision. We even gradually began to accept the fact that the patient, simply for whimsical reasons referred to as "personal preferences," had the right to refuse treatment that we thought was unequivocally beneficial. The desired model became more of a transaction between equals than a charitable caring act toward another person in need. How often this model actually reflected reality is open to question. It also may have fostered a loss of the caring attitude of the physician and moved the physician-patient relationship into a more legalistic and — too often — adversarial mode.

In retrospect, the principle of respect for self-determination (autonomy) might have come along just in the nick of time for physicians. For it was in the seventies that the great euphoria of lifesaving medical technology produced almost simultaneously a great uncertainty regarding its adverse consequences and its failures, which were many. No one knew whether the permanently disabled child who survived from the rescue of a very premature infant was in fact a success. No one knew if the rescue by renal dialysis of the nursing home patient with advanced Alzheimer's disease was in fact a success. Prolonged dying during weeks of ICU care was clearly not a success. But now we had a conceptual framework in which we didn't have to make those awesome and God-like decisions ourselves. We could simply say this is what the patient (or surrogate) wanted. There is no doubt that modern medicine presents physicians with agonizing decisions. Principlism gave physicians a way of dealing with that agony and moving on.

Principlism also made it possible to teach principles-based bioethics in medical schools in ways that were remarkably successful. Students would learn their "mantra of principles" and then be able to read the literature as it appeared in medical journals, increasingly full of articles on medical ethics, and answer questions on exams invoking the principles that they had learned. As a resident and very quickly a teacher in this area, I remember saying countless times, "I'm less interested in what decision you make than in your reasons for making that decision." Here the clever student would invoke a conflict of principles, using data, language, and logic, and then articulate arguments "why" one principle would win out over another.

It should not be surprising to us that principlism has outlived its dominance. As Toulmin reminds us, many of the concrete moral demands of care, such as the relief of pain, are pretheoretical, and clinical facts often resolve the case, with principles remaining vaguely in the background or completely unnecessary. Interestingly, Childress too addresses the imprecision of principles, urging that they are useful as guidelines and frameworks, especially when values collide, but that we can rarely understand clinical situations correctly if we look only to principled abstractions. It would be incorrect, therefore, to say that principlism has outlived its usefulness because the principles are after all identifiable sources of shared values. The hierarchy of these principles and even their subtle meaning in complex and specific cases may not be as universally shared as we once imagined, but the concepts of beneficence, respect for persons, and autonomy are in fact important touchstones of the shared morality within our somewhat diverse and complicated fabric of cultural and ethnic backgrounds.

Horizons in the 1990s

A number of forces are driving American bioethics in the 1990s to move "beyond principlism." One is the plain and simple observation that principles do not explain the full complexity of moral problems and human interaction. This reality is explicated by Rita Charon in the turn to literary approaches to values and meaning, almost a 180-degree departure from the reductionism of principles to the thick description one finds in narrative. Similarly, Jonsen and Toulmin's revival of casuistry (1988), one of the truly dramatic strokes of modern bioethics, also has contributed to a recognition of principlism's tendency toward reductionism. Casuistry is now fully resuscitated and links with the new movement in narrative to give substance to the search for meaning. "Meaning" in the medical experience seems to be the underlying, and missing, component in much of a biomedical ethics dominated by principlism that these new and more elaborate stories promise us.

The other major reason for moving away from principlism is that it hasn't really worked. First, it hasn't met all the expectations set forth by bioethics proponents and hoped for by clinicians. Second, the emphasis on autonomy has not really made decisions easier. Third, it has spawned both "the demanding and unreasonable family" and the growing demand of the public for more control over their dying than just the refusal of life-sustaining treatment. Moreover, it has created even more bureaucratic demands for signatures and uncomfortable discussions with patients and families at a time when health care is facing growing bureaucracy in every other realm as well.

Finally, a philosopher would say that principlism is too simple. Books like *Clinical Ethics* (Jonsen, Siegler, and Winslade 1986) have succeeded in making principled clinical bioethics accessible to every physician who can carry such a book in the pocket of her white coat. In a field as now well established as bioethics, we should have an intellectual elite, and the intellectual elite is dissatisfied with oversimplified principles. The variegate scholarly discussion that now ensues is valuable to the history of ideas. The unanswered question is whether practitioners and patients in the world of health care will value this discussion. Consider whether philosophical ethics has had any impact on human behavior in society. One can think of the *oeuvre* stretching from Aristotle to Rawls as only distantly, if at all, related to social decisions concerning forms of government, punishment of criminals, and treatment of underprivileged populations. Similarly, the new frontiers in bioethics could develop in a discourse among the theorists, parallel to the world of health care but with little real effect upon it. One argument against this happening is the number of new voices urging more concreteness (casuistry), more specificity (narrative), and more connectedness with communities of meaning (hermeneutics and critical thinking).

In *Ethics in an Aging Society* Moody (1992) argues that a communicative ethics based on critical theory is more useful than an ethics of principles or virtue for approaching ethical problems in an aging society. This observation is not limited to the reality of the aging society but addresses all of the limitations of principlism articulated by the authors in this volume. In the larger scheme of things, critical theory, as drawn from Habermas, insists that ethics cannot exist outside historical, political, and social realities. Here is exactly the entrée that American biomedical ethics needs to step over the barriers that principlism has set up for the clinician between clinical bedside ethics and such social justice problems as resource allocation. Although the historical framework of critical theory itself brings with it the ideology of equity and fairness, it is in theory free of ideology and thus also awkwardly free of principles.

To say that ethics should be embedded in the concrete political and interpersonal reality of the situation is still not to say how to find out what's right and what's wrong and how to get there. Indeed, injustice is so embedded in the institutions around us that we cannot assume that ethical decisions are being correctly framed. This poses a problem to physicians who have a tendency toward meliorism, namely, how to perform in an ethical way in an unjust system and an unjust society. Moody draws on Habermas to offer us something called "communicative ethics" to deal with this problem that Fleck referred to as "interstitial ethics" (Fleck 1987) and that Niebuhr might call "moral man in an immoral society" (Niebuhr 1960).

Communicative ethics says among other things simply that we can expect imperfect results from our ethical choices, but that striving for the best among imperfect results is admirable, especially when strict adherence to principles does not allow for negotiation and compromise essential to the sharing of power and the framing of decisions. In specific contextual realities, power is disbursed through communication. Furthermore, communication (negotiation and discourse) is at the heart of a process leading to ethical decision making or an ethical stance in policy. This idea speaks to the awkwardness and ineffectiveness of principles in the clinical setting as well as in the world of policy.

An Example

Autonomy-based ethics has taught our medical students and physicians in training that the families, not the physician, are the decision makers. Thus, we have created a new kind of ethical problem that didn't seem to exist ten years ago — that of the unreasonable or demanding family. In clinical settings now, we frequently hear the intern or resident report that in the case of a dying patient for whom the use of medical technology seems increasingly futile, the family is being unreasonable and insisting that "everything be done." Indeed, this very thing occurred in the now classic case of Helga Wanglie in Minnesota (Miles 1991). Every time I hear this statement, "The family insists that everything be done," I wonder the same thing: How is it that the family has become so unreasonable when just a few years ago families were clamoring for the doctors to stop intensive interventions, and the doctors were the ones who felt uneasy about termination of life support?

Many things of course have happened in the intervening decade, not the least of which has been cost-containment measures leading patients, particularly those with inadequate or no insurance, legitimately to suspect that they are being undertreated. But I don't think this is the main problem. I think the main problem is the overemphasis on autonomy in clinical practice and the physicians' resulting loss of ability to take tragic responsibility on their own shoulders and offer the family compassion instead of legalism. When the intern talks to the family outside the intensive care unit and says, "Do you want us to keep your mother alive?" this is considered the exercise of respect for patient autonomy. The really smart intern will ask, "Would your mother want us to try to keep her alive?" But in either case, the question is reductionistic and oversimplified. It presents the family with incorrect information, namely, that their relative has a chance of meaningful survival, and it implies, more importantly, that it is *their* responsibility to make that decision and to live afterward with the guilt or other emotional consequences of the decision. Thus, it is a rare family member who would stand up to the intern in that reductionist dichotomy and say, "No, pull the plug. Let her die." Instead what we have is the exchange from the physician, "Do you want us to do everything?" and the family members, of course, because they love their mother (or feel guilty that they don't, or both), reply, "Yes, of course, do everything."

Too rarely does anyone talk about what "do everything" *means*. The meaning of this statement is *not* best explicated by a checklist of medical technologies that the family wants or doesn't want. It is best explicated by setting goals for the treatment. Do everything toward what end? Is it time for her to die? Will she die comfortably? Will she suffer? Will you (doctor!) stay with us and help us with our grief? If these questions are never asked and therefore never answered, the only affirmative, meaningful, loving statement the family can make is "Do everything."

Imagine a different scenario, perhaps drawn from earlier times when the physician comes to the family, takes someone's hand or puts an arm gently around someone's shoulder, and says sadly, "I can do nothing more to prolong your mother's life, but she will not suffer, and we'll do everything to make her comfortable. I'll be with her and with you, and she will not be alone." Evaluated by simplistic standards of familiar principles, this kind of statement would be considered paternalistic, and currently, this kind of behavior is rarely taught at our teaching hospitals in the United States. The principle of patient autonomy has so far infected the practice of medicine that we now have legal advisors who would caution against such a paternalistic stance. Indeed, legislation in some states — such as the legislation in New York requiring patient or family to sign the DNR order — reinforces the more adversarial relationship rather than the more caring relationship.

If you multiply this story thousands of times across the country, you probably come to understand why health care expenditures at the end of life are so great, why (ironically) the public clamor for death with dignity has grown, and why physicians have come to develop such an uncomfortable relationship with their patients. The care of the dying patient is now too often considered an esoteric specialty only for those interested in hospice care and is rarely a required element of medical education. Nonetheless, all physicians do deal with death. What little formal education there is about the care of the dying often occurs in a medical ethics course, where they are taught the simple rules of autonomy, respect for persons, and beneficence, learning that the patient and, if not the patient, the family are the ones who make decisions. However, physicians learn nothing about what kind of communication best enables patients and families to make wise and caring decisions. It's much more complicated to talk about communicative ethics, about negotiation, about narrative, and even about meaning than it is to talk about rules and algorithms.

Conclusion

Principlism has been a kind of "safe harbor" for physicians in this last decade of rampant change in standards and bioethics, medical law, and regulations. At least with these simple principles and a simple understanding of the law, physicians could feel that they were somewhat protected from potential lawsuits and even more so from being considered unethical by their peers, supervisors, attending physicians, or anyone else in the highly public and peopled world of patient care. But now, in this complex world, we ask physicians to reestablish intimacy in their relationships with patients, to take back some of that heavy weight on their own shoulders, to ask about and perhaps internalize the patient's own sources of meaning — be they religious or philosophical — and to connect them with his or her own sense of meaning. This is asking a great deal, especially since none of it is paid for under the ICD9 codes of Medicare. Indeed that's another problem — that principlism fits in too well with medicine as a business transaction. The meaning of these profound encounters with human mortality at the beginnings and ends of life has been forgotten as the exchange has become more transient, more businesslike, and more wary or even adversarial.

In conclusion, then, my assessment of the frontier leads to a deep ambivalence. We should not throw out the baby with the bath water. The baby is our ability to create a common vocabulary with which physicians can talk to one another about moral problems. We should not underestimate the important progress that has occurred in this era of principlism. Certainly, we would rather have physicians concerned about informed consent and patient autonomy than to have them oblivious to these issues. But how much more can we expect? Is it too much to expect physicians to have the intellectual and interpersonal skills and the spiritual depth to crave a deeper and more complex understanding of the moral basis of the healing profession? Looking around us in 1992, I can give only a qualified answer.

Certainly it is necessary for some scholars in ethics to move beyond principlism. As is evidenced by this volume and by much of the most interesting literature of recent years, this movement is already occurring. From my perspective as a clinician, however, I still wonder how to translate new knowledge, new frontiers, and deeper, more complex realities into the busy daily practice of medicine. Neither the business components of medicine nor the busyness of it are likely to change in the decade ahead. Thus, if we are going to ask physicians to take part in this more complex endeavor, we will have to find a way for it to bring them personal satisfaction. Perhaps, for example, it could bring greater meaning to their work or help them feel more cultural connectedness to their communities. Or perhaps this endeavor could bring them efficiency — through a return to paternalism or delegation of some authority to collaborative negotiations. Herein lie important frontiers for both empirical and theoretical work.

Clinical practitioners and medical researchers need biomedical ethics to both cope with and understand their powers and limitations in dealing with human life and human death, with human health and disability, with suffering and with joy. They also need bioethics to understand and to cope with the future that is practically upon us in the form of new genetic diagnostic and therapeutic methods, transplantations of all sorts, electronic assistive and prosthetic devices, and new, more insistent pressures for cost containment. The questions facing patients, health care providers, and the public, who will in some way pay for all this, are deeper than just who should get this health care and how much of it. They also include the kinds of questions being raised and the attempts being made in this volume to broaden the ethics-scholarship base beyond principlism. If biomedical ethics is to remain useful to the clinician, principles cannot be cast away. But the deepening and broadening understanding of ethics that comes from feminism, from phenomenology, from hermeneutics and unitary theory, from casuistry, and from literature and narrative are all of extraordinary value.

Perhaps the most concrete and important step forward in making these somewhat abstract frameworks relevant to the clinician is to clarify two important dimensions of ethics in clinical medicine. The first, making the decisions and understanding the reasons for them, has been bioethics' sole argument and justification until recent times. The second dimension, which draws so much on literature and casuistry, is understanding the meaning of what we do. Here, we have had utter poverty in the clinical realm. One wonders what a physician thinks when faced with rules and regulations on advance directives and informed consent coming from the federal government, the state government, the hospital administration, and the medical societies. We can only assume that she feels as harassed by these regulations as she does by the paperwork required for insurance reimbursement. It all becomes part of the same bureaucratic mess. Where in all of this is the deeper meaning of morality and, indeed, the deeper meaning of the profession?

Finding this deeper meaning is the most important challenge for the next decade. The words with which we talk about new currents in bioethics are not words that are or will become very familiar to most physicians, and yet, if they understand what we are really talking about, they should find it as welcome as water to the thirsty. Some physicians have begun to react against technocracy and the loss of meaning that has occurred in the last decade. Sometimes this backlash has gone under the name of professionalism; sometimes it goes under the name of humanism. Whatever it is called, however, many clinicians from many arenas within the profession hunger for precisely this deeper, more substantive, more real, more meaningful, and perhaps, more spiritual discussion of morality.

REFERENCES

Callahan, D. 1991. *What Kind of Life: The Limits of Medical Progress*. New York: Simon and Schuster.

Cassel, C. K. 1987. "Decisions to Forgo Life-Sustaining Therapy: The Limits of Ethics." *Social Service Review* 61, no. 4 (December): 552–64.

Fleck, L. 1987. "DRGs: Justice and the Invisible Rationing of Health Care Resources." *Journal of Medicine and Philosophy* 12 (May): 165–96.

Glick, H. R. 1992. *The Right to Die: Policy Innovation and Its Consequences*. New York: Columbia University Press.

Hill, T. P., and D. Shirley. 1992. *A Good Death: Taking More Control at the End of Your Life*. Reading, Mass.: Addison Wesley.

Jonsen, A. R., M. Siegler, and W. Winslade. 1986. *Clinical Ethics: A Practical Approach to Ethical Decisions in Clinical Medicine*. 2d ed. New York: Macmillan.

Jonsen, A. R., and S. Toulmin. 1988. *The Abuse of Casuistry: A History of Moral Reasoning*. Berkeley: University of California Press.

Miles, S. H. 1991. "Informed Demand for 'Non-Beneficial' Medical Treatment." *New England Journal of Medicine* 325, no. 7 (15 August): 512–15.

Moody, H. R. 1992. *Ethics in an Aging Society*. Baltimore: Johns Hopkins University Press.

Niebuhr, R. 1960. *Moral Man and Immoral Society: A Study in Ethics and Politics*. New York: Scribners.

~ 16 ~

Beyond Principlism Is Not Enough
A Theologian Reflects on the Real Challenge for U.S. Biomedical Ethics

Richard A. McCormick

The title of my essay is important; it denotes an appropriate narrowing of expertise and focus. Specifically, the title is not "Theology's Contribution to ..." or "The Importance of Theology to..." I have in the past made several attempts in those directions (McCormick 1985; McCormick 1989). Like it or not, such attempts create the impression that one is speaking for a whole discipline and that the discipline is univocally understood and can be tapped to provide nourishment, supports, correctives, insights for bioethics. I know that is a caricature, but I fear it is not always recognized as such, even by some physicians.

"A Theologian Reflects" makes no such sprawling and universalist claims. It suggests that what is to follow represents the personal reflections of one ("a" not "the" theologian) who tries to approach and view matters from a theological perspective. But even that is too general; for there are Jewish, Muslim, Catholic, Lutheran, and numerous other theological perspectives. Furthermore, even within Catholicism there are different theologies much as there were with the evangelists. This further underlines the personal character of the following reflections.

The essays in the volume share a more or less explicit theme: a pervasive dissatisfaction with the status quo of bioethical reflection in the United States. A sense of malaise is unmistakably present and hovers over the subject like a dark cloud. Most of the dissatisfaction points to the "principles approach as the regnant paradigm." It is said to be a dilemma-oriented, problem-solving, deductive, rationalistic, individualistic, and rights-focused enterprise. This is especially clear in Renée Fox's long study in which she identifies the things persons in bioethics seem to be reaching for: less reliance on principlism; proximity to lived experience; inclusion of the imagistic; symbolic, emotional dimensions; less absolutism; greater emphasis on the self as connected to others; modification of secularism in bioethical thought; and so on. If Fox is correct — and I believe she is — U.S. bioethics of the past twenty years has powerfully reinforced the very problematic perspectives it should be challenging and correcting.

I agree that there is malaise within bioethics. So much of what is written seems tired and predictable, only marginally relevant. But I am not sure that the diagnosis goes deep enough. If it does not, then we are involved with Band-Aids. I do not mean that Fox's litany is inaccurate or undesirable. Not at all. What I do mean is that these shifts in approach are not likely to occur in any lasting way through explicit effort on the part of ethicists alone. They will be a significant aspect of bioethics only if the practice of medicine itself is changed. For that is where the malaise originates. Medicine may have been content with the bioethical enterprise for twenty years because it was left comfortably unchallenged and free to go its businesslike way.

The essays in this volume reflect on bioethics in the United States and, in one way or another, suggest the perspectival shifts that have to be made if bioethics is to be a formative leaven in the discipline(s) on which it reflects. The assumption is that if bioethics makes these shifts — "from above," so to speak — it will be much more relevant and formatively influential.

I have to wonder about that, even doubt it. The forces that are dissolving the culture of medicine as a profession have a certain independent and almost uncontrollable dynamic about them. Adjustments in bioethics will not change them. And unless they do change, medicine will continue on its present course. Indeed, one could mount a fairly persuasive argument that bioethics in the United States in the past twenty years has developed peacefully and serenely *because* it has posed no threat to the major developments in medicine of the past twenty years. That means it has been irrelevant to the major transformation occurring, namely, the displacement of the culture of medicine as a profession.

I will use Catholic hospitals as a symptom for the substance of my concern. Two facts bring the issue into focus. First, Catholic hospitals have beautiful mission statements. We read references to continuing the healing mission of Jesus through comprehensive health care. They talk about caring service for each individual, personalized patient care, the wholistic approach that weds competence and compassion. They make assertions about an option for the poor, about continuing Christ's redemptive presence. Yet, second, everywhere I go I see Catholics involved in health care who are doubtful and perplexed, asking themselves whether they ought to be in health care and wondering whether Catholic institutions are viable, whether they have a clear identity, and how they differ from non-Catholic institutions. I see a great deal of institutional navel-gazing. In sum, a gap exists between institutional purpose and aim, and personal conviction and involvement.

What is going on here? I believe that the circumstances of the United States in the late twentieth century have weakened and sometimes dissolved the culture of the Catholic health care facility, the strength and transforming power of its vision. Could it be that dissatisfaction with principlism is but a superficial response and is indicative of much deeper longings and losses? I think so. And if this is true of Catholic hospitals, it is likely all the more true of other religiously affiliated institutions and of the medical establishment in general.

Let me draw on Thomas Peters and Robert Waterman's *In Search of Excellence* to make my point (Peters and Waterman 1982). They note:

> As we worked on research of our excellent companies, we were struck by the dominant use of story, slogan, and legend as people tried to explain the characteristics of their own great institutions. All the companies we interviewed, from Boeing to McDonald's, were quite simply rich tapestries of anecdote, myth, and fairy tale.... The vast majority of people who tell stories today about T. J. Watson of I.B.M. have never met the man or had direct experience of the original more mundane reality. Two Hewlett-Packard engineers in their mid-twenties recently regaled us with an hour's worth of "Bill and Dave" (Hewlett and Packard) stories. We were subsequently astonished to find that neither had seen, let alone talked to, the founders. These days, people like Watson and A. P. Giannini at Bank of America take on roles of mythic proportions that the real persons would have been hard-pressed to fill. Nevertheless, in an organizational sense, these stories, myths, and legends appear to be very important *because they convey the organization's shared values, or culture.* (Peters and Waterman 1982:75)

Peters and Waterman then continue to highlight the importance of culture.

> Without exception, the dominance and coherence of culture proved to be an essential quality of the excellent companies.

Moreover, the stronger the culture and the more it was directed toward the marketplace, the less need was there for policy manuals, organization charts, or detailed procedures and rules. In these companies, people way down the line know what they are supposed to do in most situations because the handful of guiding values is crystal clear. (Peters and Waterman 1982:75–76)

If we ask why or how the guiding values are crystal clear, Peters and Waterman respond:

The shared values in the excellent companies are clear, in large measure, because the mythology is rich. Everyone at Hewlett-Packard knows that he or she is supposed to be innovative. Everyone at Procter & Gamble knows that product quality is the sine qua non.... "Right from the start" said the late Richard R. Deupree when he was chief executive officer, "William Procter and James Gamble realized that the interests of the organization and its employees were inseparable...."

Poorer-performing companies often have strong cultures, too, *but dysfunctional ones* [emphasis added]. They are usually focused on internal politics rather than on the customer, or...the product and the people who make and sell it. The top companies, on the other hand, always seem to recognize what the companies that set only financial targets don't know or don't deem important. The excellent companies seem to understand that *every* person seeks meaning (not just the top fifty who are in the bonus pool). (Peters and Waterman 1982:76)

And so it goes with Johnson and Johnson, Maytag, Marriott, Bechtel, Boeing, Delta, Dana, Caterpillar, Wang, 3–M, Digital Equipment, etc.

Now what do we see here? We see (1) shared values or culture, and values shared throughout the company; (2) values that are crystal clear; (3) values that are communicated by legends and stories; (4) values that give meaning (motivation and inspiration) to the work of individuals.

I realize that it is somewhat anomalous to turn to business to clarify the importance of culture in Catholic health care when one of the vexing problems of such care is that it has been transformed into a business. The point of contact, however, remains the notion of culture. Culture is essential to the flourishing of institutions, whether they be Catholic hospitals or business corporations. When the culture is dysfunctional or absent, we usually see a company in disarray. We see a Catholic hospital questioning its identity. More to the point, we see a situation where "people's only security comes from where they live on the organization chart." We see people who have jobs, not great causes.

I think this may well have happened to many Catholic hospitals. They were organized around the "greatest story ever told" (of God's engendering deed in Jesus[1] that transforms us and our world). Catholic hospitals exist to enact in the health care setting what God did in Jesus. Jesus is God's love for us in the flesh. The Catholic hospital exists, therefore, to be Jesus' love for the other in the health care setting. It has the daily vocation of telling every patient — especially the poor — and every employee how great they are, because Jesus told us how great we are and in the process empowered us. Yet I suspect this *raison d'être* has practically disappeared. If that is the case, then the heart of the Catholic health care culture is gone. And if that is the case, then persons in this context will derive their meaning, significance, and security from elsewhere, not from the great cause that defines their reason for being where they are. They will be performing a job only.

I have used the Catholic hospital as an example of the importance of culture. Something analogous can be said of the medical profession itself. It is a culture that distinguishes medicine from business. Physicians are rightly proud of it. Marvin R. Dunn, M.D., dean of the University of South Florida College of Medicine, noted that in the last ten years applications to medical school have fallen off. One of the reasons cited by Dunn was that "college students began to see medicine as more of a business than a profession" (Dunn 1992:28). For this reason, Dunn concludes, "there is probably no more important area for us [physicians] all to work together in than the preservation of these values that continue to define medicine as a true profession."

What are those values, or what I have above called a culture? Dunn puts it as follows:

> Medicine is a unique profession. More than for any other, something seems to develop within the individual before formal medical education begins and to remain even after retirement from active practice. This is the human side. It is that something which separates the physician from the computer. It is the caring and compassion that makes medicine an art as well as science. It is the capacity for ethical concern for the total individual that invites patients to share in total confidence those intimate aspects of their lives that are shared with few or none other.

Better than anyone familiar to me, Leon R. Kass has analyzed the meaning of "concern for the total individual." I will cite him at length because what he says lies close to the heart of the culture of medicine as a profession. The physician-patient *relationship* is too pale and unspecified a term to enlighten. Rather, drawing on Aristotle, Kass notes:

> The patient as beneficiary is, in a sense, the physician-at-work. The physician's being, manifested as physicianly activity, lives in the patient. Healing the patient manifests the physician's *own wholeness*, in its self-manifesting activity. As parents love their children, and teachers their students, so physicians their patients — for it is only in and through the patient that the doctor's being is actively realized, for the doctor himself.

Medicine is thus not rightly described as a profession that requires self-sacrifice and self-denial. Anyone who enters it in this spirit is courting disappointment. Neither are the deepest rewards of medicine external to the activity. Anyone who thinks that money or prestige or honor alone will make the practice rewarding is courting discontent — for what will sustain him when the coffers are full and the tributes are paid? No, medicine calls you to intrinsically self-manifesting and self-fulfilling activity, in which your good and the patient's good coincide. In each daily encounter with your patients, you will serve yourself exactly in your efforts to help others, as you energetically respond to the call for help, exercising your art that makes help possible.

But there is one more wrinkle to this self-sustaining activity of benefaction, which, as described so far, does not distinguish the unique form of doing good that is physicianly. For it seems strange to say that the hip surgeon lives in the prosthesis he has implanted or that the internist is at work in the digitalis he has sent circulating in the cardiac patient's blood. To the extent that doctors are thought to act on the human being regarded scientifically as objectifiable body, to that extent the claim of living participation in the beneficiary rings somewhat hollow. The engineer is not the benefactor of the bridge; the plumber is not the benefactor of the pipes; the physician regarded as body engineer or plumber is not the benefactor of the body — silent, indifferent, private. If one regards the patient only as objectified body, then one may *take* care *of* the patient, but one does not yet *care for* the patient. Squaring the life and work of physician as benefactor with patient as beneficiary requires a *relationship* with the patient regarded not as body but *as embodied soul*. It requires converting the private and unsharable good of well-healed bodily parts into a common and consciously sought good, which in turn requires attentive, sympathetic, and concerned speech, as always, the bond of truly human associations. (Kass 1991:553–60)[2]

It is precisely certain shared values that make medicine a profession rather than a business. There may be other ways of stating those values, but many would think that Dr. Dunn is close to the mark and that Dr. Kass is right on it. When those values (that culture) are under threat or weakened, the profession itself is threatened, weakened, as a profession.

I see the dissatisfaction with principlism (deductive, rationalistic, individualistic, rights-focused, and so forth) as a symptom of this deeper malaise: the well-founded fear that the profession itself is profoundly threatened, perhaps even already severely undermined by the forces that make up the context of its practice in the United States. Put differently, an increasing number of people judge that Dunn and Kass have described a desirable but disappearing species.

If that is true, we all will be the poorer. For that reason it is essential to identify those characteristics or aspects that powerfully shape the context of the practice of medicine. Here I will list five, though there are probably many more, some perhaps even more formative than the ones I list.

1. *Depersonalization.* Three factors are at work in the way we perceive and respond to health care problems. First, we have the growth of technology. Everything from diagnosis through acute care to billing is done by computer. Check the advertisements in any medical journal, and it becomes clear that medicine and the machine are wed. This gives efficiency but inevitably some impersonality.[3] I mean in no way to bad-mouth technology in medicine. My own life owes its continuance on several occasions to "high-tech" medicine.

Second, there is cost and cost containment. Spiraling costs are due to many factors (for example, sophistication of services, higher wages, more personnel, cost pass-along systems, paperwork, technology, inflation, fraud). In 1990 national health expenditures were projected to be 12 percent of the gross national product, and they are probably above that now. Per capita health care spending was $2,566 compared to Canada's $1,991. Seattle has more CT scanners than all of Canada (*New York Times*, 17 February 1992). A Gallup poll done for the AMA revealed that 68 percent of patients disagreed with the statement "doctors' fees are usually reasonable" (*American Medical News*, 1 June 1992, 15). Obviously the cost factor will force difficult decisions, sooner or later, soon at the latest.

Finally, we have the multiplication of public entities. By "public entities" I mean attorneys, courts, and legislatures. Thus we have the Patient Self-Determination Act of 1990 passed as part of the Omnibus Budget Reconciliation Act. We have had a series of trial cases: *Quinlan, Saikewicz, Fox, Spring, Perlmutter, Herbert, Conroy, Brophy, Cruzan.* We have *Roe v. Wade.* These are but the protruding tips of the icebergs.

Together these factors affect the very matrix of the healing profession. This matrix has roots in the conviction that patient-management decisions must be tailor-made to the individual, to the individual's condition and values. They are *personal* decisions that must fit the individual like a glove to a hand. Yet the three factors mentioned above are rather *impersonal* factors. When they begin to preprogram our treatment, they tend to depersonalize that treatment. A clear sign of this depersonalization is the constant physician complaint about loss of autonomy. John Lee Clowe, M.D., president of the AMA, stated that "based on the letters I receive from around the country, there is no question in my mind that the loss of autonomy is the most troubling trend physicians in this country face" (*American Medical News,* 1 June 1992, 7). Complaints about loss of autonomy escalated after 1983 with the introduction of Medicare's 467 diagnostic-related groups.

2. *Secularization.* The very forces that lead to depersonalization of health care can robustly support the secularization of the medical profession. By *secularization* I refer to the divorce of the profession from those values (that culture) that make health care a *human service.* Or stated somewhat more aggressively, it is an increasing preoccupation with factors that are peripheral to and distractive from wholistic human care (competition, liability, government controls, finances).

I see any number of symptoms of this drift toward secularization. One is the fact that physicians are leaving the profession. A survey of physicians done in 1989 by the Gallup Organization revealed that a considerable number of physicians definitely would not (14 percent) or probably would not (25 percent) go to medical school if they were in college now, knowing what they know about medicine (*New York Times,* 18 February 1990).

Another symptom is physician discontent with the physician-patient relationship. Dr. Paul Bearman, director of urgent care at Park Nicollett Medical Center in Minneapolis, put it this way: "The ability to have the same kind of relationship. I think that's gone. There is the feeling that you could just replace one physician with another and that's unfortunate. A lot of the really good doctors feel bad" (*New York Times,* 20 February 1990). Dr. William Roper, deputy director of domestic policy in the White House, stated: "I am worried about the growing disenchantment of the average doctor....I fear that the loss of faith by doctors will make them less caring and compassionate" (*New York Times,* 18 February 1990). Perhaps it already has. Of 1,500 people polled by Gallup in 1989, 67 percent said that doctors are too interested in making money, and 57 percent agreed that "doctors don't care about people as much as they used to" (*New York Times,* 18 February 1990).

Behind such an erosion of the physician-patient relationship is the loss of a culture of compassion and care. It is being replaced by a business ethos. As Lawrence Altman and Elizabeth Rosenthal summed it up: "The image of the dedicated physician toiling long hours for the good of his patients is fading fast, replaced by salaried doctors who work 9 to 5" (*New York Times,* 18 February 1990). Many physicians feel that what they do is "a job."

When medicine is reduced to a business, physicians begin acting like businesspeople. As Dr. Edmund Pellegrino has observed, they claim the same rights as the businessperson — that is, to do business with whom they choose. Medical knowledge is viewed as something that belongs to the physician and that can be dispensed on her own terms in the marketplace, and illness is seen as no different from any other need that requires a service (Pellegrino 1987:1939–40). It is this ethos that James Gorman bashes in his wonderful tongue-in-cheek piece "The Doctor Won't See You Now" (Gorman 1992).[4]

I am not interested in assigning blame for this secularization of medicine. Physicians would doubtless point to their eroded autonomy (controls), diminished prestige, increased liability exposure, reduced compensation, and so forth. Others would lay the blame squarely on the profession. I shall not referee this dispute here. I simply want to note the fact of secularization and the replacement of the professional culture by the business ethos.

Once the profession is secularized, physicians will begin to make secularized judgments. One such is that the physician is free to not treat AIDS patients. Thirty percent of the physicians polled by the AMA made such a choice. I can only view this as extremely ominous. Another, in my opinion, is the refusal to treat Medicaid patients.

Another judgment that could easily convey a full-blown secularization is the following: "I will not impose my values on my patient." Of course, there is a perfectly healthy and orthodox understanding of this statement. It is: In designing patient management regimes, I will take appropriate account of the patient's background, education, age, values, preferences. The noxious and secularized reading is this: I will do anything the patient prefers and requests. Here the physician is reduced to a technological tool of the patient, conscripted to do the patient's bidding for a price.

It is easy to see why the secularization of medicine feeds off of (I do not say "caused" because it is unclear which caused which) an absolutized notion of patient autonomy. When autonomy is absolutized, very little thought is then given to the values that ought to inform and guide the use of autonomy. Given such a vacuum, the sheer fact that the choice is the patient's tends to be viewed as the sole right-making characteristic of the choice. That trivializes human choice. It is no coincidence that the notorious Jack Kevorkian is drum major for an absolutized autonomy. "In my view the highest principle in medical ethics — in any kind of ethics — is personal autonomy, self-determination. What counts is what the patient wants and judges to be a benefit or a value in his or her own life. That's primary" (*Free Inquiry*, 1991:14). Stop. Period. No qualifications. As Leon Kass notes: "The autonomy argument kicks out all criteria for evaluating the choice, save that it be uncoerced" (Kass 1991:22). And it is no coincidence that Kevorkian regards medicine as a "strictly secular endeavor." It should be entirely separate from religious ethics. His example: a Catholic doctor should be prepared to provide an atheistic woman with an abortion (*American Medical News*, 10 February 1992, 3). Behold the indissoluble union of a secularized medicine with absolutized autonomy that trumps every other consideration. In this system Kevorkian has become what he provides: a machine.

3. *The emergence of public morality*. Nearly everyone has heard the term *public morality* and is vaguely conscious of the need for it. But what does the term mean? It suggests that the pursuit of the basic goods that define our well-being has increasingly been shifted from private one-on-one acts and has been put into the public sphere. That means that bioethics will have to say much more at the level of policy making than it has. Until quite recently it has been much more concerned with the level of individual decision. "But," as Daniel Callahan correctly notes, "on a national scale those decisions are going to be over-shadowed by large structural moral and political decisions. It is these decisions that will eventually shape the individual decisions" (Callahan 1980:1232).

I will begin by stating what public morality is not. First, it is not simply public participation in the directions and priorities of medical practice, research, and health care. If public morality is understood in this way, it easily becomes a merely formal affair, a matter of structuring dialogue to include representative participants.

Second, it is not merely law or public policy. One of the prime tests of law is its own "possibility," as John Courtney Murray words it, or its feasibility, "that quality whereby a proposed course of action is not merely possible but practicable, adaptable, depending on the circumstances, cultural ways, attitudes, traditions of a people" (Murray

1960:166). Public policy must, therefore, take account of some very pragmatic considerations in a rather utilitarian way. Reducing public morality to public policy would be to undermine public morality.

A clearer grasp of the meaning of public morality becomes possible when we consider the contemporary context of health care delivery. Individual decisions will, of course, remain important. But increasingly, institutions mediate the services of physician to patient. Such institutions have become partners in health care delivery. Thus we have group practice, third-party carriers, legislative and administrative controls (e.g., Food and Drug Administration).

Groups (whether universities, insurance companies, or the government) have interests and concerns other than the immediate good of the patient. Thus the government has a legitimate interest in population control, in reducing welfare rolls, in control of illegitimacy, in the advancement of diagnostic, therapeutic, preventive medicine, in balancing the budget, in protecting life. Teaching and research hospitals have a concern for the health of future generations.

This suggests that whenever other values (than the patient's) are the legitimate concern of the mediator of health care, the good of the individual patient becomes one of several values in competition for priority. It further suggests that the individual is in danger of being subordinated to these values.

As I understand the term, *public morality* is the pursuit of these other values without violating the needs and integrity of the individual. It is a harmonizing of public concerns with individual needs. These "other values and concerns" constitute the public dimension of biomedicine because they represent concerns other than and beyond the individual. In Callahan's words: "Ways will have to be found to balance that ethic [patient-centered] off against the legitimate interests of the public."

Callahan has summarized this matter splendidly. He argues that the allocation of resources, the development of a just health care delivery system, the adjudication of the rights and claims of competing groups "are and will be the important moral problems of the future." These problems will "force biomedical ethics to move into the mainstream of political and social theory, beyond the model of the individual decision maker, and into the thicket of important vested and legitimate private and group interests" (Callahan 1980:1232). Establishing the proper balance between individual patient-centered concerns and other legitimate interests is what I mean by the term *public morality.*

When groups with other (than the individual's) concerns mediate biomedicine, the medical-research establishment is thereby deeply inserted into the value perspectives of society at large, and these perspectives and priorities begin to shape it. One need not be a Cassandra to note that in the United States top cultural priorities are technology, efficiency, and comfort. This means that these priorities will unavoidably penetrate the "medical-research complex" and shape its directions. It requires no stretch of the imagination to see how deleteriously such values can affect the professional culture of medicine.

4. *The market-driven health care system.* By *market-driven* I mean institutions whose existence and policies are heavily dictated by the economic factor. In such an atmosphere, one thing is clear: the institution is financially viable, or it does not survive ("No margin, no mission").

Telltale indicia all around us point to the ascendancy, even primacy, of the economic factor and, perhaps especially, the competitive environment. Hospitals have marketing directors. They experience pressures from HMOs, which will increasingly feel pressure from PPOs. Health care institutions must train a keen institutional eye on diagnostic-related groups. Between 1980 and 1986, 414 hospitals closed. Predictions vary, but some estimates foresee the closure of 700 more by 1995. Increasingly hospitals are forced into joint ventures and mergers. Essential services (e.g., trauma centers) do not support themselves. The dumping syndrome is alive and well, even if in subtle and changing ways. Acquisition decisions, hiring practices, and incentive proposals are often closely market related.

This litany could be continued almost indefinitely, but that is unnecessary. Above I pointed to cost-containment concerns and related them to depersonalization. My focus is somewhat different here. When institutions are swept into preoccupation with their financial status, their sense of mission can be swallowed up in the process. And when that happens, the culture of the profession can be severely tested. The professional culture of medicine should find reinforcement in institutions, not threats. A symptom of my concern here is the growing literature on the fiscal responsibilities of physicians, and on physicians as fiscal gatekeepers. This issue is much more intense now than it ever was in the past.

5. *The crisis of nursing.* It is obvious that nurses are an essential part, probably the most important part, of hospital care and health care more generally. What is not so obvious is that if there is a nursing crisis, that has the potential of affecting negatively the culture of medicine.

Why so? Physicianly care is care of the person, as Kass pointed out. Therefore, it combines the collaborative contributions of many people: physicians, nurses, pastoral care people, paramedical personnel. If one element is in crisis, the whole collaborative team will be affected. Nurses are an especially valuable adjunct in this collaboration. So often they bring, besides their technical competence, a special presence, communication, support, shared faith, empathy. Quite simply they often make the difference between healing and mere fixing.

The crisis is a shortage of nurses. There are many reasons for this. One of the key dissatisfactions of nurses is the absence of satisfying professional relationships with physicians (Aiken and Mullinix 1987). Some others are small financial rewards compared to responsibilities; limited autonomy in clinical situations; little involvement in hospital management decisions regarding standards of practice and support services; disarray in titling and educational preparation of nurses (the American Nursing Association wants all nurses to have the four-year baccalaureate degree, but two-thirds enter practice with an associate degree or a diploma); Medicare's prospective payment system, wherein economic incentives to reduce the length of hospital stays mean the same care must be given in less time; unpopular working hours and shift rotations and absence of adequate support personnel — and all of this at the very time of the proliferation of alternative health delivery plans that provide nurses with new career opportunities.[5]

I have mentioned five aspects or characteristics that make up the context of the practice of medicine in the United States today: depersonalization, secularization, the emergence of public morality, the market-driven system, and the crisis of nursing. These are obviously interrelated and overlapping. Thus the crisis of nursing is clearly related to the secularization of medicine. Depersonalization and secularization are related, as are the emergence of public morality and market-driven health care.

My interest, however, is that cumulatively these forces are capable of, indeed are, undermining the culture that makes medicine a profession. Contemporary medicine has gone a long way toward becoming a business and a business that is heavily self-interested. Everybody from physicians, nurses, administrators, politicians, bioethicists to patients (now called "consumers") is screaming bloody murder about this. But on it goes. As I noted at the outset, the problem is the displacement of the culture of medicine as a profession.

Let me appeal to a symbol to illustrate my point. As I write, the National Conference of Catholic Bishops is in the process of updating the *Ethical and Religious Directives for Catholic Health Facilities.* One can predict what the ultimate product will look like. It will state basic values to which we are committed (for example, sanctity of life), and it will hammer these out in more concrete directives about abortion, experimentation, care of the dying, transplantation, and so on. The bishops will vote on these directives, and they will become official policy — as if such guidance and directives were responding to the real problems of Catholic health care institutions. They are not. These institutions exist in a climate that dispossesses them of their culture. They are losing their souls so to speak. *That* is the problem that should rivet our attention.

Something similar can be said of the field of bioethics. If it simply makes strategic adjustments, it will continue to march, in a disciplined and orderly way to be sure, parallel to the truly formative developments in the field. If, on the other hand, those forces that have been dissolving the culture of the medical profession can be honestly faced and effectively dealt with, then we might be pleasantly surprised to see the adjustments called for in this volume occur almost spontaneously, "from below" so to speak. For a genuine professional culture would be in place to suggest, nourish, support, even demand such adjustments.

Can these forces be faced and dealt with effectively? I honestly do not know. It may be unduly pessimistic to put it this way, but major cultural shifts or conversions (and that is what is called for here) so often occur only via catastrophe and suffering. Is it excessive to believe that until we feel *painfully, corporately*, and *personally* the results of the dissolution of the professional culture in medicine, nothing will change? In this sense truly helpful revisions in bioethics may be painful, because changes in the forces that shape medicine will condition them.

Let me return to my title, "A Theologian Reflects." One may legitimately wonder what the reflections presented above have to do with theology. In my view, a great deal.

Medicine has what some have called its own "internal" morality. Philosopher Robert Sokolowski notes that the good of the medical art is the health of the individual or community. He continues:

> In acting according to his art the physician also seeks the good of the patient. Because the art of medicine aims at something that is a good for the patient, the doctor, in the exercise of his art, seeks the medical good of the patient as his own good. He pursues professionally what is good for another.... The nature of his art...makes him, in the good exercise of his art, not only a good doctor but also essentially a good moral agent, one who seeks the good of another formally as his own. The doctor's profession essentially makes him a good man, provided he is true to his art and follows its insistence. (Sokolowski 1989:269)

This morality internal to the medical profession is even more resplendent when viewed through the eyes of Christian theology. In the Christian understanding, the encounter of persons has a certain structure. It is the categorical moment for the faithful activity in love that describes the very being of the "new creature." It is literally our way of loving God in this context. It is the vertical in the horizontal, or, as Joseph Sittler puts it, "Love is the function of faith horizontally just as prayer is the function of faith vertically" (Sittler 1958:64). This is true of both the curing and the caring dimensions of health care. If we do not view health care in this way, we interpret and restrict its reality short of the depths of faith. The "Decree on the Apostolate of the Laity" of Vatican II, after noting that Christ made the commandment of love his own and endowed it with new meaning, states: "For he wanted to identify himself with his brethren as the object of this love when he said, 'as long as you did it for one of these, the least of my brethren, you did it for me' " (Abbott 1966:498). But if this profound structure of the health care encounter is to be lived, "certain fundamentals must be observed. Thus attention is to be paid to the image of God in which our neighbor has been created, and also to Christ the Lord to whom is really offered whatever is given to a needy person" (Abbott 1966:499).

If the medical encounter is viewed and lived in this way, it would be both guided by and generative of the moral dispositions and perspectives implied in Christ's phrase "as I have loved you." One need not understand this as a psychological "immediacy." Physicians as well as others have to live with the incomplete and fragmentary character of their relationships. The same is true of patients. Only a rather inflated religious romanticism would expect a direct, immediate I-Thou encounter in every human relation. I am speaking rather of the profoundest ontological structure of the encounter, fully disclosed in and by Christ, a structure we perceive only dimly (in faith), but one that ought to be the organizing shape and power of our responses. This is nothing more nor less than the encounter to which Christ enjoined his followers. This is exactly what the "Decree on the Apostolate of the Laity" meant when it urged professional people to remember that in fulfilling their secular duties of daily life, "they do not disassociate union with Christ from that life." It further urged professionals to "see Christ in all men whether they be close to us or strangers" (Abbott 1966:493).

If health care personnel view their profession in this way, I believe we can reasonably predict three important results. First, we may see growth in those dispositions that nourish, protect, and support the medical encounter as a truly human (not merely technological) one: compassion, honesty, self-denial, and generosity.

Second, we may reasonably expect that a profession deeply penetrated with persons of such faith and such dispositions will be transformed. The "Decree on the Apostolate of the Laity" states of persons of faith that "their behavior will have a penetrating impact, little by little, on the whole circle of their life and labors" (Abbott 1966:505). It regards this as the "penetrating and perfecting of the temporal sphere." I take it as indisputable that, in a time of high technology and growing impersonality in health care, this would be a truly desirable leavening influence. Faith creates sensitivities in the believer beyond natural capacities. It bestows sensitivity to "dimensions of possibility" not otherwise suspected.

Third, this "penetrating and perfecting of the temporal sphere" will be guided by the phrase "as I have loved you." Therefore it will be permeated with the ultimacy and absoluteness of the God-relationship, and the corresponding relativizing of other human goods. In health care delivery this can be very important.

The characteristic temptation of the ethos of the medical profession is to idolize life and the profession's ability to preserve it. The manifestation of this is the abandonment of patients when cure is no longer possible and death is imminent. For many physicians death is defeat. ("No one dies on my shift.") This can skew and distort the ministry of health care, decontextualize its instrumentalities, technologize its value judgments, and bloat its practitioners — to say nothing of limitlessly expanding its cost.

If medicine is indeed being transformed into a business, then the theologian must view this as a disaster. It involves a crucial displacement and disharmony at the heart of the medical art. What is supposed to be a privileged encounter, indeed a graced one (a source of healing and growth for both physician and patient), has become a means. The theologian views the physician encounter with the patient as the physician encounter with Christ. Precisely for that reason, the theologian legitimately expects the three results mentioned above.

When, however, the crucial encounter of physician with patient is displaced into a business context, not only is the professional ethos (compassion, honesty, self-denial, generosity) exposed to erosion, but we all will be deprived of the transforming effect of faith alive in a physician.

To the theologian that is unacceptable.

NOTES

1. I borrow this wording from Sittler 1958.
2. *American Medical News* (May 4, 1992) reported a statement of Kevin Sullivan, a consultant to medical groups, on physician performance standards: "Quality improvement is a tool for achieving business objectives. It is a means

to an end." This elicited a scathing response from David L. Wishart, in the June 22 issue. He noted that the Sullivan approach "puts the business cart before the service horse." And in an analysis close to Kass he stated: "The rewards to the practitioner come as a consequence of the satisfaction of the patient and those who support him (third parties)."

3. Several New York hospitals have hired carefully trained impostors to play patient roles in an effort to improve doctors' ability to communicate. The program originated as a "response to concerns that today's doctors are more adept with technology and jargon than with compassion" (*New York Times,* 4 June 1992).

4. It is also this ethos that prompted journalist J. Taylor Buckley to say of his stay at a Helsinki hospital: "A stay in the surgical hospital of Helsinki last month provided ample proof that at least Finland's brand of subsidized, universal care would never fly here. For one thing, their approach is far too mercy-driven and personal-care oriented to merit consideration as a possible replacement for a free-market arrangement like ours. Having people in health jobs because they are dedicated is scary anathema to our rich tradition of economic incentives and government bungling" (*USA Today,* 19 May 1992).

5. I take this list from Aiken and Mullinix 1987.

REFERENCES

Abbott, Walter, ed. 1966. *Documents of Vatican II.* New York: America.

Aiken, Linda H., and Connie Flynt Mullinix. 1987. "The Nurse Shortage: Myth or Reality?" *New England Journal of Medicine* 317:641–45.

Buckley, J. Taylor. 1992. *USA Today,* 19 May.

Callahan, Daniel. 1980. "Shattuck Lecture: Contemporary Biomedical Ethics." *New England Journal of Medicine* 302:1232.

Dunn, Marvin R. 1992. *American Medical News,* 1 June: 28.

Gorman, James. 1992. "The Doctor Won't See You Now." *New York Times,* 12 January.

Kass, Leon R. 1991. "Suicide Made Easy." *Commentary,* December: 22.

———. 1991. "The Care of the Doctor." *Perspectives in Biology and Medicine* 34 (Summer): 553–60.

McCormick, Richard A. 1989. "Theology and Bioethics." *Hastings Center Report* 19 (March/April): 5–10.

———. 1985. "Theology and Bioethics: Christian Foundations." In *Theology and Bioethics,* ed. Earl E. Shelp, 95–114. Dordrecht: D. Reidel.

Murray, John Courtney. 1960. *We Hold These Truths.* New York: Sheed and Ward.

Pellegrino, Edmund D. 1987. "Altruism, Self-Interest, and Medical Ethics." *Journal of the American Medical Association* 258:1939–40.

Peters, Thomas J., and Robert H. Waterman, Jr. 1982. *In Search of Excellence: Lessons from America's Best-Run Companies.* New York: Harper and Row.

Sittler, Joseph. 1958. *The Structure of Christian Ethics*. New Orleans: Louisiana State University Press.

Sokolowski, Robert. 1989. "The Art and Science of Medicine." In *Catholic Perspectives on Medical Ethics*, ed. Edmund D. Pellegrino, John P. Langan, and John Collins Harvey. Dordrecht: Kluwer Academic Publishers.

Wishart, David L. 1992. *American Medical News*, 22 June: 25.

Afterword

James P. Wind

The essays in this book are the latest communication in a conversation that has been evolving for centuries. For longer than historians can trace, women and men have been gathering to deal with the mysteries of human health and illness. The bones and stones from the paleolithic era are silent, but they bear traces of the earliest medical care. Holes cut into ancient skulls remind us of some of the earliest human surgery, the trepanations, or openings, drilled into human heads. The purpose of these holes puzzles us. Was it to heal? To release a spirit trapped within mortal remains? Scholars speculate, but we cannot know for certain. Still, as one ponders the fragments from prehistory, one can imagine early humans gathered around a body, carrying out a complex practice, and struggling together to interpret symptoms, to solve a problem, to perform a good and right act.

Somewhere in these ancient origins, we find the precursors to a practice of reflection about medical action that has come to take on very sophisticated characteristics in our age. Over the centuries, the conversations have taken different forms and have featured different participants. Shamans and medicine men and women orchestrated elaborate healing rituals in primitive societies. Egyptian papyri tell of physician-priests who gathered to discern the appropriate magical cure for their patients. In Greece, schools of would-be physicians gathered around great healers like Hippocrates, and deliberations about care and the nature of the good physician became more frequent. The great physician Galen gathered students around him in Rome during the second century of our era and began, in systematic fashion, to dissect human bodies and experiment on monkeys, pigs, and dogs in order to improve human ability to care for the sick and cure their illnesses.

And so we could proceed, if this were a historical essay on the development of the reflective practice of medicine, pausing to note all the great teachers and reflectors, people like Vesalius in the Renaissance period or Osler in the modern era. But to do so would be to turn away from the significance of this latest conversation. For now, it is sufficient to remind ourselves that this conversation is part of a great tradition or argument about how we care for the needs of the sick and dying. As late- or post-moderns tempted to forget our stories (one of the problems that runs like an undercurrent through the essays in this volume), we need to place ourselves in this long history, seeing our hospital ethics committees and bioethics institutes as the latest temporary solutions to an age-old problem. Revisiting our past may allow us to see our own situation more clearly and to discover a larger possible repertoire of commitments and responses to human need.

A Matter of Principles? needs to be located within that context, and the continuities and discontinuities between these late-twentieth-century voices and all of their predecessors must be noted. But that is another project.

A Matter of Principles? is a book about present circumstances that seeks to have a practical impact. Its authors gather in a kind of case conference, but this time the patient is not a particular person with a serious malady but a practice that affects millions of patients around the world. On the table here is the way Americans think about and talk about what they do in the pursuit of health. *Principlism,* a strange-sounding neologism, is this patient's name, and perhaps it is apt that it should ring oddly upon our ears, because it represents a world filled with new names and realities that few, save the experts, can comprehend.

In 1990, the Park Ridge Center convened a most unusual case conference to examine this most unusual patient. Men and women, physicians and scholars from a range of disciplines, representatives from Europe, Asia, and Latin America gathered to test a diagnosis that the reigning approach to the ethical problems of modern medicine was inadequate and was causing something analogous to the iatrogenic disease that can occur when physicians intervene. In this case, the attempt to construct a practice of ethical reflection based on a handful of shared principles seemed to be having side effects that were harmful to patients, caregivers, and society at large.

Taken as a whole, the essays seem to confirm the diagnosis. To be sure, this volume includes the voices of those who defend a principles-based approach to bioethics. And it is clear that many of the achievements of the past thirty years (roughly the life span of the new discipline) are the results of the principlists' labors. The volume also made room for those who would modify the principlists' canon by adding one or more new principles to the short list — compassion, for example, or the preferential option for the poor.

But the book's cumulative weight indicates grave concern about the state of health of U.S. bioethics. The majority of the participants in this case conference worry that principlism arbitrarily limits the ethical playing field. They are concerned that, in the day-to-day practice of bioethics, the inner realities of medical experience are ignored, or worse, injured. Both physicians and patients bring distinct, particular worlds into health care situations. And principles can gloss over those realities, when what is needed is a deep entering into them. Depersonalized forms of care, patients who become disembodied selves during treatment and medical conversations, and health care professionals who are trained without attention to the dispositions, habits, and character required to accompany a patient into the liminal state of illness — all these seem to be outcomes of a medical practice and a technological and functional rationality that apply a handful of principles to our variegated and contradictory realities.

A central concern here is the changing nature of the patient-physician relationship. New words or metaphors are employed to comprehend it: *accommodation, contract, care of strangers.* Does principlism further the erosion of the human relationships and senses of self that are underneath all the behaviors, techniques, policies, and institutions of modern health care? These authors, as a whole, think so. They worry that principlism reduces humans (both givers and receivers of care) to much less than they really are and that those reductions are unhealthy.

Principlism, of course, is not the sole cause of these changes. These authors acknowledge that secularism, bureaucratic organizations, complex technologies, professionalism, pluralism, and commodification of life are not the inventions of bioethics. Rather, they are major social dynamics that permeate modern health care and bioethical reflection. But principlism does not counter these forces as strongly as these authors would like.

These essays warn about a blindness to context that seems endemic to U.S. bioethics. They note how individual-centered principlism is, how it slights the real needs of human communities, and how it serves the interests of the medical-industrial complex and fails to challenge its preoccupations with costly and profitable forms of care at the expense of basic care for all or prevention of illness in the first place. Not enough questions are asked about medical indigence or power relations between physicians and patients.

Of special interest here is how voices from outside the U.S. call for focus on community, for compassion, and for attention to the macrosocial realities that are the context of our health care practices. The U.S. bioethical focus on quandaries and individual cases seems habitually to leave out the crushing realities of poverty, sexism, racism, and classism that give rise to so many of the problems that bring patients through the doors of our hospitals and clinics. Preoccupied with the quandaries we meet in individual confrontations with our new technologies, we fail to focus our attention and energies on the larger questions about the nature of a good society, about justice in its largest sense, about what is needed for our communities to become places that foster health.

This case conference did more than try to identify principlism's problems, however. Alongside the diagnoses that this approach failed to go deeply enough into either the internal or the external realities of contemporary medical experience came numerous proposals for remedying the maladies of bioethics. A few authors suggested radically different perspectives as starting points. Begin, they propose, by looking through the lenses of the liberation theologians, of feminists, of those from other cultural or religious settings. Others suggested different approaches to ethical inquiry — some quite old, others very new. Attend to virtue, practice casuistry, conduct careful phenomenological investigations, listen to the narratives of the actors in our medical dramas, enter into the hermeneutical circle of medical experience.

What I find interesting in these varied proposals is that although they would take us in a variety of directions, they all share a desire for "something more," for a wider playing field. They sense that more is going on in our medical experience and in our reflection on it than we recognize. Even principlism's defenders and modifiers acknowledge this need and propose strategies to meet it.

Proponents of the alternative approaches suggest that an adequate bioethics must break through the abstract world of theory and draw nearer to actual clinical experience, which has something more to offer. Here, I find Richard Zaner's image of the Grand Duchess waiting in the wings to be provocative. He employs that image to justify postponing both the task of settling the question of the usefulness of ethical principles and the question of the religious or spiritual nature of clinical experience. Just as one must wait until the right moment at the party before the Grand Duchess makes her entrance, so these matters, he claims, cannot be adequately addressed until we have honored medical experience by discovering all that is really going on within it.

Zaner's scholarly modesty is laudable, but I wonder about his hesitance to let the Duchess enter the room. His own essay, along with several others in this volume, take us several steps "beyond principlism." The book is not just a call for moving beyond a current state of affairs. It is a demonstration that bioethics is moving — a sign that the Grand Duchess may have slipped into the room ahead of schedule. Zaner's and his colleagues' probing of the "soft" aspects, or underside, of clinical experience takes us far beyond considerations of autonomy, beneficence, nonmaleficence, and justice. The world they disclose is one where people lose their everyday lives, where the routines that people use to make sense of their lives collapse. In this liminal world, strangers come together and are forced to trust each other in the midst of great uncertainty and danger. All the conventional borders in life break down as patients and physicians share intimacies that are taboo in the everyday world. This is an arena of confrontation with power and vulnerability, of help sought and promises made. It is a world where the mystery of human suffering rises up in all its complexity. In this world, individuals encounter themselves with a clarity that is impossible in the to and fro of everyday life — they confront their own mystery and mortality. They also meet the other — the stranger in the adjacent bed, the stranger in the hospital uniform, but also the other in their own bodies, and the other that is the larger unknown that transcends the coping strategies and therapies of modern health care. For each person who becomes a patient, a unique experience unfolds that cannot be packaged neatly within the typifying language of principlism. The patient needs something more.

Which brings me to religion. And again, the Grand Duchess is already in the room.

As patient and physician pursue their quests for health or healing, they find themselves tripping over the ultimate questions embedded in their shared experience. More than solving ethical problems, these strangers search for ways to see and make sense of what is happening. They find themselves in the presence of what theologian Paul Tillich once called "ultimate concerns" — concerns about their identities and destinies, their purposes and meaning. Do they have reason to hope? Is there a trustworthy presence that can anchor them as they descend into the netherworld of illness and suffering?

Tillich, writing in the fifties, attempted to widen our understanding of what religion was. In *Theology of Culture*, he made a series of important assertions that can help us locate religion in the experiences that concern all the authors of this volume. "Religion is not a special function of man's spiritual life, but it is the dimension of depth in all of its functions." Tillich went on to provide some pointers that indicate where we might pay special attention: "the religious aspect points to that which is ultimate, infinite, unconditional" in human life. This aspect manifests itself "in all creative functions" of our life. The realms of medicine and health, with their paradoxical experiences of human excellence and human failure, of confronting limits and of occasionally transcending them, are rich zones for finding this aspect. The surgeon's knife, the patient's cry, the nurse's soothing touch, the radiologist's pinpoint delivery of the X-ray, the pharmacologist's brilliant combination of chemicals are all places where this aspect of the human spirit reveals itself. Responding to the reality of the ultimate in human life requires something more than principles.

The perspectives and methods that together point the way beyond principlism provide something more. They take us in directions that Tillich would recognize. Ultimate concern permeates the clinic, hospital boardroom, and bedside situation. Tillich expected to find it "manifest in the moral sphere as the unconditional seriousness of the moral demand." But he looked in other places, too. "Ultimate concern is manifest in the realm of knowledge as the passionate longing for ultimate reality. . . . Ultimate concern is manifest in the aesthetic of the human spirit as the infinite desire to express ultimate meaning" (Tillich 1959:5–8).

H. Richard Niebuhr, a contemporary of Tillich's, found another way to make the same important point when he wrote that the real question to be asked "in every moment of decision and choice" was, "What is going on?" (Niebuhr 1963:60). Finding both the conventional deontological and teleological approaches to ethical reasoning inadequate, Niebuhr felt that the real challenge was to do what was fitting to all that was taking place in a given situation. For him, that meant setting the individual situation in its full historical and social context. But more than that, responsible selves needed to discern that they were also functioning in larger theological or religious contexts — those of absolute dependence and sin and salvation.

Although participants in this case conference do not go as far toward explicit theological claims as Niebuhr did, they assert that far more is going on in our bioethics cases than the principlists' approaches let us see. Hidden in these situations are larger historical and social realities, like patterns of economic injustice and dynamics of racial and sexual oppression. Deeper within them are encounters with human finitude and fallenness. Doctors don't always know what to do. They lose their will. They put other needs — including their own well-being — ahead of patients' needs. Patients exploit doctors and present illnesses that are signs of careless and irresponsible living. As fellow travelers, physicians and their patients find, sometimes together and sometimes separately, that they must depend on powers and forces beyond their control, whether those be governmental, medical, economic, or social. In short, all our autonomy claims notwithstanding, each of us finds, in the world of medicine, that we cannot control our own destiny, that we need something more.

Our public languages of rights and duties, our ethical principlist short-hands do not do justice to these larger parts of the smaller stories told in our bioethics cases. Other languages are needed. These essays conspire to make room for us to listen to the other languages being spoken in the world of medical experience. But still more is needed than just listening to all the languages currently being spoken — although that challenge is daunting enough. We must turn to methods and perspectives that make use of other languages — religious, cultural, and philosophical — that gravitate toward these larger dimensions. Otherwise, we will miss the greater significance embedded within the individual moments of our lives.

Recently, theologian James B. Wiggins generalized about contemporary understandings of religion. While scholars divide themselves into many camps when they consider this topic, he nonetheless felt that "all agree that religion has to do with universal life experiences and the ways in which sense is made of those experiences and meaning is attached to them. These universal experiences constitute the field from which the perennial human effort to make sense of the world (or deny that sense in some instances) arises: birth, death; joy, sorrow; knowledge, ignorance; success, failure; love, hate; suffering, relief; body, spirit" (1992:398).

Wiggins's list of religious experiences is also simultaneously a list of medical realities. It is also the list that the authors of *A Matter of Principles?* seek to respond to. The Duchess is clearly in the room, and she does not look at all like what we expected. Now, after thirty years during which even the bioethicists who brought theological and religious perspectives to their tasks tiptoed around lest they introduce her too soon, perhaps we are ready to recognize her presence and hear what she has to say. The more we listen, the more we will be led to delve into the same mystery that caused our prehistoric ancestors first to gather around a body and attempt to do something — was it medical, was it religious, or was it both? — that was right and good.

REFERENCES

Niebuhr, H. Richard. 1963. *The Responsible Self.* New York: Harper and Row.
Tillich, Paul. 1959. *Theology of Culture,* ed. Robert C. Kimball. New York: Oxford University Press.
Wiggins, James B. 1992. "Religion." In *A New Handbook of Christian Theology,* ed. Donald W. Musser and Joseph L. Price, 397–402. Nashville: Abingdon.

CONTRIBUTORS

Márcio Fabri dos Anjos, Ph.D., is professor of moral theology at the Instituto de Teologia Morale and director of the Alfonsianum Instituto, São Paulo, Brazil.

Courtney S. Campbell, Ph.D., is assistant professor of religious studies at Oregon State University, Corvallis.

Christine K. Cassel, M.D., is chief of the Section of General Internal Medicine, University of Chicago Medical Center, and professor of medicine in the Pritzker School of Medicine.

Rita Charon, M.D., is assistant professor of clinical medicine, Department of Medicine, in the College of Physicians and Surgeons of Columbia University, New York.

James F. Childress, Ph.D., is Kyle Professor of Religious Studies and professor of medical education at the University of Virginia, Charlottesville.

Larry R. Churchill, Ph.D., is professor and chair of social medicine at the University of North Carolina at Chapel Hill.

James F. Drane, Ph.D., is the Russell B. Roth Professor of Clinical Ethics at Edinboro University, Edinboro, Pennsylvania.

Edwin R. DuBose, Ph.D., is senior associate for religious ethics and clinical practice, Park Ridge Center for the Study of Health, Faith, and Ethics, Chicago.

Renée C. Fox, Ph.D., is Annenberg Professor of the Social Sciences at the University of Pennsylvania, Philadelphia.

Christine E. Gudorf, Ph.D., is professor of religious studies, Florida International University, Miami.

Ronald P. Hamel, Ph.D., is senior associate for theology, ethics, and clinical practice, Park Ridge Center for the Study of Health, Faith, and Ethics, Chicago.

Henk ten Have, M.D., Ph.D., is professor of medical ethics and chair of the Department of Ethics, Philosophy and History at the University of Nijmegen, The Netherlands.

Albert R. Jonsen, Ph.D., is chair of the Department of Medical History and Ethics, School of Medicine, University of Washington, Seattle.

Drew Leder, Ph.D., is associate professor of philosophy at Loyola University, Baltimore.

Richard A. McCormick, S.J., S.T.D., is the John A. O'Brien Professor of Christian Ethics at the University of Notre Dame, Notre Dame, Indiana.

Laurence J. O'Connell, Ph.D., S.T.D., is president and CEO of the Park Ridge Center for the Study of Health, Faith, and Ethics, Chicago.

Pinit Ratanakul, Ph.D., is director of the Center of Human Resources Development at Mahidol University, Bangkok, Thailand.

Cheryl J. Sanders, Ph.D., is professor of Christian ethics in the School of Divinity at Howard University, Washington, D.C.

Stephen Toulmin, Ph.D., is the Henry Luce Professor at the Center for Multiethnic and Transnational Studies, University of Southern California, Los Angeles.

James P. Wind. Ph.D., is program director, Religion Division, Lilly Endowment, Inc., Indianapolis, Indiana.

Richard M. Zaner, Ph.D., is the Ann Geddes Stahlman Professor of Medical Ethics at Vanderbilt University School of Medicine.

Index